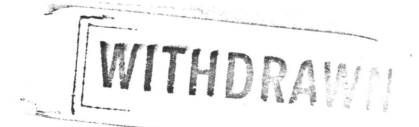

Dental Care and Oral Health

SOURCEBOOK

SIXTH EDITION

Dental Care and Oral Health
SOURCEBOOK

SIXTH EDITION

Basic Consumer Health Information about Caring for the Mouth and Teeth, Including Facts about Dental Hygiene and Routine Care Guidelines, Fluoride, Sealants, Cavities, Root Canals, Extractions, Implants, Veneers, Dentures, and Orthodontic and Orofacial Procedures

Along with Information about Periodontal (Gum) Disease, Canker Sores, Dry Mouth, Temporomandibular Joint and Muscle Disorders (TMJ), Oral Cancer, and Other Conditions That Impact Oral Health, Suggestions for Finding and Financing Care, a Glossary of Related Terms, and Directories of Additional Resources

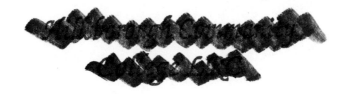

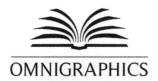

OMNIGRAPHICS

615 Griswold, Ste. 520, Detroit, MI 48226

Table of Contents

Part II: Visiting Your Dentist's Office

Part III: Dental Care for Infants and Children

Part IV: Orthodontic, Endodontic, Periodontic, and Orofacial Conditions and Procedures

Part V: Oral Diseases and Disorders

Part VI: Health Conditions That Affect Oral Health

Part VII: Finding and Financing Oral Health in the United States

Part VIII: Additional Help and Information

Preface

About This Book

Oral health is essential to overall health. Good oral health includes more than maintaining healthy teeth and gums. Oral health also involves avoiding craniofacial conditions that can affect the face and mouth. These conditions can lead to systemic health problems such as infections, immune disorders, cancer, or heart and lung disease. Although, there has been significant improvement in the oral health of Americans due to increasingly effective prevention and treatment efforts, some challenges remain and new concerns have emerged.

Dental Care and Oral Health Sourcebook, Sixth Edition offers information about mouth and tooth care guidelines for effective hygiene, nutrition, and decay prevention. Facts about tooth pain, dental fillings, orthodontia, and other endodontic treatments and dental implants are provided. Facial trauma and cleft palate treatments are also discussed. Disorders such as temporomandibular joint and muscle (TMJ) disorder, mouth sores, jaw problems, tongue disorders, and health conditions, such as bad breath, that impact oral health are addressed. The book concludes with guidelines for finding and financing dental care, a glossary of dental care terms, and directories with further information about dental care and oral health services.

How to Use This Book

This book is divided into parts and chapters. Parts focus on broad areas of interest. Chapters are devoted to single topics within a part.

Part I: Taking Care of Your Mouth and Teeth begins by outlining key steps for dental health and provides an overview on the anatomy of the mouth. Information on procedures and products used to clean teeth and remove dental plaque is provided. The impact of nutrition and fluoride is described along with details about mouth injuries. Oral health for older adults is also discussed.

Part II: Visiting Your Dentist's Office explains common dental procedures, such as dental imaging, fillings, sedation, and dental drills, besides information on routine dental visits and overcoming dental phobia. It also talks about dental caries in primary and permanent teeth and prevalence of total and untreated dental caries among youth. Details about rebuilding and reshaping teeth, having a tooth pulled, as well as denture choices are also provided.

Part III: Dental Care for Infants and Children offers strategies for initiating and maintaining healthy primary teeth. Fluoride treatments and sealants with adequate calcium intake are addressed. Other specific concerns for children, such as teething, using a pacifier, childhood bruxism, weaning a child from a bottle, and the impact of sugar on children's oral health, are also explained. It also discusses preventing oral injuries and tooth decay in children and the importance of routine dental care visits.

Part IV: Orthodontic, Endodontic, Periodontic, and Orofacial Conditions and Procedures provides information about treatment for endodontic conditions, periodontal (gum) disease, and dental implants. Facial trauma and corrective jaw surgery are also discussed.

Part V: Oral Diseases and Disorders provides information about various diseases and disorders that affect the oral health, such as bad breath, burning mouth syndrome, cleft palate, dentinogenesis imperfecta, jaw problems, mouth sores, oral cancer, thrush, tongue disorders, and so on.

Part VI: Health Conditions That Affect Oral Health describes specific medical conditions that cause—or result in—oral complications, including cancer treatment, celiac disease, diabetes, heart disease, immune system disorders, organ transplantation, osteoporosis, and the use of tobacco products.

Part VII: Finding and Financing Oral Health in the United States provides information on oral healthcare status and factors that impact access to oral healthcare. It reviews average dental expenses for dental care and includes suggestions for finding low-cost dental care.

Specific information about school-based oral health services is also provided.

Part VIII: Additional Help and Information provides a glossary of terms related to dental care and oral health. Directories of local dental schools and other dental care and oral health resources are also included.

Bibliographic Note

This volume contains documents and excerpts from publications issued by the following U.S. government agencies: Benefits.gov; Centers for Disease Control and Prevention (CDC); Centers for Medicare and Medicaid Services (CMS); ChildCare.gov; Early Childhood Learning and Knowledge Center (ECLKC); Effective Health Care Program; Genetic and Rare Diseases Information Center (GARD); Health Resources and Services Administration (HRSA); National Cancer Institute (NCI); National Human Genome Research Institute (NHGRI); National Institute of Dental and Craniofacial Research (NIDCR); National Institute of Diabetes and Digestive and Kidney Diseases (NIDDK); National Institute of Neurological Disorders and Stroke (NINDS); National Institute on Aging (NIA); National Institute on Deafness and Other Communication Disorders (NIDCD); National Institute on Drug Abuse (NIDA) for Teens; National Institutes of Health (NIH); *NIH News in Health*; NIH Osteoporosis and Related Bone Diseases—National Resource Center (NIH ORBD—NRC); Office of Disease Prevention and Health Promotion (ODPHP); Office of Head Start (OHS); Office on Women's Health (OWH); U.S. Department of Health and Human Services (HHS); U.S. Environmental Protection Agency (EPA); and U.S. Food and Drug Administration (FDA).

It may also contain original material produced by Omnigraphics and reviewed by medical consultants.

About the Health Reference Series

The *Health Reference Series* is designed to provide basic medical information for patients, families, caregivers, and the general public. Each volume takes a particular topic and provides comprehensive coverage. This is especially important for people who may be dealing with a newly diagnosed disease or a chronic disorder in themselves or in a family member. People looking for preventive guidance, information about disease warning signs, medical statistics, and risk factors for health problems will also find answers to their questions in the *Health*

Reference Series. The *Series*, however, is not intended to serve as a tool for diagnosing illness, in prescribing treatments, or as a substitute for the physician/patient relationship. All people concerned about medical symptoms or the possibility of disease are encouraged to seek professional care from an appropriate healthcare provider.

A Note about Spelling and Style

Health Reference Series editors use *Stedman's Medical Dictionary* as an authority for questions related to the spelling of medical terms and the *Chicago Manual of Style* for questions related to grammatical structures, punctuation, and other editorial concerns. Consistent adherence is not always possible, however, because the individual volumes within the *Series* include many documents from a wide variety of different producers, and the editor's primary goal is to present material from each source as accurately as is possible. This sometimes means that information in different chapters or sections may follow other guidelines and alternate spelling authorities. For example, occasionally a copyright holder may require that eponymous terms be shown in possessive forms (Crohn's disease vs. Crohn disease) or that British spelling norms be retained (leukaemia vs. leukemia).

Medical Review

Omnigraphics contracts with a team of qualified, senior medical professionals who serve as medical consultants for the *Health Reference Series*. As necessary, medical consultants review reprinted and originally written material for currency and accuracy. Citations including the phrase "Reviewed (month, year)" indicate material reviewed by this team. Medical consultation services are provided to the *Health Reference Series* editors by:

Dr. Vijayalakshmi, MBBS, DGO, MD
Dr. Senthil Selvan, MBBS, DCH, MD
Dr. K. Sivanandham, MBBS, DCH, MS (Research), PhD

Our Advisory Board

We would like to thank the following board members for providing initial guidance on the development of this series:

- Dr. Lynda Baker, Associate Professor of Library and Information Science, Wayne State University, Detroit, MI

- Nancy Bulgarelli, William Beaumont Hospital Library, Royal Oak, MI

- Karen Imarisio, Bloomfield Township Public Library, Bloomfield Township, MI

- Karen Morgan, Mardigian Library, University of Michigan-Dearborn, Dearborn, MI

- Rosemary Orlando, St. Clair Shores Public Library, St. Clair Shores, MI

Health Reference Series *Update Policy*

The inaugural book in the *Health Reference Series* was the first edition of *Cancer Sourcebook* published in 1989. Since then, the *Series* has been enthusiastically received by librarians and in the medical community. In order to maintain the standard of providing high-quality health information for the layperson the editorial staff at Omnigraphics felt it was necessary to implement a policy of updating volumes when warranted.

Medical researchers have been making tremendous strides, and it is the purpose of the *Health Reference Series* to stay current with the most recent advances. Each decision to update a volume is made on an individual basis. Some of the considerations include how much new information is available and the feedback we receive from people who use the books. If there is a topic you would like to see added to the update list, or an area of medical concern you feel has not been adequately addressed, please write to:

Managing Editor
Health Reference Series
Omnigraphics
615 Griswold, Ste. 520
Detroit, MI 48226

Part One

Taking Care of
Your Mouth and Teeth

Chapter 1

Steps to Dental Health

Healthy teeth and gums make it easy for you to eat well and enjoy good food. Several problems can affect the health of your mouth, but good care should keep your teeth and gums strong as you age.

How to Clean Your Teeth and Gums

There is a right way to brush and floss your teeth. Every day:

- Gently brush your teeth on all sides with a soft-bristle brush and fluoride toothpaste.

- Use small circular motions and short back-and-forth strokes.

- Brush carefully and gently along your gum line.

- Lightly brush your tongue to help keep your mouth clean.

- Clean around your teeth with dental floss. Careful flossing removes plaque and leftover food that a toothbrush cannot reach.

- Rinse after you floss.

This chapter contains text excerpted from the following sources: Text in this chapter begins with excerpts from "Taking Care of Your Teeth and Mouth," National Institute on Aging (NIA), National Institutes of Health (NIH), June 1, 2016; Text under the heading "CDC DentalCheck Mobile App for Dental Healthcare Personnel" is excerpted from "CDC DentalCheck Mobile App," Centers for Disease Control and Prevention (CDC), June 18, 2019.

Tooth Decay

Teeth are covered in a hard, outer coating called "enamel." Every day, a thin film of bacteria called "dental plaque" builds up on your teeth. The bacteria in plaque produce acids that can harm enamel and cause cavities. Brushing and flossing your teeth can prevent decay, but once a cavity forms, a dentist has to fix it.

Use fluoride toothpaste to protect your teeth from decay. If you are at a higher risk for tooth decay (for example, if you have a dry mouth because of a condition you have or medicines you take), you might need more fluoride. Your dentist or dental hygienist may give you a fluoride treatment during an office visit, or they may tell you to use a fluoride gel or mouth rinse at home.

Gum Disease

Gum disease begins when plaque builds up along and under your gum line. This plaque causes infections that hurt the gum and bone that hold your teeth in place. Gum disease may make your gums tender and more likely to bleed. This problem, called "gingivitis," can often be fixed by brushing and flossing every day.

A more severe form of gum disease, called "periodontitis," must be treated by a dentist. If not treated, this infection can ruin the bones, gums, and other tissues that support your teeth. Over time, your teeth may have to be removed.

To prevent gum disease:

- Brush your teeth twice a day with fluoride toothpaste.
- Floss once a day.
- Visit your dentist regularly for a checkup and cleaning.
- Eat a well-balanced diet.
- Quit smoking. Smoking increases your risk for gum disease.

Dentures

Sometimes, false teeth (dentures) are needed to replace badly damaged teeth. Partial dentures may be used to fill in one or more missing teeth. Dentures may feel strange at first. In the beginning, your dentist may want to see you often to make sure the dentures fit. Over time, your gums will change shape, and your dentures may need to be adjusted or replaced. Be sure to let your dentist handle these adjustments.

Be careful when wearing dentures, because it may be harder for you to feel hot foods and drinks or notice bones in your food. When learning to eat with dentures, it may be easier if you:

- Start with soft, nonsticky food
- Cut your food into small pieces
- Chew slowly using both sides of your mouth

Keep your dentures clean and free from food that can cause stains, bad breath, or swollen gums. Brush them every day with a denture care product. Take your dentures out of your mouth at night, and soak them in water or a denture cleansing liquid.

Dry Mouth

Dry mouth happens when you do not have enough saliva, or spit, to keep your mouth wet. It can make it hard to eat, swallow, taste, and even speak. Dry mouth can accelerate tooth decay and other infections of the mouth. Many common medicines can cause this problem.

There are things you can do that may help. Try sipping water or sugarless drinks. Do not smoke, and avoid alcohol and caffeine. Sugarless hard candy or sugarless gum that is a little tart may help. Your dentist or doctor might suggest using artificial saliva to keep your mouth wet.

Oral Cancer

Cancer of the mouth can grow in any part of the mouth or throat. It is more likely to happen in people over the age of 40. A dental checkup is a good time for your dentist to look for signs of oral cancer. Pain is not usually an early symptom of the disease. Treatment works best before the disease spreads. Even if you have lost all of your natural teeth, you should still see your dentist for regular oral cancer exams.

You can lower your risk of getting oral cancer in a few ways:

- Do not use tobacco products, such as cigarettes, electronic cigarettes, chewing tobacco, snuff, pipes, or cigars.

- If you drink alcohol, do so only in moderation.

- Use lip balm with sunscreen.

Finding Low-Cost Dental Care

Dental care can be costly. Medicare does not cover routine dental care, and very few states offer dental coverage under Medicaid.

You may want to check out private dental insurance. Make sure you are aware of the cost and what services are covered. The following resources may help you find low-cost dental care:

- Some dental schools have clinics where students get experience by treating patients at a reduced cost. Qualified dentists supervise the students.

- Dental hygiene schools may offer supervised, low-cost care as part of the training experience for dental hygienists.

- Call your county or state health department to find dental clinics near you that charge based on your income.

CDC DentalCheck Mobile App for Dental Healthcare Personnel

Dental healthcare personnel can use the mobile application, CDC DentalCheck, to periodically assess practices in their facility and ensure they are meeting the minimum expectations for safe care.

Key Features

- Check Yes/No to acknowledge adherence to office policies or observed practices.

- Review basic infection prevention principles and link to full recommendations and source documents for dental health care settings.

- Export or save results and notes for records management.

The infection prevention coordinator and other staff trained in infection prevention are encouraged to use this app at least annually to assess the status of their administrative policies and practices, and also engage in direct observation of personnel and patient-care practices.

Chapter 2

Anatomy of the Mouth

The mouth, or oral cavity, is the first part of the digestive tract. It is adapted to receive food by ingestion, break it into small particles by mastication, and mix it with saliva.

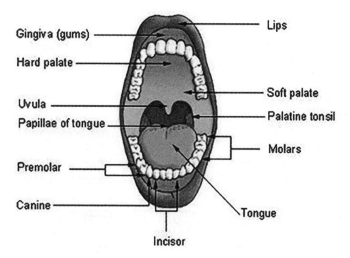

Figure 2.1. *Parts of the Mouth*

This chapter contains text excerpted from the following sources: Text in this chapter begins with excerpts from "Mouth," Surveillance, Epidemiology, and End Results Program (SEER), National Cancer Institute (NCI), July 1, 2002. Reviewed July 2019; Text under the heading "Anatomy of the Lips, Mouth, and Oral Region" is excerpted from "Anatomy of the Lips, Mouth, and Oral Region," National Human Genome Research Institute (NHGRI), January 18, 2009. Reviewed July 2019.

The lips, cheeks, and palate form the boundaries. The oral cavity contains the teeth and tongue, and it receives secretions from the salivary glands.

Lips and Cheeks

The lips and cheeks help hold food in the mouth and keep it in place for chewing. They are also used in the formation of words for speech. The lips contain numerous sensory receptors that are useful for judging the temperature and texture of foods.

Palate

The palate is the roof of the oral cavity. It separates the oral cavity from the nasal cavity. The anterior portion, the hard palate, is supported by bone. The posterior portion, the soft palate, is skeletal muscle and connective tissue. Posteriorly, the soft palate ends in a projection called the "uvula." During swallowing, the soft palate and uvula move upward to direct food away from the nasal cavity and into the oropharynx.

Tongue

The tongue manipulates food in the mouth and is used in speech. The surface is covered with papillae that provide friction and contain the taste buds.

Teeth

A complete set of deciduous (primary) teeth contains 20 teeth. There are 32 teeth in a complete permanent (secondary) set. The shape of each tooth type corresponds to the way it handles food.

Anatomy of the Lips, Mouth, and Oral Region

The appearance of the lips varies with facial movement. Smiling and crying can alter dramatically the shape of the upper lip, as do pursing or pouting. Therefore, the lips must be assessed when the subject has a relaxed (neutral) face: the eyes are open, the lips make gentle contact, and the teeth are slightly separated. The neck, jaw, and facial muscles should not be stretched nor contracted, and the face should be positioned using the Frankfurt horizontal (a line joining the orbitale and the porion).

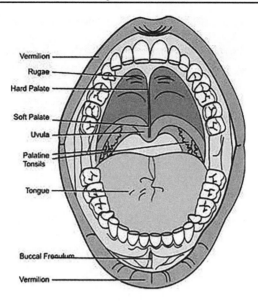

Figure 2.2. *Features of the Oral Cavity*

Lips

The lips are the structures that surround the oral aperture. In the central region, their superior border corresponds to the inferior margin of the base of the nose. Laterally, their limits follow the alar sulci and the upper and lower lips join at the oral commissures. The inferior limit of the lips in the central region is the mentolabial sulcus. Anatomically, the philtrum and its pillars are a part of the upper lip. The surface of the lip is comprised of four zones: hairy skin, vermilion border, vermilion, and oral mucosa. The normal shape of the lips varies with age, and it is influenced by ethnicity.

Vermilion

The vermilion is the red part of the lips (Figure 2.2). It is covered with a specialized stratified squamous epithelium, which is in continuity with the oral mucosa of the gingivolabial groove. Confusingly, the vermilion itself is also often referred to as the lips.

Vermilion Border

The vermilion border is the rim of paler skin that demarcates the vermilion from the surrounding skin.

Cupid's Bow

The Cupid's bow is the contour of the line formed by the vermilion border of the upper lip. In a frontal view, this line resembles an archer's bow, which curves medially and superiorly from the commissures to the paramedian peaks located at the bases of the pillars of the philtrum (crista philtrae) with an inferior convexity lying between those peaks. The philtrum is the vertical groove in the midline of the upper lip bordered by these lateral pillars (ridges).

Oral Mucosa

Stratified squamous nonkeratinized epithelium covering of the inner aspect of the oral cavity.

Mouth

The mouth is the oral aperture that opens into the oral cavity proper. The opening is bounded by the upper and lower vermilion. The cavity comprises the alveolar arches with gums and teeth, the hard and soft palate, and the tongue, anchored to the floor of the mouth (Figure 2.2). The oral cavity leads into the oropharynx, bounded by the tonsillar pillars. Standards exist for measuring the length and height of the oral aperture.

Oral Commissure

The oral commissure is the place where the lateral aspects of the vermilion of the upper and lower lips join. The cheilion is the anthropological landmark located at this site (see Figure 2.2).

Labial Fissure

Slit-like space between the lips; the oral vestibule.

Oral Cavity

The oral cavity is the space bounded superiorly by the hard and soft palates, laterally by the alveolar processes of the maxillary bone, and inferiorly by the tongue (see Figure 2.2).

Alveolar Ridge

The alveolar ridge is the U-shaped bony crests of the upper and lower jaw in which the teeth are situated.

Hard Palate

The hard palate is the bony anterior two-thirds of the roof of the mouth separating the nasal cavity from the oral cavity. The boundary of the hard and soft palates can be determined by palpation.

Soft Palate (Velum Palatinum)

The soft palate, or the velum palatinum is the posterior one-third of the palate comprises of a fibromuscular fold of soft tissue suspended from the hard palate and separating the nasal and oral cavities.

Uvula

The uvula is a conical projection of soft tissue extending inferiorly from the posterior edge of the middle of the soft palate (see Figure 2.2).

Gingiva (Gums)

Gingiva, or gums, is a dense fibrous tissue that is covered by mucous membrane overlying the alveolar ridge in which the teeth are situated.

Buccal Frenulum

The buccal frenulum is a thin fold of soft tissue extending from the gingiva of the mid-anterior alveolar ridge to the inner surface of the medial part of the upper or lower lip (see Figure 2.2).

Lingual Frenulum

The lingual frenulum is a thin fold of soft tissue extending from the floor of the mouth to the base of the tongue.

Tongue

The tongue is a muscular organ of deglutition, speech, and taste, and it is covered with epithelium and bound to the floor of the mouth.

Teeth

Teeth are hard dental structures that are located on the alveolar ridges and situated in the gingiva. In humans, teeth have two stages, the primary (deciduous) and the secondary (permanent, adult).

Chapter 3

Taking Care of Your Teeth

Chapter Contents

Section 3.1

Preventing Tooth Decay and Gum Disease

This section includes text excerpted from "Take Care of
Your Teeth and Gums," Office of Disease Prevention and Health
Promotion (ODPHP), U.S. Department of Health and
Human Services (HHS), June 26, 2018.

Healthy habits, including brushing and flossing, can prevent tooth decay (cavities) and gum disease. Tooth decay and gum disease can lead to pain and tooth loss.

You can prevent most problems with teeth and gums by taking these steps:

- Brush your teeth two times a day with a fluoride toothpaste.

- Floss between your teeth every day.

- Visit a dentist regularly for a checkup and cleaning.

- Cut down on sugary foods and drinks.

- Do not smoke or chew tobacco.

- If you drink alcohol, drink only in moderation.

What Causes Tooth Decay and Gum Disease

Plaque is a sticky substance that forms on your teeth. When plaque stays on your teeth too long, it can lead to tooth decay and gum disease. Brushing and flossing help get plaque off your teeth so your mouth can stay healthy.

Taking care of your teeth and gums is especially important if you:

- Have diabetes

- Have cancer

- Are an older adult

- Are pregnant

Take Action

Follow these tips for a healthy, beautiful smile.

Brush Your Teeth

Brush your teeth two times every day. Use a toothbrush with soft bristles and toothpaste with fluoride. Fluoride is a mineral that helps protect teeth from decay.

- Brush in circles, and use short, back-and-forth strokes.

- Take time to brush gently along the gum line.

- Brush your teeth for about two minutes each time.

- Do not forget to brush your tongue.

- Get a new toothbrush every three to four months. Replace your toothbrush sooner if it is wearing out.

Floss Every Day

Floss every day to remove plaque and any food between teeth that your toothbrush missed. Rinse your mouth with water after you floss. If you are not sure how to floss, ask the dentist or dental assistant to show you at your next visit.

Get Regular Checkups at the Dentist

Visit a dentist once or twice a year for a checkup and cleaning. Get checkups even if you have no natural teeth and have dentures. If you have problems with your teeth or mouth, see a dentist right away.

What If I Do Not Like Going to the Dentist?

Some people get nervous about going to the dentist. Try these tips to help make your visit to the dentist easier:

- Let your dentist know that you are feeling nervous.

- Choose an appointment time when you will not feel rushed.

- Take headphones and a music player on your next visit.

What If I Do Not Have Insurance?

Even if you do not have dental insurance, you can get dental care.

Cut Down on Sugary Foods and Drinks

Choose low-sugar snacks, such as vegetables, fruits, and low-fat or fat-free cheese. Drink fewer sugary sodas and other drinks that can lead to tooth decay.

Quit Smoking

People who use tobacco in any form (cigarettes, cigars, pipe, e-cigarettes, smokeless tobacco) are at higher risk for gum disease and oral (mouth) cancer.

Drink Alcohol Only in Moderation

Drinking a lot of alcohol can increase your risk of oral cancer. If you choose to drink, have only a moderate amount. This means no more than one drink a day for women or two drinks a day for men.

Take Care of Your Children's Teeth

If you have kids, help them learn good habits for a healthy mouth. Start cleaning your child's teeth as soon as they come in.

Section 3.2

The Use and Handling of Toothbrushes

This section includes text excerpted from "Use and Handling of Toothbrushes," Centers for Disease Control and Prevention (CDC), March 25, 2016.

How Should Toothbrushes Be Cared For?

The mouth is home to millions of germs. In removing plaque and other soft debris from the teeth, toothbrushes become contaminated with bacteria, blood, saliva, oral debris, and toothpaste. Because of this contamination, a common recommendation is to rinse one's toothbrush thoroughly with tap water following brushing. Limited research has suggested that even after being rinsed visibly clean, toothbrushes can remain contaminated with potentially pathogenic organisms. Various means of cleaning, disinfecting, or sterilizing toothbrushes between uses have been developed, but no published research documents that brushing with a contaminated toothbrush has led to the recontamination of a user's mouth, oral infections, or other adverse health effects.

Recommended toothbrush care:

- Do not share toothbrushes. Toothbrushes can have germs on them, even after rinsing, that could raise the risk of infection, especially for people with immune suppression.

- After brushing, rinse your toothbrush with tap water until it is completely clean, let it air-dry, and store it in an upright position. If more than one brush is stored in the same holder, do not let them touch each other.

- You do not need to soak toothbrushes in disinfecting solutions or mouthwash, which may actually spread germs under the right conditions.

- You do not need to use dishwashers, microwaves, or ultraviolet devices to disinfect toothbrushes. These methods may damage the toothbrush.

- Avoid covering toothbrushes or storing them in closed containers, which can cause the growth of bacteria.

- Replace your toothbrush every three to four months, or sooner if the bristles look worn out. This is because a worn-out toothbrush may not work as well, not because it might carry more germs.

How Should Toothbrushes Be Handled in Group Settings Such As in Schools?

Tooth brushing in group settings should always be supervised to ensure that toothbrushes are not shared and that they are handled properly. The likelihood of toothbrush cross-contamination in these environments is very high, either through children playing with them or toothbrushes being stored improperly. In addition, a small chance exists that toothbrushes could become contaminated with blood during brushing. Although the risk for disease transmission through toothbrushes is minimal in group settings, it is a potential cause for concern. Therefore, officials in charge of tooth-brushing programs in these settings should evaluate their programs carefully.

Recommended measures for hygienic tooth brushing in schools:

- Ensure that each child has her or his own toothbrush and that it is clearly labeled. Do not allow children to share or borrow toothbrushes.

- To prevent cross-contamination of the toothpaste tube, ensure that a pea-sized amount of toothpaste is dispensed onto a piece of wax paper before dispensing any onto the toothbrush.

- After the children finish brushing, ensure that they rinse their toothbrushes thoroughly with tap water, allow them to air-dry, and store them in an upright position so they cannot contact those of other children.

- Provide children with paper cups to use for rinsing after they finish brushing. Do not allow them to share cups, and ensure that they dispose of the cups properly after a single use.

Do Toothbrushes Spread Germs?

The Centers for Disease Control and Prevention (CDC) is unaware of any adverse health effects directly related to toothbrush use, although people with bleeding disorders or who are severely immunosuppressed may suffer trauma from tooth brushing and may need to seek alternate means of oral hygiene.

Section 3.3

The Benefits of Daily Cleaning between Teeth

This section includes text excerpted from "Don't Toss the Floss!" *NIH News in Health*, National Institutes of Health (NIH), November 2016.

You may have seen or heard news stories suggesting that you can forget about flossing, since scientists lack solid evidence that you will benefit from cleaning between your teeth with a sturdy string. But, many dentists may beg to differ. They have seen the teeth and gums of people who floss regularly and those who have not. The differences can be striking.

"Every dentist in the country can look in someone's mouth and tell whether or not they floss," says Dr. Tim Iafolla, a dental health expert at the National Institutes of Health (NIH). Red or swollen gums that bleed easily can be a clear sign that flossing and better dental habits are needed. "Cleaning all sides of your teeth, including between your teeth where the toothbrush cannot reach, is a good thing," Iafolla says.

If dentists—and maybe even your personal experience—suggest that regular flossing keeps your mouth healthy, then why the news reports? It is because long-term, large-scale, carefully controlled studies of flossing have been somewhat limited.

Researchers have found modest benefits from flossing in small clinical studies. For instance, an analysis of 12 well-controlled studies found that flossing plus toothbrushing reduced mild gum disease, or gingivitis, significantly better than toothbrushing alone. These same studies reported that flossing plus brushing might reduce plaque after 1 or 3 months better than just brushing.

But there is no solid evidence that flossing can prevent periodontitis, a severe form of gum disease that is the leading cause of tooth loss in adults. Periodontitis can arise if mild gum disease is left untreated. Plaque may then spread below the gum line, leading to breakdown of bone and other tissues that support your teeth. Periodontitis develops slowly over months or years. Most flossing studies to date, however, have examined only relatively short time periods.

Another research challenge is that large, real-world studies of flossing must rely on people accurately reporting their dental cleaning habits. And people tend to report what they think is the "right" answer when it comes to their health behaviors—whether flossing, exercising, smoking, or eating. That is why well-controlled studies (where researchers closely monitor flossing or perform the flossing) tend to show that flossing is effective. But, real-world studies result in weaker evidence.

"The fact that there hasn't been a huge population-based study of flossing doesn't mean that flossing's not effective," Iafolla says. "It simply suggests that large studies are difficult and expensive to conduct when you are monitoring health behaviors of any kind."

While the scientific evidence for flossing benefits may be somewhat lacking, there is little evidence for any harm or side effects from flossing, and it is low cost. So why not consider making it part of your daily routine?

Talk to your dentist if you have any questions or concerns about your teeth or gums. If flossing is difficult, the dentist may recommend other ways to remove plaque between teeth, such as with a water flosser or interdental cleaners. "If you need help learning how to floss, or if you do not think you are doing it right, your dentist or hygienist will be happy to show you how," Iafolla says. "It helps to know the proper technique."

Chapter 4

Nutrition Impacts Oral Health

Tooth development begins in the fetus as early as six weeks of age, when the basic material that makes up teeth starts to form. The impact of nutrition on oral health and dental development begins in the womb, with the mother's nutritional status and eating patterns playing a vital role in the process. Studies have shown that adequate nutrition is a key factor in defining the health of teeth and periodontal tissues and in maintaining salivary secretions at their optimum. Early nutritional imbalances can lead to developmental malformations of the dentition, while malnutrition can result in enamel hypoplasia (thin tooth enamel), poor periodontal health, increased risk of oral infectious disease, and the early onset of dental erosion.

Importance of Balanced Diet

Nutrition plays a vital role in boosting the body's immune system and preventing infections and inflammations. Malnutrition—deficiencies of essential nutrients, such as vitamins and minerals—can have a negative impact on general health and result in cavities and gum disease. Gum disease may start as gingivitis, an inflammation of the gums usually caused by bacterial infection which, if unchecked, may progress to periodontal disease, a condition that affects the supporting tissues of the teeth.

"Nutrition Impacts Oral Health," © 2017 Omnigraphics. Reviewed July 2019.

Some Important Micronutrients

Studies show that nutrition and oral health are interrelated. Poor nutrition can cause oral and dental problems and, conversely, problems with oral health can trigger nutritional deficiencies. Food habits and eating patterns greatly impact the decay resistance of teeth in children and teens, and a well-balanced diet is an important factor in maintaining periodontal health in the adults and elderly.

A number of micronutrients (vitamins and minerals) are critical to the maintenance of healthy teeth and gums. These include:

Vitamin D (Calciferol)

Vitamin D plays a vital role in maintaining musculoskeletal health by aiding in calcium absorption. Its direct effect on bone metabolism makes it an essential nutrient in preventing tooth loss and maintaining periodontal health. Vitamin D is also involved in certain immunoregulatory pathways and reduces the risk of periodontitis or inflammation of periodontal tissues. Dietary sources of vitamin D include fish-liver oils, fatty fish, mushrooms, egg yolks, liver, and fortified foods, such as breakfast cereals, milk, and orange juice. The vitamin is also synthesized in the skin by the action of ultraviolet radiation of the sun on certain sterols (substances in many plants that help lower cholesterol).

Vitamin C (Ascorbic Acid)

Vitamin C is essential for maintaining the integrity of the connective tissue and dentine, the hard material that makes up much of a tooth. It is also necessary for the proper functioning of the immune system. The deficiency of vitamin C can lead to scurvy, a disease characterized by gingivitis (spongy, bleeding gums). Rich sources of vitamin C include citrus fruits—such as oranges, limes, and grapefruit—green leafy vegetables, tomatoes, and berries.

Choosing a Healthy Diet

- Fruits and vegetables are especially important in maintaining good oral health. Salads are ideal, as chewing raw vegetables stimulates the secretion of saliva, which helps to wash acid and food remnants from the mouth.

- Nuts are also good. Their low carbohydrate content reduces the risk of cavities. In addition to providing such benefits as minerals and vitamins, they also serve as rich sources of proteins that are important for maintaining overall health.

- Dairy products, such as milk, cheese, and yogurt, are excellent sources of proteins, as well as calcium, a mineral that is critical for the development and maintenance of healthy teeth and periodontal tissue.

- Lean meat, eggs, legumes, and green leafy vegetables, such as collards and spinach, are also rich sources of calcium and can help to build strong teeth and maintain good oral health.

Fluoridated Water and Oral Health

Drinking fluoridated water is highly beneficial for maintaining healthy teeth. Fluoride helps prevent tooth decay, and water washes away food debris in the mouth. The presence of food particles encourages the growth of bacteria that break down the sugars in food to release acids. These acids wear away the mineralized oral tissues, including enamel (the hard protective covering of the teeth), cementum (the exterior surface of the roots), and dentine. Water not only removes food residue in the mouth, but also dilutes the acid produced by cavity-causing bacteria.

Drinking water also prevents dehydration and xerostomia (dry mouth, or insufficient saliva). Saliva is an important factor in maintaining the integrity of oral structures. It helps lubricate, chew, and digest food; kill microorganisms in food; dilute sugars; and buffer acid in the mouth. Saliva also helps remineralize tooth enamel with calcium and phosphorous. Insufficient salivary secretions can increase the risk of gingivitis, dental cavities, and oral thrush, a fungal infection of the mouth.

Foods to Avoid for Better Oral Health

The connection between sugar and cavities has been studied for a long time, and it has been established that fermentable carbohydrates and sugars play a major role in the development of dental cavities. These cariogenic (cavity-causing) foods are acted upon by bacteria in the mouth, such as streptococci and lactobacilli, and are converted to acids. The acids demineralize teeth by dissolving calcium and phosphorus and causing tooth erosion. Normally, the demineralization of teeth is offset by remineralization with saliva, which is saturated with calcium and phosphorus. But if the acidic environment in the mouth persists, it interferes with the remineralization process, leading to tooth decay. Although cariogenic foods include a variety of sugars, such as glucose, lactose, fructose, and maltose—either naturally occurring or added to food—sucrose (table sugar) is by far the most cariogenic of all.

Avoiding high-sugar food, such as candies, confectionery, and sugar-sweetened drinks, is undoubtedly the most important prophylactic measure in controlling tooth decay and maintaining good oral health. While acids resulting from bacterial fermentation of sugars in the mouth are a major cause cavities, dietary acids can also, to some extent, contribute to decay by lowering pH below critical levels. Thus, foods and drinks with lower pH can cause teeth erosion. Vinegar-containing foods, as well as acids, naturally occurring in fruit or added to candies and sports drinks, can promote cavities and should be consumed in smaller amounts or eliminated from the diet entirely.

References

1. Touger-Decker, Riva, and Cor van Loveren. "Sugars and Dental Caries," *American Journal of Clinical Nutrition (AJCN)*, October 2003.

2. "The Best and Worst Foods for Your Teeth," *Health Encyclopedia*, University of Rochester Medical Center (URMC), 2016.

Chapter 5

Fluoride Prevents Tooth Decay

Chapter Contents

Section 5.1

The Process of Tooth Decay

This section includes text excerpted from "The Tooth Decay Process:
How to Reverse It and Avoid a Cavity," National Institute of Dental
and Craniofacial Research (NIDCR), July 2018.

What Is inside Our Mouths?

Our mouths are full of bacteria. Hundreds of different types live on
our teeth, gums, tongue, and other places in our mouths. Some bacteria
are helpful. But, some can be harmful, such as those that play a role
in tooth decay process.

Tooth decay is the result of an infection with certain types of bacteria that use sugars in food to make acids. Over time, these acids can
make a cavity in the tooth.

What Goes on inside Our Mouths All Day?

Throughout the day, a tug of war takes place inside our mouths.

On one team are dental plaque—sticky, colorless film of bacteria plus
foods and drinks that contain sugar or starch (such as milk, bread, cookies,
candy, soda, juice, and many others). Whenever we eat or drink something
that contains sugar or starch, the bacteria use them to produce acids.
These acids begin to eat away at the tooth's hard outer surface, or enamel.

On the other team are the minerals in our saliva (such as calcium
and phosphate) plus fluoride from toothpaste, water, and other sources.
This team helps enamel repair itself by replacing minerals lost during
an "acid attack."

Our teeth go through this natural process of losing minerals and
regaining minerals all day long.

How Does a Cavity Develop?

When a tooth is exposed to acid frequently—for example, if you
eat or drink often, especially foods or drinks containing sugar and
starches—the repeated cycles of acid attacks cause the enamel to continue to lose minerals. A white spot may appear where minerals have
been lost. This is a sign of early decay.

Tooth decay can be stopped or reversed at this point. Enamel can
repair itself by using minerals from saliva, and fluoride from toothpaste or other sources.

But, if the tooth decay process continues, more minerals are lost. Over time, the enamel is weakened and destroyed, forming a cavity. A cavity is permanent damage that a dentist has to repair with a filling.

How Can We Help Teeth Win the Tug of War and Avoid a Cavity?
Use Fluoride

Fluoride is a mineral that can prevent tooth decay from progressing. It can even reverse, or stop, early tooth decay.

Fluoride works to protect teeth. It

- Prevents mineral loss in tooth enamel and replaces lost minerals

- Reduces the ability of bacteria to make acid

You can get fluoride by:

- Drinking fluoridated water from a community water supply; about 74 percent of Americans served by a community water supply system receive fluoridated water

- Brushing with a fluoride toothpaste

If the dentist thinks your child needs more fluoride, she or he may:

- Apply a fluoride gel or varnish to tooth surfaces

- Prescribe fluoride tablets

- Recommend using a fluoride mouth rinse

Section 5.2

Water Fluoridation Basics

This section includes text excerpted from "Water
Fluoridation Basics," Centers for Disease Control and
Prevention (CDC), May 14, 2019.

The mineral fluoride occurs naturally on earth and is released from
rocks into the soil, water, and air. All water contains some fluoride.
Usually, the fluoride level in water is not enough to prevent tooth
decay; however, some groundwater and natural springs can have naturally high levels of fluoride.

Fluoride has been proven to protect teeth from decay. Bacteria in
the mouth produce acid when a person eats sugary foods. This acid eats
away minerals from the tooth's surface, making the tooth weaker and
increasing the chance of developing cavities. Fluoride helps to rebuild
and strengthen the tooth's surface, or enamel. Water fluoridation prevents tooth decay by providing frequent and consistent contact with
low levels of fluoride. By keeping the tooth strong and solid, fluoride
stops cavities from forming and can even rebuild the tooth's surface.

Community water fluoridation is the process of adjusting the
amount of fluoride found in water to achieve optimal prevention of
tooth decay.

Although other fluoride-containing products, such as toothpaste,
mouth rinses, and dietary supplements, are available and contribute to the prevention and control of tooth decay, community water
fluoridation has been identified as the most cost-effective method of
delivering fluoride to all, reducing tooth decay by 25 percent in children and adults.

Benefits: Strong Teeth

Fluoride benefits children and adults throughout their lives. For
children younger than the age of eight, fluoride helps strengthen the
adult (permanent) teeth that are developing under the gums. For
adults, drinking water with fluoride supports tooth enamel, keeping teeth strong and healthy. The health benefits of fluoride include
having:

- Fewer cavities

- Less severe cavities

- Less need for fillings and removing teeth
- Less pain and suffering because of tooth decay

History of Fluoride in Water

In the 1930s, scientists examined the relationship between tooth decay in children and naturally occurring fluoride in drinking water. The study found that children who drank water with naturally high levels of fluoride had less tooth decay. This discovery was important because, during that time, most children and adults in the United States were affected by tooth decay. Many suffered from toothaches and painful extractions—often losing permanent teeth, including molars, even as teenagers.

After much scientific research, in 1945, the city of Grand Rapids, Michigan, was the first to add fluoride to its city water system in order to provide residents with the benefits of fluoride.

Since 1945, hundreds of cities have started community water fluoridation and in 2012, nearly 75 percent of the United States served by community water systems had access to fluoridated water. Because of its contribution to the dramatic decline in tooth decay over the past 70 years, the Centers for Disease Control and Prevention (CDC) named community water fluoridation as 1 of 10 great public-health achievements of the 20th century.

Cost: Saves Money, Saves Teeth

Community water fluoridation has been shown to save money, both for families and the healthcare system. The return on investment for community water fluoridation varies with the size of the community, increasing as the community size increases. Community water fluoridation is cost-saving, even for small communities. The estimated return on investment for community water fluoridation (including productivity losses) ranged from $4 in small communities of 5,000 people or less to $27 in large communities of 200,000 people or more.

Fluoride in Water

In 2012, more than 210 million people, or 75 percent of the U.S. population, were served by community water systems that contain enough fluoride to protect their teeth. However, approximately 100 million Americans still do not have access to water with fluoride. Because it is so beneficial, the United States has a national goal for 80 percent of

Americans to have water with enough fluoride to prevent tooth decay by 2020.

Section 5.3

Bottled Water and Fluoride

This section includes text excerpted from "Bottled Water," Centers for Disease Control and Prevention (CDC), July 10, 2013. Reviewed July 2019.

Consumers drink bottled water for various reasons, including as a taste preference or as a convenient means of hydration. Bottled water may not have a sufficient amount of fluoride, which is important for preventing tooth decay and promoting oral health.

Some bottled waters contain fluoride, and some do not. Fluoride can occur naturally in source waters used for bottling, or it can be added.

Does Bottled Water Contain Fluoride?

Bottled water products may contain fluoride, depending on the source of the water. Fluoride can be naturally present in the original source of the water, and many public water systems add fluoride to their water. The U.S. Food and Drug Administration (FDA) sets limits for fluoride in bottled water, based on several factors, including the source of the water. Bottled water products labeled as deionized, purified, demineralized, or distilled have been treated in such a way that they contain no or only trace amounts of fluoride unless they specifically list fluoride as an added ingredient.

How Can I Find Out the Level of Fluoride in Bottled Water?

The FDA does not require bottled water manufacturers to list the amount of fluoride on the label unless the manufacturer has added fluoride within set limits. Contact the bottled water's manufacturer to ask about the fluoride content of a particular brand.

Who Regulates Fluoride in Bottled Water

The U.S. Environmental Protection Agency (EPA) regulates public drinking water (tap water), and the FDA regulates bottled water products under the authority of the Federal Food, Drug, and Cosmetic Act.

As set forth in 21 Council on Foreign Relations (CFR) 165.110, the FDA has established standards for the maximum amount of naturally occurring fluoride or added fluoride allowed in bottled drinking water.

If bottled water meets specific standards of identity and quality set forth by the FDA, and the provisions of the authorized health claim, manufacturers may include the following health claim: "Drinking fluoridated water may reduce the risk of dental caries or tooth decay."

Section 5.4

Private Well Water and Fluoride

This section includes text excerpted from "Private Wells,"
Centers for Disease Control and Prevention (CDC),
July 10, 2013. Reviewed July 2019.

My Home Gets Its Water from a Private Well. What Do I Need to Know about Fluoride and Groundwater from a Well?

Fluoride is present in virtually all waters at some level, and it is important to know the fluoride content of your water, particularly if you have children. To find out the fluoride concentration in your well water, it would need to be analyzed by a laboratory. Your public health department should be able to advise you on how to have your home well water tested.

What Should I Do If the Water from My Well Has Less Than the Recommended Level of Fluoride for Preventing Tooth Decay?

The recommended fluoride level in drinking water for good oral health is 0.7 mg/L (milligrams per liter). If fluoride levels in your drinking water are lower than 0.7 mg/L, your child's dentist or pediatrician should evaluate whether your child could benefit from daily fluoride supplements. Their recommendation will depend on your child's risk of developing tooth decay, as well as exposure to other sources of fluoride, such as drinking water at school or day care and fluoride toothpaste. It is not currently feasible to add fluoride to an individual residence's well.

What Should I Do If the Water from My Well Has Fluoride Levels That Are Higher Than the Recommended Level for Preventing Tooth Decay?

In some regions of the United States, community drinking water and home wells can contain levels of naturally occurring fluoride that are greater than the level recommended by the U.S. Public Health Service for preventing tooth decay. The EPA currently has a nonenforceable recommended guideline for fluoride of 2.0 mg/L that is set to protect against dental fluorosis. If your home is served by a water system that has fluoride levels exceeding this recommended guideline, the EPA recommends that children eight years of age and younger be provided with alternative sources of drinking water.

What Should I Do If My Well Water Was Measured as Having Too Much Fluoride?

It is unusual to have the fluoride content of water be 4 mg/L or higher. If a laboratory report indicates that you have such a high fluoride content, it is recommended that you retest the water. You should collect at least four samples over four weeks (one sample each week) and compare the results. If one sample is above 4 mg/L and the other samples are less than 4 mg/L, then the high value may have been an error. If the results for all the samples show levels greater than 4 mg/L, you may want to consider alternate sources of water for drinking and cooking or installing a device to remove the fluoride from your home water source. Physical contact with water with high fluoride content, such as through bathing or washing dishes, is safe since fluoride does not pass through the skin.

Section 5.5

Questions about Community Water Fluoridation

This section includes text excerpted from "Community Water Fluoridation," Centers for Disease Control and Prevention (CDC), April 1, 2016.

What Is Community Water Fluoridation?

Almost all water contains some naturally occurring fluoride, but it is usually at levels too low to prevent tooth decay. Many communities adjust the fluoride concentration in the water supply to a level known to reduce tooth decay and promote good oral health (often called the "optimal level"). This practice is known as "community water fluoridation" and reaches all people who drink that water. Given the dramatic decline in tooth decay during the past 70 years since community water fluoridation was initiated, the Centers for Disease Control and Prevention (CDC) named fluoridation of drinking water to prevent dental caries (tooth decay) as 1 of 10 great public health interventions of the 20th century.

Does My Public Water System Add Fluoride to the Water?

The best way to find the fluoride level of your local public water system is to contact your water utility provider. Consumers can find the name and contact information of the water utility on the water bill. The U.S. Environmental Protection Agency (EPA) requires that all community water systems provide each customer with an annual report on water quality, including the fluoride content. If you live in one of the states that participate in the CDC's My Water's Fluoride program, you can find information on the fluoridation status of your water system online at My Water's Fluoride.

If I Am Drinking Water with Fluoride, Why Do I Also Need to Brush with Toothpaste That Contains Fluoride?

Both drinking water and toothpaste with fluoride provide important and complementary benefits. Fluoridated water keeps a low level of fluoride in saliva and dental plaque all day. The much higher concentration of fluoride in toothpaste offers additional benefit. Fluoride slows the activity of bacteria that cause decay and combines with enamel on the tooth surface to make it stronger and better able to resist decay. Together, the two sources offer more protection than using either one alone.

Given That We Get Fluoride from Other Sources, Should Communities Still Fluoridate Water to Prevent Tooth Decay?

Yes. Consuming fluoridated water and other beverages and foods prepared or processed with fluoridated water is still important for the prevention of decay in a community. Ingesting fluoridated water throughout the day maintains a low level of fluoride in saliva and plaque that enhances the remineralization of weakened tooth surfaces. Community water fluoridation has been identified as the most cost-effective method of delivering fluoride to all members of the community regardless of age, educational attainment, income level, and the availability of dental care. In studies conducted after other fluoride products, such as toothpaste, were widely available, scientists found additional reductions in tooth decay—up to 25 percent—among people with community water fluoridation when compared to those without fluoridation.

Has the Safety of Community Water Fluoridation Been Evaluated?

The safety and effectiveness of fluoride at levels used in community water fluoridation have been thoroughly reviewed by multinational scientific and public-health organizations (United States, Canada, Australia, New Zealand, Great Britain, and the World Health Organization (WHO)) using evidence-based reviews and expert panels. These panels include scientists with expertise in various health and scientific disciplines, including medicine, biophysics, chemistry, toxicological pathology, oral health, and epidemiology.

Experts have weighed the findings and quality of the available evidence and concluded that there is no association between water fluoridation and any unwanted health effects other than dental fluorosis.

Are There Any Harmful Health Effects Due to Community Water Fluoridation?

The safety and effectiveness of community water fluoridation continue to be supported by scientific evidence produced by independent scientists and summarized by panels of experts. The independent, nongovernmental Community Prevention Task Force (CPSTF) has noted that the research evidence does not demonstrate that community water fluoridation results in any unwanted health effects other than dental fluorosis, a condition that causes primarily cosmetic changes in the appearance of tooth enamel.

Will Using a Home Water Filtration System Take the Fluoride Out of My Home's Water?

The removal of fluoride from water is a difficult water treatment action. Most point-of-use treatment systems for homes that are installed on single faucets use activated carbon filtration, which will not remove the fluoride ion. Other treatment systems (such as reverse osmosis, ion exchange, or distillation systems to reduce fluoride levels) vary in their effectiveness to reduce fluoride. Check with the manufacturer of the individual product.

Will Boiling or Freezing Reduce the Fluoride Level in the Water?

Fluoride is not released from water when it is boiled or frozen. One exception would be a water distillation system. These systems heat water to boiling point and then collect the water vapor as it evaporates. Water distillation systems are typically used in laboratory installations. For home use, these systems can be expensive and may present safety and maintenance concerns.

Will Water Fluoridation Result in Pipe Corrosion or Increased Lead in Drinking Water?

Water fluoridation will not increase pipe corrosion or cause lead to leach from pipes and household plumbing fixtures. Although lead in public drinking water is typically found to be very low or is below laboratory detection, there are locations where old lead pipes, solder, or plumbing fixtures in old homes may experience leaching of lead into the water. Claims by some that fluoride might result in increased lead leaching from pipes and fixtures have not been substantiated in the peer-reviewed literature.

What Did the 2015 Report from the Cochrane Oral Health Group Say about the Effectiveness of Water Fluoridation?

The Cochrane review found that water fluoridation is effective in reducing cavities in the primary and permanent teeth in children. It found that water fluoridation resulted in fewer teeth affected by cavities (about 2 primary teeth and 1 permanent tooth), compared to communities that did not have water fluoridation. These differences indicated that the initiation of water fluoridation could result in decreases of up to 35 percent in cavities in children. In addition, water fluoridation resulted in higher percentages of children without any cavities.

Cochrane's restrictive methodology for including studies in their analyses excluded the majority of studies done after 1975. Although valid, peer-reviewed studies clearly document the effectiveness of community water fluoridation in children and adults even after the use of fluoride toothpaste became widespread, these studies were not considered by Cochrane. As a result, Cochrane found insufficient information available to determine if water fluoridation had an impact in an environment where fluoride products, such as toothpaste, are now widely used.

Another factor that impacted Cochrane's assessment of the evidence is that their methodology favors randomized controlled trials (RCTs). While RCTs are a preferred study design for studies comparing different clinical treatments among individual patients, this research design is often not feasible for interventions that occur on a community level, such as community water fluoridation.

Section 5.6

Fluoride Products for Dental Care

This section includes text excerpted from "Other Fluoride Products,"
Centers for Disease Control and Prevention (CDC), March 8, 2019.

In the United States, water fluoridation is not the only form of fluoride delivery that is effective in preventing tooth decay in people of all ages. Use the information listed below to compare the other fluoride products that may lower the risk for tooth decay, especially for people who are at a higher risk for decay.

Although all of these products reduce tooth decay, combined use with fluoridated water offers protection greater than any of these products used alone.

Fluoride Toothpaste
Form

Concentrations of fluoride in toothpaste sold in the United States range from 1,000 to 1,500 ppm.

Use

Most people report brushing their teeth at least once per day, but more frequent use can offer additional protection. Fluoride in toothpaste is taken up directly by the dental plaque and demineralized enamel, and it also increases the concentration of fluoride in saliva.

Availability

Fluoride toothpaste is available over-the-counter (OTC) and makes up more than 95 percent of toothpaste sales in the United States.

Recommendations

For most people (children, adolescents, and adults) brushing at least twice a day—when you get up in the morning and before going to bed—with a fluoride toothpaste—is recommended.

Advice for Parents

For children aged six years and younger, some simple recommendations are advised to reduce the risk of dental fluorosis.

- Supervise brushing to discourage swallowing toothpaste.

- Place only a small pea-size amount of fluoride toothpaste on your child's toothbrush.

- For children younger than two, consult first with your doctor or dentist regarding the use of fluoride toothpaste

Fluoride Mouth Rinse
Form

Fluoride mouth rinse is a concentrated solution intended for daily or weekly use. The most common fluoride compound used in mouth rinse is sodium fluoride. OTC solutions of 0.05 percent sodium fluoride (230 ppm fluoride) for daily rinsing are available for use by persons older than 6 years of age. Solutions of 0.20 percent sodium fluoride (920 ppm fluoride) are used in supervised, school-based weekly rinsing programs. Other concentrations are also available.

Use

Rinses are used daily or weekly for a prescribed amount of time. The fluoride from mouth rinse is retained in dental plaque and saliva to help prevent tooth decay.

Availability

Mouth rinses intended for home use can be purchased OTC. Higher-strength mouth rinses for those at high risk of tooth decay must be prescribed by a dentist or physician.

Recommendations

For children younger than six years of age, consult first with your doctor or dentist regarding the use of mouth rinse because dental fluorosis could occur if such mouth rinses are repeatedly swallowed. Because fluoride mouth rinse has resulted in only limited reductions in tooth decay among schoolchildren, especially as their exposure to other sources of fluoride has increased, its use should be targeted to individuals or groups at a high risk for decay.

Fluoride Supplements
Form

Tablets, lozenges, or liquids (including fluoride–vitamin preparations) are available. Most supplements contain sodium fluoride as the active ingredient. Tablets and lozenges are manufactured with 1.0, 0.5, or 0.25 mg fluoride.

Use

Fluoride supplements can be prescribed for children at a high risk for tooth decay and whose primary drinking water has a low fluoride concentration. To maximize the topical effect of fluoride, tablets and lozenges are intended to be chewed or sucked for 12 minutes before being swallowed.

Availability

All fluoride supplements must be prescribed by a dentist or physician.

Recommendations

For children younger than six years of age, the dentist, physician, or other healthcare provider should weigh the risk for tooth decay without fluoride supplements, the decay prevention offered by supplements, and the potential for dental fluorosis. Consideration of the child's other sources of fluoride, especially drinking water, is essential in determining this balance. Parents and caregivers should be informed of both the benefit of protection against tooth decay and the possibility of dental fluorosis.

Fluoride Gel and Foam
Form

Fluoride gel is often formulated to be highly acidic (pH of approximately 3.0). Products available in the United States include gel of acidulated phosphate fluoride (1.23% [12,300 ppm] fluoride), gel or foam of sodium fluoride (0.9% [9,040 ppm] fluoride), and self-applied (i.e., home use) gel of sodium fluoride (0.5% [5,000 ppm] fluoride) or stannous fluoride (0.15% [1,000 ppm] fluoride).

Use

In a dental office, fluoride gel is applied for one to four minutes. For home-use fluoride gel, follow the instructions provided on the prescription.

Availability

Most fluoride gel and foam applications are delivered in a dental office by a dental professional. These higher strength products, if used in the home, must be prescribed by a dentist or physician.

Recommendations

Because these applications are relatively infrequent, generally at 3 to 12 month intervals, fluoride gel poses little risk for dental fluorosis, even among patients younger than six years of age. Routine use of professionally applied fluoride gel or foam likely provides little benefit to persons not at a high risk for tooth decay, especially those who drink fluoridated water and brush daily with fluoride toothpaste.

Fluoride Varnish

Form

Varnishes are available as sodium fluoride (2.26% [22,600 ppm] fluoride) or difluorsilane (0.1% [1,000 ppm] fluoride) preparations.

Use

High-concentration fluoride varnish is painted by dental or other healthcare professionals directly onto the teeth. Fluoride varnish is not intended to adhere permanently; this method holds a high concentration of fluoride in a small amount of material in close contact with the teeth for many hours. Varnishes must be reapplied at regular intervals with at least two applications per year required for effectiveness.

Availability

All fluoride varnish must be applied by a dentist or other healthcare provider.

Recommendations

No published evidence indicates that professionally applied fluoride varnish is a risk factor for dental fluorosis, even among children younger than six years of age. Proper application technique reduces the possibility that a patient will swallow varnish during its application and limits the total amount of fluoride swallowed as the varnish wears off the teeth over several hours.

Although it is not currently cleared for marketing by the U.S. Food and Drug Administration (FDA) as an anticaries agent, fluoride varnish has been widely used for this purpose in Canada and Europe since the 1970s. Studies conducted in Canada and Europe have reported that fluoride varnish is as effective in preventing tooth decay as professionally applied fluoride gel.

Chapter 6

Dental Plaque

Dental Plaque and Its Causes

Plaque is a clear, sticky substance that builds upon and between teeth. Unlike other parts of the body, teeth do not have surfaces that follow a systemic cycle of shedding and renewal. This provides a rich area for microorganisms to breed, creating a biofilm, an ecosystem of thousands of species of colonizing bacteria that attach themselves to the enamel of the tooth. The biofilm, or plaque, is composed of a heterogeneous arrangement of bacterial cells, polysaccharides, proteins, and salt.

Plaque can form all over teeth, but it is found most often in the crevices of the molars. It tends to feel fuzzy or rough to the touch and is often difficult to see with the naked eye.

Problems Caused by Plaque

The bacteria in plaque live on sugars in the food that we eat. The fermentation of sugar produces acid byproducts that corrode teeth enamel and can subsequently result in a cavity. Unhindered, plaque may solidify into a hard substance called "tartar" or "calculus." As the tartar and plaque progress further, the gums can become red and swollen and bleed when brushing. This is a condition known as "gingivitis," an early-stage periodontal disease. If not treated properly, gingivitis

---

"Dental Plaque," © 2017 Omnigraphics. Reviewed July 2019.

may develop into periodontitis, a condition that is characterized by receding gums, infection, and damage to the bones supporting the teeth. Untreated, periodontitis can eventually result in the loss of teeth.

Plaque Identification

Plaque is identified using two procedures:

- A disclosing tablet is chewed for 30 seconds, and the mouth is rinsed with water. The tablet leaves a pink dye on the plaque that can easily be seen.

- The mouth is rinsed with a special fluorescent solution and then rinsed gently with water. An ultraviolet light is shone on the teeth, revealing the existing plaque in a bright orange-yellow color. The advantage of this method is that it does not cause visible stains on teeth.

How to Deal with Dental Plaque

You cannot get rid of plaque completely on your own, but it can be prevented through proper dental hygiene:

- The best way to prevent dental plaque is to brush and floss daily. Brush your teeth once in the morning and again at night with fluoridated toothpaste. This dislodges the plaque and prevents the buildup of tartar.

- Use an interdental cleaner to remove plaque from hard-to-reach places where it is difficult to clean with a toothbrush.

- In addition to freshening breath, mouthwash can be useful in removing food debris, but do not depend on mouth rinses alone to keep plaque at bay. Brushing and flossing is essential.

- Eat healthy, balanced meals and limit snacks that may provide an environment for the bacteria in plaque.

- Make use of a sealant. If necessary, a dentist will cover teeth with a substance that forms a clear coating of plastic preventing the growth of bacteria and acids.

- Chewing sugar-free gum after meals can help prevent plaque by producing saliva, which washes away the acid present in the mouth after eating or drinking. Do not overuse chewing gum, though, because it may cause bruxism (tooth grinding) and problems in the joints of the jaw.

- Schedule regular visits to the dentist for a thorough oral examination and professional cleaning.

Failing to brush and floss is the single most common cause of plaque buildup that can lead to gingivitis and periodontitis later. Following a daily regimen of oral hygiene, combined with regular check-ups by a dentist, is the best way to prevent plaque and make sure teeth remain strong and healthy for a lifetime.

References

1. "Dental Plaque Identification at Home," A.D.A.M., Inc., August 23, 2016.

2. "What Is Plaque?" Delta Dental, March 2012.

3. Szalay, Jessie. "What Is Plaque?" LiveScience, August 26, 2014.

4. Laura, Manonelles. "What Is Tooth Plaque?" Propdental, May 16, 2014.

5. Hicks, Rob. "5 Bad Habits That Lead to Plaque on Your Teeth," WebMD, January 28, 2015.

Chapter 7

Mouth Injuries

What Are Mouth Injuries?

Mouth injuries are wounds or cuts on the lips, teeth, tongue, jaw, inner cheeks, and floor or roof of the mouth. These injuries often occur while playing sports or during other physical activity, and children tend to incur them more than adults. When mouth or dental injuries take place, there can be excessive bleeding, since a lot of blood vessels are concentrated in the mouth area. Though most of these types of injuries are minor and can be treated at home, severe cuts or bruises may call for professional medical attention.

Types of Mouth Injuries

- **Minor injuries.** Minor mouth injuries include cuts, bruises, and wounds that can be treated at home or that heal over time without treatment. Minor cuts are generally caused by playing, sports, or other daily activities. Even during routine activities like eating or sleeping a person may accidentally bite her or his tongue and cause a minor injury, but these normally heal over time without treatment.

- **Major injuries**. Major injuries in the mouth require evaluation by a doctor, since they can affect the tonsils, soft palate (the fleshy area at the back of the roof of the mouth), or the throat.

"Mouth Injuries," © 2017 Omnigraphics. Reviewed July 2019.

When a child falls with a pointed object in her or his mouth, it may lead to a major mouth injury, which can affect deeper tissues in the head or neck.

- **Upper and lower lip cuts.** Upper lip cuts usually occur when a person falls, which can cause a tear in the connective tissue between the upper lip and gum called "frenulum." A suture is not always necessary, as this tear may heal on its own, although bleeding can recur during the healing process. A lower lip cut may take place during a fall when the lip is caught between the upper and lower teeth. In serious cases, sutures might be required.

Stitches may also be required for an injury to the mouth or lips that causes a loose flap of tissue, called a "gaping wound." If the frenulum tears, it may require stitches or, if minor, it could heal on its own over time.

- **Dental injuries.** An injury to a tooth, which often occurs during a fall or sports activity, can cause it to crack, break off, lose color or be chipped. The tooth can also be displaced from its original position (dental luxation) or jammed into the gum (intruded). Other causes of dental injuries include grinding of the teeth, orthodontic procedures that cause mouth sores, and piercings in the mouth. A medical professional should evaluate all such injuries.

Symptoms of Mouth and Dental Injuries

Symptoms of mouth and dental injuries include bleeding, pain, laceration of tissue, tooth damage, swelling, bruising, tissue loss, and loose tissue flaps.

Treatment for Mouth and Dental Injuries

Most minor mouth injuries can be treated at home using some of the remedies listed below.

Stop the bleeding. To stop bleeding from the inner lip or tissue that connects the inner lip with the gum, apply pressure to the bleeding site with sterile gauze or a clean cloth for ten minutes. Be careful reexamining the site, or bleeding may start again. Similarly, bleeding from the tongue can be stopped by pressing on the area with sterile gauze or a clean cloth. Applying a piece of ice or popsicle to the affected area may also help.

Reduce pain in the mouth. Pain in the mouth can be reduced with nonprescription medicines, such as:

- A topical medication, such as Orabase, Anbesol, or Ulcerease

- Pain relievers, such as acetaminophen (Tylenol)

- Nonsteroidal anti-inflammatory drugs like ibuprofen (Advil or Motrin) or naproxen (Aleve or Naprosyn)

It is wise to read the instructions carefully before consuming nonprescription medicines and only recommended doses are advisable. If a person is pregnant, allergic to certain medicines, or has been advised not to take certain medicines, a doctor should be consulted before treatment.

Promote healing. Rinsing the mouth with warm salt water after every meal can promote the healing of many types of mouth wounds. Saltwater can be made by mixing 1 cup (250 ml) of warm water with 1 tsp. (5g) of salt.

Recommended Diet

After a mouth or dental injury, a diet of soft foods is recommended in order to avoid disrupting the healing process.
Suggestions for soft foods include:

- Dairy products, such as milk, yogurt, ice-cream, and cheese

- Fluids, such as milkshakes and sherbets, to avoid dehydration

- Eggs and tender or ground meats

- Fruits and vegetables that are well-ripened, or baked or mashed

Things to be avoided include:

- Citrus fruits and salty or spicy food that may cause stinging

- Alcoholic beverages

- Smoking or using other tobacco products

When Must a Doctor Be Consulted for Mouth Injuries?

A doctor needs to be consulted if there is a major injury or if the following symptoms are observed:

- Loose flaps of tissue or a gaping wound
- Severe pain
- Bleeding that won't stop
- Swelling, redness, tenderness, or evidence of infection in the affected area
- Severe toothache or one that persists for two weeks or interferes with daily activities
- Fever
- Cuts that are caused by a dirty or rusty object
- A tooth that is knocked out or torn out of its socket

Prevention of Mouth and Dental Injuries

Most mouth and dental injuries can be prevented by being careful and protecting oneself. Some suggestions:

- Get regular dental checkups to prevent tooth and gum problems.
- Wear a mouth guard to prevent injuries while playing sports.
- Follow instructions after an orthodontic procedure, and follow up with a medical professional if pain persists.

Children are particularly susceptible to mouth and dental injuries. Here are some steps parents can take to reduce the likelihood of such injuries:

- Make children aware of the dangers of playing or running with objects in their mouths.
- Teach children not to chew or suck on sharp or pointed objects.
- Be sure children wear mouth guards or face masks while playing sports.
- Teach children to sit while eating or drinking, especially while eating food on a stick.
- Discourage eating while riding in a car.

References

1. "Mouth and Dental Injuries: Topic Overview," WebMD, September 9, 2014.

2. "Cuts and Wounds of the Mouth and Lips," Stanford Children's Health, n.d.

3. Schmitt, Barton. "Should Your Child See a Doctor," Seattle Children's Hospital, n.d.

Chapter 8

Oral Health for Older Adults

Chapter Contents

Section 8.1

Adult Oral Health Problems

This section includes text excerpted from "Adult Oral Health,"
Centers for Disease Control and Prevention (CDC), July 13, 2016.

The baby boomer generation is the first where the majority of people will keep their natural teeth over their entire lifetime. This is largely because of the benefits of water fluoridation and fluoride toothpaste. However, threats to oral health, including tooth loss, continue throughout life.

The major risks for tooth loss are tooth decay and gum disease that may increase with age because of problems with saliva production; receding gums that expose "softer" root surfaces to decay-causing bacteria; or difficulties flossing and brushing because of poor vision, cognitive problems, chronic disease, and physical limitations.

Although more adults are keeping their teeth, many continue to need treatment for dental problems. This need is even greater for members of some racial and ethnic groups—about three in four Latinx and non-Latinx Black adults have an unmet need for dental treatment, as do people who are poor. These individuals are also more likely to report having poor oral health.

In addition, some adults may have difficulty accessing dental treatment. For every adult 19 years of age or older without medical insurance, there are 3 who do not have dental insurance.

Oral Health Problems

Oral health problems in adults include the following:

- **Untreated tooth decay.** More than 1 in 4 (27%) adults in the United States have untreated tooth decay.

- **Gum disease.** Nearly half (46%) of all adults 30 years of age or older show signs of gum disease; severe gum disease affects about 9 percent of adults.

- **Tooth loss.** Complete tooth loss among adults between the ages of 65 to 74 has steadily declined over time, but disparities exist among some population groups. If left untreated, cavities (tooth decay) and periodontal (gum) disease can lead to tooth loss.

- **Oral cancer.** Oral cancers are most common in older adults, particularly in people older than 55 years of age who smoke and are heavy drinkers.

  - People treated for cancer who have chemotherapy may suffer from oral problems, such as painful mouth ulcers, impaired taste, and dry mouth.

- **Chronic diseases.** Having a chronic disease, such as arthritis, heart disease or stroke, diabetes, emphysema, hepatitis C, a liver condition, or being obese, may increase an individual's risk of having missing teeth and poor oral health.

  - Patients with weakened immune systems, such as those infected with human immunodeficiency virus (HIV) and other medical conditions (organ transplants) and who use some medications (e.g., steroids), are at higher risk for some oral problems.

  - Chronic disabling diseases such as jaw joint diseases (temporomandibular disorders (TMD)); autoimmune conditions, such as Sjögren syndrome, and osteoporosis, affect millions of Americans and compromise oral health and functioning, more often among women.

Oral Health Tips

You can keep your teeth for your lifetime. Here are some things you can do to maintain a healthy mouth and strong teeth.

- Drink fluoridated water and brush with fluoride toothpaste.

- Practice good oral hygiene. Brush your teeth thoroughly, and floss between the teeth to remove dental plaque.

- Visit your dentist on a regular basis, even if you have no natural teeth or have dentures.

- Do not use any tobacco products. If you smoke, quit.

- Limit alcoholic drinks.

- If you have diabetes, work to maintain control of the disease. This will decrease the risk for other complications, including gum disease.

- If your medication causes dry mouth, ask your doctor for a different medication that may not cause this condition. If dry mouth cannot be avoided, drink plenty of water, chew sugarless gum, and avoid tobacco products and alcohol.

- See your doctor or dentist if you have sudden changes in taste and smell.

- When acting as a caregiver, help older individuals brush and floss their teeth if they are not able to perform these activities independently.

Section 8.2

Older Adults' Oral Health: Myths and Facts

This section includes text excerpted from "Older Adults and Oral Health," National Institute of Dental and Craniofacial Research (NIDCR), November 2017.

Tooth Decay (Cavities)

Myth: Only school kids get cavities.

Fact: Tooth decay can develop at any age. Tooth decay is not just a problem for children. It can happen as long as you have natural teeth. Dental plaque—a sticky film of bacteria—can build up on teeth. Plaque produces acids that, over time, eat away at the tooth's hard outer surface and create a cavity.

Even teeth that already have fillings are at risk. Plaque can build up underneath a chipped filling and cause new decay. And if your gums have pulled away from the teeth (called "gum recession"), the exposed tooth roots are also vulnerable to decay.

But, you can protect your teeth against decay. Here is how:

- Use toothpaste that contains fluoride. Fluoride can prevent tooth decay and also heal early decay. And, it is just as helpful for adults as it is for children. Be sure to brush twice daily. This will help remove dental plaque that forms on teeth. Drinking fluoridated water also helps prevent tooth decay in adults.

- Floss regularly to remove plaque from between teeth. Or use a special brush or wooden or plastic pick recommended by a dental professional.

- See a dentist for routine checkups. If you are at a higher risk for tooth decay (for example, if you have a dry mouth because of medicines you take), the dentist or dental hygienist may give you a fluoride treatment, such as a varnish or foam during the office visit. Or, the dentist may tell you to use a fluoride gel or mouth rinse at home.

Gum Diseases

Myth: Gum disease is just a part of growing older.

Fact: You can prevent gum disease—it does not have to be a part of getting older.

Gum (periodontal) disease is an infection of the gums and surrounding tissues that hold teeth in place. Gum disease develops when plaque—is allowed to build up along and under the gum line.

The two forms of gum disease are:

- Gingivitis, a mild form that is reversible with good oral hygiene. In gingivitis, the gums become red, swollen, and bleed easily.

- Periodontitis, a more severe form that can damage the soft tissues and bone that support the teeth. In periodontitis, gums pull away from the teeth and form spaces (called "pockets") that become infected. The body's immune system fights the bacteria as the plaque spreads and grows below the gum line. Bacterial toxins and the body's natural response to infection start to break down the bone and connective tissue that hold teeth in place. If not treated, the bones, gums, and tissue that support the teeth are destroyed. The teeth may eventually become loose and have to be removed.

The good news is that gum disease can be prevented. It does not have to be a part of growing older. With thorough brushing and flossing and regular professional cleanings by a dentist, you can reduce your risk of developing gum disease as you age.

And if you have been treated for gum disease, sticking to a proper oral hygiene routine and visiting the dentist for regular cleanings can minimize the chances it will come back.

Here are some things you can do:

- Brush your teeth twice a day (with a fluoride toothpaste).
- Floss regularly to remove plaque from between teeth. Or, use a special brush or wooden or plastic pick recommended by a dental professional.
- Visit a dentist for routine checkups.
- Do not smoke or use chewing tobacco or snuff.
- Eat a well-balanced diet.

If you smoke, you are at a higher risk for developing periodontitis than a nonsmoker. In fact, smoking is one of the most significant risk factors for gum disease.

Here is why:

- Smoking may impair blood flow to the gums, reducing the amount of oxygen and nutrients to the tissues and make them more vulnerable to infection.
- Chemicals in tobacco smoke cause inflammation and cell damage, and they can weaken the immune system.
- Nicotine is toxic to cells that make new connective tissue, and it also increases the production of an enzyme that breaks down tissue.

Smoking can also lower the chances that treatment for periodontitis will be successful and can lengthen the time it takes for treatments to work.

Dry Mouth

Myth: Dry mouth is a natural part of the aging process. You just have to learn to live with it.

Fact: Dry mouth is not a part of the aging process itself; it is important to find the cause of dry mouth so you can get relief.

Dry mouth is the feeling that there is not enough saliva in the mouth. Common causes of dry mouth in older adults include side effects of certain medications and dehydration. Dry mouth can make it hard to chew, swallow, or even talk. Having less saliva also increases the risk of developing tooth decay or fungal infections in the mouth since saliva helps keep harmful germs in check.

If you have dentures, dry mouth can make them uncomfortable, and they may not fit as well. Without enough saliva, dentures can also rub against the gums or the roof of the mouth and cause sore spots.

It is important to know that dry mouth is not part of the aging process itself. However, many older adults take medications that can dry out the mouth. And, older adults are also more likely to have certain conditions that can lead to oral dryness.

Here are some causes of dry mouth:

- **Side effects of medicines.** Hundreds of medicines can cause the salivary glands to make less saliva. Medicines for high blood pressure, depression, and bladder control problems often cause dry mouth.

- **Dehydration.** Older adults are more prone to dehydration than younger people.

- **Disease.** Diabetes, Sjögren syndrome, and human immunodeficiency virus /acquired immunodeficiency syndrome (HIV/AIDS) can cause dry mouth.

- **Radiation therapy (RT).** The salivary glands can be damaged if they are exposed to radiation during cancer treatment.

- **Chemotherapy.** Drugs used to treat cancer can make saliva thicker, causing the mouth to feel dry.

- **Nerve damage.** Injury to the head or neck can damage the nerves that tell salivary glands to make saliva.

If you think you have dry mouth, see a dentist or physician. She or he can try to determine what is causing your dry mouth and what treatments might be helpful. For example, if dry mouth is caused by a medicine, the physician might change your medicine or adjust the dosage.

The dentist or physician also might suggest that you keep your mouth wet by using artificial saliva, sold in most drugstores/pharmacies. Some people benefit from sucking sugarless hard candy or chewing sugarless gum.

Oral Cancer

Myth: If you do not use chewing tobacco, you do not need to worry about oral cancer.

Fact: It is not just smokeless tobacco ("dip" and "chew") that can increase your chances of getting oral cancer.

Tobacco use of any kind, including cigarette smoking, puts you at risk. Heavy alcohol use also increases your chances of developing the disease. And using tobacco plus alcohol poses a much greater risk than using either substance alone.

The likelihood of oral cancer increases with age. Most people with these cancers are older than 55 years of age when the cancer is found.

Also, recent research has found that infection with the sexually transmitted human papillomavirus (HPV) has been linked to a subset of oral cancers.

It is important to catch oral cancer early because treatment works best before the disease has spread. Pain is usually not an early symptom of the disease. So be on the lookout for any changes in your mouth, especially if you smoke or drink.

If you have any of the following symptoms for more than two weeks, be sure to see a dentist or physician:

- A sore, irritation, lump, or thick patch in the mouth, lips, or throat

- A white or red patch in the mouth

- A feeling that something is caught in the throat

- Difficulty chewing or swallowing

- Difficulty moving the jaw or tongue

- Numbness in the tongue or other areas of the mouth

- Swelling of the jaw that causes dentures to fit poorly or become uncomfortable

- Pain in one ear without hearing loss

Most often, these symptoms do not mean cancer. An infection or other problem can cause the same symptoms. But, it is important to get them checked out because if it is cancer, it can be treated more successfully if it is caught early.

Section 8.3

Helping Older Adults with Brushing

This section includes text excerpted from "Brushing," National
Institute of Dental and Craniofacial Research (NIDCR), August 2018.

If you regularly help someone with oral healthcare, this section is
for you. It offers practical suggestions about how to provide guidance
or direct care, as well as tips that may make the job easier. Oral health
is important for people of all ages. A healthy mouth helps people enjoy
their food, chew better, eat well, and avoid pain and tooth loss. With
good oral hygiene and regular visits to the dentist, older adults can
maintain their oral health into their later years.

Brushing

If the person you care for can brush but needs some help or guidance:

- **Encourage self-care.** If the person you care for has problems
  with memory or judgment, she or he might need reminders. For
  example, leave the toothbrush and toothpaste on the sink. Or,
  apply toothpaste and hand them the toothbrush, or brush your
  teeth at the same time.

- **Encourage thorough brushing.** Thorough brushing and
  flossing are essential for removing dental plaque, a sticky film
  of bacteria. Plaque buildup can cause tooth decay, gum disease,
  and bad breath.

- **Guide the toothbrush.** Help them brush by placing your hand
  very gently over the person's hand and guiding the toothbrush.

- **Adapt the toothbrush, or try different types of
  toothbrushes.** Make the toothbrush easier to use, or try a
  power or multiple-sided toothbrush.

If the person you care for is unable to brush, you need to brush her
or his teeth.

Getting Started

- Choose a location, such as a kitchen or dining room, that allows
  plenty of space to work. Make sure you have good lighting. Place

61

the toothbrush, toothpaste, dental mirror, towel, bowl, and a glass of water within reach.

• Make sure the person you care for is seated in a chair or is upright in bed. Then, choose a position for yourself where you can see all surfaces of the teeth and gums. This may mean sitting or standing to the front or side, or behind the person.

• Ease the person you care for into the situation through conversation, and be patient as she or he gets used to you providing care.

• Use the "tell-show-do" approach. Tell what will happen, show it, and then do the oral care as you have explained.

• Have a dental care routine. Use the same technique at the same time and place every day.

• Be creative. If behavior problems arise, use favorite objects or music for comfort.

• Seek the advice of a dental professional for additional suggestions.

Visiting the Dentist

The person you care for should have regular dental appointments. Professional cleanings are just as important as brushing and flossing at home. Regular exams can identify problems early, before they cause unnecessary pain. Before each appointment, make sure to have a list of current medications, known allergies, and any insurance or billing information.

At these visits, the dentist or dental hygienist can suggest an oral hygiene routine that may make it easier for the person you care for. The dentist may also prescribe a special toothpaste or mouthwash to help prevent tooth decay or a mouthwash to fight germs that cause gum disease. Follow the dentist's instructions for use.

Part Two

Visiting Your Dentist's Office

Chapter 9

Routine Dental Visits and Overcoming Dental Phobia

Routine Dental Checkup

It is generally recommended that most people visit a dentist every six months for a routine dental checkup. Routine dental checkups usually include teeth cleaning, visual and physical exams, and sometimes dental x-rays.

Teeth Cleaning

A dental hygienist is a medical professional who specializes in teeth cleaning. This process involves removing tartar, a hard mineral that accumulates on teeth over time. The hygienist uses a small metal tool to scrape tartar off the tooth surface. The hygienist then flosses the teeth and polishes teeth with a small rotating tool and tooth polishing compound. The hygienist may also apply a fluoride treatment to teeth. While cleaning the teeth, the hygienist also looks for evidence of tooth decay, cavities, gum disease, and other dental problems.

"Routine Dental Visits and Overcoming Dental Phobia," © 2017 Omnigraphics. Reviewed July 2019.

Dental X-Rays

Sometimes a routine dental checkup includes the creation of dental x-rays. These special images allow dentists and other medical professionals to see inside the teeth and the bones of the face. X-rays are an important part of good dental health and are used for identifying, diagnosing, and monitoring dental problems.

Dental Exam

The dental exam is usually performed by a dentist. The exam typically includes a visual examination of the teeth and mouth as well as a review of x-ray images. The dentist looks for possible problems with a person's bite and assesses any need for tooth restoration, removal, or replacement. For people who use dentures, the dentist and/or hygienist will check the fit of devices and discuss any problems or necessary adjustments. The dentist may provide recommendations on improving dental health, instructions on effective flossing and brushing, or other information. Dental exams sometimes also include a physical examination of the jaw, the area under the jaw, the soft tissue inside the mouth, the tongue, and the neck. These exams are done to check for signs of certain oral diseases and some types of cancer.

Dental Impressions

In some cases, dentists will order the creation of a dental impression. A bite impression is created by having the patient bite down on a special paper or other soft material that records the places where upper and lower teeth meet when the mouth is closed. This type of impression is useful in fitting tooth fillings, crowns, caps, and dentures.

Another type of dental impression is used to create a mold or model of a person's teeth and mouth tissue. These impressions are created by filling a U-shaped tray with special gelatin or paste, which is then placed over the arch of teeth and held for a few minutes. Once the impression material has partially hardened, the tray is removed. The resulting mold is used to create a cast of the teeth for the purpose of evaluating bite or making a custom mouth guard.

Dental Phobia

Although it is fairly safe to say that very few people enjoy dental visits, some people suffer from a severe form of anxiety known as "dental phobia." For these people, a visit to the dentist can be a cause of extreme stress, fear, or panic. People who live with dental phobia generally avoid visiting a dentist, often for extended periods of time. The discomfort of tooth pain, broken teeth, or serious gum disease can seem more tolerable than seeking dental treatment for those with dental phobia. As a result, people with dental phobia are at a much higher risk for premature tooth loss and other health problems related to lack of dental care. Oral health has been linked to health conditions as diverse as diabetes, heart disease, and lung infections.

Causes of Dental Phobia

Phobias develop for a variety of reasons and it can be difficult to trace the origin of a fear that many people consider unreasonable. Among people with dental phobia, the reasons for fear can be different for each person. The most commonly expressed reason for avoiding dental care is a fear of pain. This fear is somewhat more common among older people whose early experiences with dental treatment occurred before modern advancements in dental sedation and pain management. Others express a fear of not being in control of a situation in which they are expected to remain still while someone works on their teeth and they are unable to anticipate what is happening. Some people are unable to tolerate the physical closeness with other people that are required as a hygienist or dentist works on their teeth.

Symptoms of Dental Phobia

Anyone might feel anxious before a visit to the dentist, but for some people, a pending dental visit produces feelings of terror and panic. People with dental phobia often describe their experiences during the time before a dental visit in similar terms: feeling tense, inability to sleep, feeling physically ill, trouble breathing, chest pains, vomiting, uncontrollable crying, and/or fear that builds as the time of the visit gets closer. During a dental procedure, people with dental phobia may also panic or have difficulty breathing. Sometimes the sight of dental instruments or dental staff can induce a panic attack.

Overcoming Dental Phobia

Dental phobia can be successfully treated and managed in a way that allows people to receive the dental care they need. Fear management begins with open communication with the dentist, hygienist, and other office staff. Modern dentistry offers many advancements and techniques that can be of great help to people with dental phobia. The first among these techniques is the presentation and maintenance of the dental office environment, including the waiting room. A comfortable, soothing environment can help people with milder forms of dental anxiety feel more calm and confident. The use of artwork, background music, and color schemes can gently influence a person's first impression of the dental office as a safe place. Attention to details, such as keeping dental instruments out of sight as much as possible and providing distractions, such as headphones or personal television screens for patients can also help manage anxieties.

Dental phobia can also be alleviated somewhat through the use of continued communication. Dentists and hygienists may provide descriptions of procedures and outline what will be done before beginning while responding to any questions or concerns that the patient may have. In some cases, alternative sedation may be offered to those with dental phobia. The dentist might prescribe an antianxiety medication to be taken earlier in the day of the dental visit. Inhalation sedation techniques (sometimes referred to as "laughing gas") can help people relax before any procedures are begun. Sedation via intravenous medication (IV sedation) is another option for people with dental phobia. IV sedation usually results in deeper sedation that can be achieved through other means. Advances in dental equipment have produced tools engineered to be smaller and quieter than older equipment, and some modern dental drills include an emergency "stop" button that can be operated by the patient. This particular advancement has helped many with dental phobia to feel more in control of their experience during dental visits. Some people with dental phobia find it helpful to bring a friend or relative with them to dental visits. This companion acts as an advocate, providing comfort and a feeling of safety for the person with dental phobia. In any case of dental phobia, communicating with the dental office staff is crucial to ensuring the needs of the patient are met.

References

1. "Oral Care," WebMD, November 14, 2014.

2. "Test and Procedures: Dental Exam," Mayo Clinic, February 14, 2015.

3. "What Is Dental Anxiety and Phobia?" Aetna, September 18, 2013.
4. "What Can Help?—Ways of Tackling Dental Fears," Dental Fear Central, 2016.

Chapter 10

Dental Caries (Cavities)

Chapter Contents

Section 10.1

What Are Dental Caries?

This section includes text excerpted from "Tooth Decay," National Institute of Dental and Craniofacial Research (NIDCR), April 2019.

Tooth decay (dental caries) is damage to a tooth that can happen when decay-causing bacteria in your mouth make acids that attack the tooth's surface, or enamel. This can lead to a small hole in a tooth, called a "cavity." If tooth decay is not treated, it can cause pain, infection, and even tooth loss.

People of all ages can get tooth decay once they have teeth—from childhood through the senior years.

Young children are at risk for "early childhood caries," sometimes called "baby bottle tooth decay," which is severe tooth decay in baby teeth.

Because many older adults experience receding gums, which allows decay-causing bacteria in the mouth to come into contact with the tooth's root, they can get decay on the exposed root surfaces of their teeth.

Causes

When decay-causing bacteria come into contact with sugars and starches from foods and drinks, they form an acid. This acid can attack the tooth's enamel and cause it to lose minerals.

This can happen if you eat or drink often, especially food and drinks containing sugar and starches. The repeated cycles of these "acid attacks" will cause the enamel to continue to lose minerals. Over time, the enamel is weakened and then destroyed, forming a cavity.

Symptoms

In early tooth decay, there are not usually any symptoms. As tooth decay advances, it can cause a toothache (tooth pain) or tooth sensitivity to sweets, hot or cold. If the tooth becomes infected, an abscess, or pocket of pus, can form and cause pain, facial swelling, and fever.

Diagnosis

Tooth decay can be found during a regular dental check-up. Early tooth decay may look like a white spot on the tooth. If the decay is more advanced, it may appear as a darker spot or a hole in the tooth. The dentist can also check the teeth for soft or sticky areas or take an x-ray, which can show decay.

Treatment

Dentists commonly treat cavities by filling them. A dentist will remove the decayed tooth tissue and then restore the tooth by filling it with a filling material.

Helpful Tips

Here are some things you can do to prevent tooth decay:

- Use fluoride, a mineral that can prevent tooth decay from progressing, and even reverse, or stop, early tooth decay. You can get fluoride by

  - Brushing with a fluoride toothpaste
  - Drinking tap water with fluoride
  - Using a fluoride mouth rinse

- Have a good oral hygiene routine. Brush teeth twice a day with a fluoride toothpaste and regularly clean between teeth with floss or another interdental (between-the-teeth) cleaner.

- Make smart food choices that limit foods high in sugars and starches. Eat nutritious and balanced meals and limit snacking.

- Do not use tobacco products, including smokeless tobacco. If you currently use tobacco, consider quitting.

- See a dentist for regular checkups and professional cleanings.

Section 10.2

Dental Caries (Cavities) in Primary and Permanent Teeth

This section includes text excerpted from the following sources: Text under the heading "Dental Caries in Primary (Baby) Teeth" is excerpted from "Dental Caries (Tooth Decay) in Children Age 2 to 11," National Institute of Dental and Craniofacial Research (NIDCR), July 2018; Text under the heading "Dental Caries in Permanent (Adult) Teeth" is excerpted from "Dental Caries (Tooth Decay) in Adults (Age 20 to 64)," National Institute of Dental and Craniofacial Research (NIDCR), July 2018.

Dental Caries in Primary (Baby) Teeth

Overall dental caries in the baby teeth of children 2 to 11 declined from the early 1970s until the mid-1990s. From the mid-1990s until the most recent National Health and Nutrition Examination Survey (NHANES), this trend has reversed: a small but significant increase in primary decay was found. This trend reversal was more severe in younger children.

Prevalence

- 42 percent of children 2 to 11 have had dental caries in their primary teeth.

- Black and Hispanic children and those living in families with lower incomes have more decay.

Dental Caries in Permanent (Adult) Teeth

Dental caries, both treated and untreated, in all adults age 20 to 64 declined from the early 1970s until the most recent National Health and Nutrition Examination Survey. The decrease was significant in all population subgroups. In spite of this decline, significant disparities are still found in some population groups.

Note: Approximately 5 percent of adults age 20 to 64 have no teeth. This survey applies only to those adults who have teeth.

Prevalence

- 92 percent of adults 20 to 64 have had dental caries in their permanent teeth.

- White adults and those living in families with higher incomes and more education have had more decay.

Unmet Needs

- 26 percent of adults 20 to 64 have untreated decay.

- Black and Latinx adults, younger adults, and those with lower incomes and less education have more untreated decay.

Severity

- Adults 20 to 64 have an average of 3.28 decayed or missing permanent teeth and 13.65 decayed and missing permanent surfaces.

- Latinx subgroups and those with lower incomes have more severe decay in permanent teeth.

- Black and Latinx subgroups and those with lower incomes have more untreated permanent teeth.

Section 10.3

Prevalence of Total and Untreated Dental Caries among Youth

This section includes text excerpted from "Prevalence of Total and Untreated Dental Caries among Youth: United States, 2015–2016," Centers for Disease Control and Prevention (CDC), July 25, 2018.

What Was the Prevalence of Total and Untreated Dental Caries in Youth for 2015 to 2016?

The prevalence of total dental caries (untreated and treated) in primary or permanent teeth among youth aged 2 to 19 years was 45.8 percent (Figure 10.1). Prevalence increased with age, going from 21.4 percent among youth aged 2 to 5 to 50.5 percent among those aged 6 to 11 to 53.8 percent among those aged 12 to 19.

The prevalence of untreated caries in primary or permanent teeth among youth aged 2 to 19 years was 13 percent. The prevalence among youth aged 2 to 5 (8.8%) was lower than it was among youth aged 6 to 11 (15.3%) and 12 to 19 (13.4%).

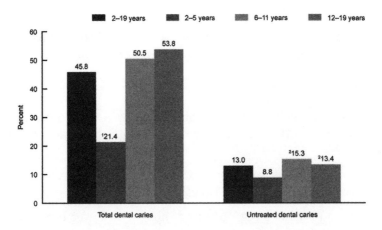

Figure 10.1. *Prevalence of Total Dental Caries and Untreated Dental Caries in Primary or Permanent Teeth among Youth Aged 2 to 19 Years, by Age: United States, 2015 to 2016* (Source: National Center for Health Statistics (NCHS), National Health and Nutrition Examination Survey (NHANES), 2015–2016.)

[1] *Significant linear trend with increasing age.*
[2] *Significantly different from youth aged 2 to 5 years.*
Notes: Total dental caries include untreated and treated caries.

Did the Prevalence of Total and Untreated Dental Caries Differ among Youth by Race and Hispanic Origin for 2015 to 2016?

Among youth aged 2 to 19 years, the prevalence of total dental caries was highest for Hispanic youth (57.1%) compared with non-Hispanic Black (48.1%), non-Hispanic Asian (44.6%), and non-Hispanic White (40.4%) youth (Figure 10.2). However, the difference between the prevalence of Hispanic youth and non-Hispanic Black youth did not reach statistical significance. Prevalence of total dental caries was also higher among non-Hispanic Black than among non-Hispanic White youth.

The prevalence of untreated dental caries was highest among non-Hispanic Black (17.1%) youth compared with Hispanic

(13.5%), non-Hispanic White (11.7%), and non-Hispanic Asian (10.5%) youth. However, the difference between the prevalence of non-Hispanic Black youth and Hispanic youth did not reach statistical significance.

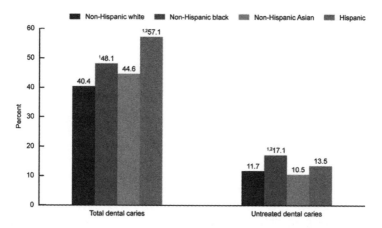

Figure 10.2. *Prevalence of Total Dental Caries and Untreated Dental Caries in Primary or Permanent Teeth among Youth Aged 2 to 19 Years, by Race and Hispanic Origin: United States, 2015 to 2016* (Source: National Center for Health Statistics (NCHS), National Health and Nutrition Examination Survey (NHANES), 2015–2016.)

[1] *Significantly different from non-Hispanic White youth.*
[2] *Significantly different from non-Hispanic Asian youth.*
Notes: Total dental caries include untreated and treated caries.

Were There Differences in the Prevalence of Total and Untreated Dental Caries among Youth by Income Level for 2015 to 2016?

The prevalence of total dental caries decreased as family income levels increased, from 56.3 percent for youth from families living below the federal poverty level to 34.8 percent for youth from families with income levels greater than 300 percent of the federal poverty level (Figure 10.3).

The prevalence of untreated dental caries decreased from 18.6 percent for youth from families living below the federal poverty level to 7 percent for youth from families with incomes greater than 300 percent of the federal poverty level.

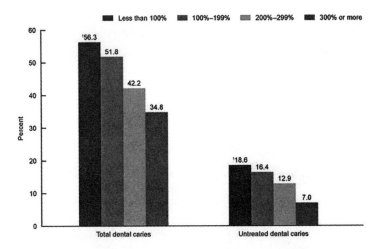

Figure 10.3. *Prevalence of Total Dental Caries and Untreated Dental Caries in Primary or Permanent Teeth among Youth Aged 2 to 19 Years, by Federal Poverty Level: United States, 2015 to 2016* (Source: National Center for Health Statistics (NCHS), National Health and Nutrition Examination Survey (NHANES), 2015 to 2016.)

[1] Significant decreasing linear trend.
Notes: Total dental caries include untreated and treated caries.

What Are the Trends in Total and Untreated Dental Caries in Youth from 2011 to 2012 through 2015 to 2016?

A decrease was seen in the prevalence of total dental caries (from 50 to 45.8%) in youth from 2011 to 2012 through 2015 to 2016. However, this decline was not statistically significant.

For untreated dental caries, the prevalence was 16.1 percent for 2011 to 2012, with the percentage increasing to 18 percent for 2013 to 2014, and then declining to 13 percent for 2015 to 2016 (Figure 10.4).

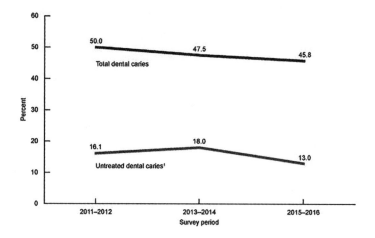

Figure 10.4. *Trends in Prevalence of Total Dental Caries and Untreated Dental Caries in Primary or Permanent Teeth among Youth Aged 2 to 19 Years: United States, 2011 to 2012 through 2015 to 2016* (Source: National Center for Health Statistics (NCHS), National Health and Nutrition Examination Survey (NHANES), 2015 to 2016.)

[1] Significant quadratic trend from 2011 to 2012 to 2015 to 2016.
Notes: Total dental caries include untreated and treated caries.

Chapter 11

Dental Imaging

What Is Dental Imaging?

Dental imaging refers to the practice of creating pictures of a person's mouth and teeth using x-rays. X-rays, also known as "radiographs," are electromagnetic waves of energy that can pass through many materials including bones and teeth. Because different materials absorb x-rays to varying degrees, x-rays are used to show the internal composition of things that are not normally visible. X-rays provide dentists with a way to see inside a person's teeth and jawbone without surgery or other invasive procedures. X-rays are an important part of good dental care and are the most commonly used form of radiograph technology.

Dentists use x-rays to identify, diagnose, and monitor dental health issues for their patients. Dental x-rays allow dentists and other medical professionals to see details of teeth, bones, and mouth tissue. X-rays are used to examine the roots of teeth and their position within the jaw, locate cavities, diagnose dental diseases and other problems, and monitor the development of teeth.

Dental Imaging Procedures

Dental x-rays are classified into two groups: intraoral and extraoral. To create intraoral x-rays, technicians place an x-ray film inside

"Dental Imaging," © 2017 Omnigraphics. Reviewed July 2019.

a person's mouth. Extraoral x-rays are created using a film that is located outside the mouth.

Intraoral x-rays result in highly detailed images and are the most common form of dental imaging. There are four main types of intraoral dental x-rays that are used to examine different aspects of the teeth and mouth. Intraoral x-ray procedures are painless and quick, usually taking only a few seconds to complete.

- Bite-wing x-rays are used to see examine the crowns of teeth in the back of the mouth, including the molars and bicuspids. To create bite-wing x-ray images, the technician asks the patient to bite down on a device that holds the x-ray film while the image is created.

- Periapical x-rays are used to examine one or two teeth in full, including the entire length of the tooth from the crown to root. The procedure for periapical x-rays is similar to that of bite-wing x-rays.

- A full-mouth radiographic survey, or FMX, is a set of intraoral x-rays that includes images of every tooth from crown to root, including supporting tissue. An FMX survey is created using both bite-wing and periapical x-rays.

- Occlusal x-rays are used to produce images that are larger than other types of dental imaging, including the full arch of teeth in either the upper or lower jaw. Occlusal x-rays are most often used to monitor the dental health of children.

Extraoral x-rays provide fewer details than intraoral x-rays, and are generally used to create images that provide a broad view of a person's teeth, jaw, and skull. Dentists use extraoral x-rays to monitor the growth of teeth, the position of teeth in relation to the bones of the jaw and face, and the position of teeth relative to each other within the jawbone. There are five main types of extraoral x-rays.

- Panoramic x-rays allow dentists and other medical professionals to create a single image of the entire mouth, including all the teeth and upper and lower jaws. Panoramic x-rays are created using a machine that directs x-rays forward from behind the head, while the film is gradually moved from one side of the face to the other. The panoramic x-ray machine holds a fixed position and the film moves on a fixed path. The procedure requires people to be positioned with attachments that hold the head and jaw in place for the duration of the x-ray. The procedure is safe, painless, and typically takes only a few minutes to complete.

- Cephalometric projections are extraoral x-rays that provide a view of the entire side of a person's head. These images are used to examine a person's profile and the location of their teeth in relation to the jaw. These x-rays are most often used by orthodontists in planning treatment strategies.

- Cone-beam computed tomography (CT) is a type of extraoral x-ray that is used to create three-dimensional images of a person's entire head. During this procedure, a person stands or sits without moving while the x-ray machine moves around their head. These images are most often used to determine treatment strategies for people who need dental implants.

- Standard CT is a type of dental imaging procedure that is usually conducted at a hospital or a radiologist's office. The procedure usually requires a person to lie down while the image is created. These images are similar to cone-beam computed tomography and are used for similar purposes.

- Digital radiography is a type of dental imaging that replaces standard x-ray film with a tablet computer or other type of sensor. Digital x-ray images are created and stored as computer files. These images can then be viewed on screen or printed.

Radiation and Radiation Dose

X-ray images are created through the use of emitted radiation (electromagnetic energy waves). The radiation dose is the measurement of the amount of energy that is absorbed when a person is exposed to x-rays. Dental and medical x-rays emit extremely small doses of radiation. Excessive absorption of radiation can cause health problems, and people working with x-rays or those who are exposed to many x-rays over time should take precautions to protect themselves.

Modern x-ray machines are built to limit the amount of emitted radiation to the smallest possible effective dose. Dental x-ray machines generally emit radiation in a narrow beam that is less than three inches in diameter. Very little radiation is emitted outside of this beam. Modern x-ray film has also been engineered to produce images using the smallest possible amount of radiation. Film holders keep x-ray films in place without the need for people to directly handle the film. Digital radiography further reduces the emitted radiation dose by as much as 80 percent. X-ray procedures commonly include the use of lead shields or aprons that cover patients from the neck to the knees. A lead collar is also sometimes used for further protection of people with thyroid disease or other specific health concerns. Lead blocks emitted radiation, and therefore, protects the body from harm. To limit exposure to x-ray radiation over time, x-ray technicians typically leave the procedure room and operate x-ray machines remotely.

Dental Radiology and Pregnancy

Pregnant women and their fetuses are considered to be at a higher risk of physical damage from excessive radiation exposure over time. Although dental x-rays expose people to extremely small doses of radiation, it is common practice to protect pregnant women with lead aprons when creating dental x-rays.

References

1. "Radiation Protection of Patients: Dental Radiology—X Rays," International Atomic Energy Agency (IAEA), 2013.

2. "Treatments and Procedures: Types of Dental X-Rays," Cleveland Clinic Foundation, 2015.

3. "Types of X-Rays," Aetna, 2013.

Chapter 12

Tooth Pain

What Are Toothaches?
Causes of Toothaches

Toothaches are primarily caused by tooth decay, which may initially result in pain when eating sweet, cold, or hot food. Decay can irritate the tooth's pulp—the inner core of teeth that contains nerves and connective tissue—stimulating the nerves and resulting in pain.

Other causes of toothache include infection, bleeding gums, tooth trauma, grinding teeth, an abnormal bite, gum disease, and the emergence of new teeth (in babies and young children). Sinus problems, ear infections, temporomandibular joint disorders (TMJ/TMD), and tension in the facial muscles could also cause toothaches, generally accompanied by headaches. In some cases, pain surrounding the teeth and jaws could indicate an underlying heart disorder, such as angina.

Symptoms of a Toothache

Since toothache pain can be caused by a number of dental and medical conditions, the symptoms can only be diagnosed after a complete evaluation by a dentist. You may notice pus in the region of a toothache as a result of an abscess that is caused by an infection. An abscess could also be the result of gum disease, usually characterized by inflamed tissues and bleeding gums.

"Tooth Pain" © 2017 Omnigraphics. Reviewed July 2019.

Consult a dentist if you have the following symptoms:

- Fever

- Difficulty breathing or swallowing

- Swelling in the region of a tooth

- Discharge of foul-tasting fluid

- Continuous pain

Alleviating Pain in an Emergency

It is important to consult a dentist for a toothache, since leaving the condition untreated might lead to serious complications later.

If you are unable to consult a dentist right away, the self-care procedure below may help provide temporary relief:

- Use warm water to rinse your mouth.

- Floss gently to remove food particles that are stuck in your teeth.

- Take on over-the-counter (OTC) medication, such as ibuprofen or acetaminophen, for pain relief.

- Do not apply aspirin directly to the affected tooth, since this may burn the gum tissue.

- Apply an OTC antiseptic with benzocaine to the tooth or gums for pain relief. Clove oil (eugenol) applied to the gums may also help numb the pain. Rub the oil directly on the surface or soak a cotton swab with the oil and apply it to the tooth.

- Apply cold compresses to the cheek to reduce pain and swelling.

How a Dentist Helps

A dentist will determine the location and cause of the tooth pain with an oral examination. She or he will look for redness, swelling, and other visible indications of the cause. An x-ray exam will help the dentist confirm an impacted tooth, decay, bone disorder, or other problems.

Depending on the underlying cause, antibiotics and pain relievers are typically prescribed to improve the healing of the toothache. An advanced infection at the time of examination may require the extraction of the tooth or root canal surgery, which involves the removal of the infected pulp from within the teeth.

Preventing Tooth Pain

The best way to prevent tooth pain is to practice regular oral hygiene. Failure to brush and floss after meals significantly increases the risk of developing cavities and the resulting toothaches.

Use the following tips to help prevent tooth pain:

- Brush at least twice a day, after meals and snacks.

- Floss daily to help prevent gum disease.

- Visit a dentist regularly for professional cleaning and an oral examination.

Hypersensitive Teeth
Causes of Sensitivity

If you experience sharp, temporary pain when consuming a hot beverage or eating ice cream, when breathing through the mouth, or when brushing or flossing, you may have a condition known as "sensitive teeth." Sensitive teeth can be caused by tooth decay, cracks in teeth, worn tooth enamel, exposed tooth roots, receding gums, periodontal disease, and overly aggressive brushing.

Symptoms of Sensitivity

The crowns of the teeth are covered by a strong protective layer of enamel. Below the gum line is a layer known as the "cementum" that covers the teeth and protects the root. Another layer called "dentin" covers the teeth underneath the enamel and the cementum. Dentin is less dense than enamel and cementum and has tubules that reach the core of the teeth. When the layers covering the dentin wear off, the tubules are exposed, allowing sensitivity to occur when hot or cold food stimulates the cells and nerves within the teeth.

Periodontal disease—a disease of the gums—may also lead to hypersensitive teeth. If left untreated, periodontal disease can result in the separation of gum tissue from the tooth, leaving pockets for bacteria to invade. The layers of the tooth can then erode, leaving the root exposed. Regular dental checkups are highly recommended for the prevention, detection, and early treatment of periodontal disease and other problems.

Treatment of Sensitivity

An evaluation by a dentist is essential to diagnose hypersensitivity and rule out other causes of tooth pain. Based on the circumstances, a dentist might recommend the following:

- **Desensitizing toothpaste:** Compounds present in desensitizing toothpaste block nerve impulses from causing pain. Several applications of the paste may be necessary for noticeable effects to be felt. Choose a toothpaste that carries the American Dental Association's (ADA) Seal of Acceptance, which ensures compliance with the ADA's criteria for safety and effectiveness.

- **Fluoride:** Fluoride gel, possibly with a desensitizing agent, may be applied to sensitive areas of the teeth by the dentist as an in-office treatment. Fluoride may also be prescribed for use at home.

- **Bonding:** Sensitive and exposed root surfaces are sometimes treated by applying bonding resin under local anesthesia.

- **Surgical gum graft:** Healthy gum tissues extracted from elsewhere in the mouth are grafted onto exposed root surfaces to protect them and reduce sensitivity.

- **Root canal:** If other treatments do not work and sensitivity is severe and persistent, root canal surgery may be recommended. This procedure involves replacing infected pulp in the teeth with an inert material to eliminate sensitivity.

Preventing Teeth Sensitivity

Proper oral hygiene is essential to avoid teeth sensitivity. Brush twice per day using a soft-bristled toothbrush and fluoridated toothpaste. Floss on a daily basis. Do not use extremely abrasive toothpaste, and avoid aggressive and excessive brushing and flossing. Talk to your dentist about a mouth guard if you grind your teeth. Tooth-grinding can fracture teeth and lead to sensitivity.

Limit the intake of acidic foods and drinks, such as carbonated beverages, citrus fruits, yogurt, and wine. They can erode enamel over time and cause sensitivity. Use a straw to consume acidic liquids to prevent contact with teeth. After consuming acidic food and drinks, neutralize acidity levels in your mouth by drinking milk or water.

Do not brush immediately after consuming acidic substances because the acid softens the enamel, which could erode easily when brushing.

Cracked Teeth

Under the outer layer of enamel that surrounds the teeth, there is a hard layer of dentin. The dentin covers an inner core that is made of pulp. The pulp contains tissue, blood vessels, and nerves. When a tooth is cracked, chewing irritates the pulp and this causes pain. The pulp may become damaged to the extent that it does not heal completely. Extensive cracks may also lead to infection of the pulp, which can spread to the bone and gums.

It can sometimes be difficult to breathe cold air or consume hot or cold food with a cracked tooth. Bite on a clean piece of moist gauze to relieve the pain until you reach the dentist's office. Do not apply aspirin to tooth surfaces to relieve pain. It could cause burns.

Symptoms

Cracked teeth often cause erratic pain when chewing, when releasing pressure after biting, or when teeth are exposed to extremes in temperature. The pain may be intermittent, so a dentist may have difficulty determining which tooth is affected. It may be wise to consult an endodontist, a specialist in treating dental pulp, if you experience the symptoms of a cracked tooth.

Treatment

The treatment for cracked teeth depends on the location and type of damage that has occurred. Do not delay seeing a dentist. With proper treatment, cracked teeth can often be repaired to restore normal function.

- **Craze lines:** Tiny cracks on the outer enamel of the teeth generally do not require treatment. They are very common and do not usually cause pain.

- **Chipped teeth:** Chipped teeth are a common result of dental injuries. Chips can often be reattached or bonded with a tooth-colored filling. A crown can also be set over the tooth, if necessary.

- **Fractured cusp:** The surface of a tooth may break off—often around a filling—and result in a fractured cusp. The fracture does not damage the pulp in most cases and does not usually cause pain. Treatments for the condition generally include fillings and crowns.

- **Vertical crack:** In a vertically cracked tooth, the crack extends from the chewing surface down to the root. The tooth may not be broken, but the crack can eventually spread. Early diagnosis is necessary in order to save the tooth in such cases. If the crack does not extend to the pulp, root canal surgery can save the tooth, but if the crack extends below the gum line, the tooth will likely need to be extracted.

- **Split tooth:** A cracked tooth may progress in time into a split tooth, one that has separate segments that can divide into two portions. A split tooth generally cannot be saved fully, but proper endodontic treatment may be able to save part of it. An examination to evaluate the extent of damage will determine how much of the tooth can be saved.

- **Vertical root fracture:** This is a fracture on the tooth that extends from the root upwards to the chewing surface. Symptoms and signs are usually minimal and might not be immediately noticeable. Such fractures are most often detected when the bone and gum near the site get infected. Treatment often involves the extraction of the tooth, but endodontic treatment may help in retaining a portion of the tooth.

Healing

Broken teeth do not heal like a broken bone. Cracked teeth may worsen and break off in spite of treatment, resulting in loss of teeth. A crown could provide maximum protection but is not appropriate in all cases. The specific kind of treatment you receive is important because with proper intervention cracked teeth can be repaired to provide years of normal chewing function. Consult an endodontist to benefit from the best intervention in your case.

Prevention

You may not be able to prevent cracked teeth entirely, but here are some steps you can take to help make your teeth less vulnerable to cracks:

- Do not chew very hard food substances, like ice or unpopped popcorn kernels. And do not make a habit of chewing on hard objects, such as pens.

- Try not to clench or grind your teeth.

- If you clench or grind your teeth while sleeping, talk to your dentist about a retainer or mouth guard.
- When playing contact sports, wear a mouth guard or protective mask.

Tooth Abscess

A tooth abscess is a pus deposit caused by a bacterial infection. Abscesses can occur in any region of the tooth for a number of different reasons. A periodontal abscess usually occurs in the gums next to a decayed root. Periapical abscesses form at the tip of a tooth's root, usually due to an untreated cavity or previous dental work. A dentist will drain the pus and treat the infection with medication. In order to save the tooth, a root canal procedure might be necessary, but in some cases, the tooth may need to be extracted. It is risky to leave a tooth abscess untreated since it can lead to life-threatening complications.

Symptoms

Some of the symptoms of a tooth abscess include:

- Severe and persistent throbbing pain radiating to the neck or ear.
- Sensitivity to heat and cold.
- Sensitivity to pressure when biting or chewing.
- Fever, chills, nausea, or vomiting.
- Swelling in the face or cheek.
- Tender and swollen lymph nodes in the face or neck.
- Foul-smelling and salty-tasting fluid in the mouth.

When to Consult a Dentist

When the above symptoms occur, you must consult a dentist immediately. If you have swelling in the face accompanied by a fever and you cannot reach a dentist, go to an emergency room. Difficulty in breathing or swallowing indicates that the infection is advanced and has spread further into the jaws and other regions of the body.

Risk Factors

The risk of developing a tooth abscess is significantly increased with poor oral hygiene. Failing to brush and floss regularly can not only result in tooth decay and gum disease but may also invite bacteria that could lead to abscesses and their serious complications. The risk of abscesses is also increased by a high-sugar diet. The regular consumption of sweets and sugary carbonated beverages can result in cavities that might later develop into abscesses.

Complications

Although a rupture in a tooth abscess may reduce pain significantly, it is essential to seek medical treatment. The pus may not drain completely, or the infection may spread to other areas of the body, like the neck or the head. Sepsis—a life-threatening condition—may develop if an abscess is left untreated and allowed to proliferate. And a weakened immune system could spread the infection from a tooth abscess even more quickly.

Diagnosis

- **Dental examination:** A dentist will first make a thorough oral examination to confirm a tooth abscess.

- **Tapping the teeth:** An abscess is usually present at the tip of the root, and a slight tap will induce pain.

- **X-ray:** An x-ray will confirm the presence of an abscess and allow the dentist to evaluate the spread of the infection.

- **Computed Tomography (CT) scan:** If the abscess has spread, a CT scan will help the dentist determine the extent of infection.

Treatment

These are some of the procedures a dentist will likely follow to treat a tooth abscess:

- **Drain the abscess:** The dentist will make an incision in the abscess, drain the pus, then wash the area with saline.

- **Root canal:** A root canal can treat infection and help save a tooth. The dentist drills into the tooth and removes the pulp. The empty chamber is then filled with inert material and sealed. Finally, a crown may be set on the tooth for protection.

- **Tooth extraction:** If the tooth cannot be saved, the dentist will extract the tooth and treat the abscess by draining it and treating the infection.

- **Prescribing antibiotics:** An infection that is limited to the area of the abscess may not require antibiotics, but a dentist will recommend antibiotics if the infection has spread to adjoining areas. Antibiotics will also be prescribed if you have a weakened immune system.

Phantom Tooth Pain

Phantom pain—also called "atypical facial pain," "neuropathic oro-facial pain," or "atypical odontalgia"—presents as pain in a tooth or teeth without a specific cause. It usually begins after extraction or following an endodontic procedure, and in time the pain can spread to other parts of the face.

The pain is termed "atypical" because it is dissimilar to normal tooth pain. Typical pain comes and goes and is aggravated by biting or chewing or by touch and pressure. It can be attributed to identifiable causes, such as decay, periodontal disease, or injury. Treatment usually relieves the pain.

Phantom pain, on the other hand, is a throbbing and constant pain at the site of an extraction or root canal that is not affected by hot or cold food substances or by biting or chewing. Local anesthetics and other pain treatments may or may not provide relief, and the intensity of pain may vary from mild to severe. This presents an inexplicable situation to the dentist, who might attempt more treatment that provides no symptomatic improvement.

Causes

Since the causes of phantom tooth pain remain unclear, it is termed "idiopathic." It is more common in women than in men, and it tends to occur more often in middle-aged and older people. Research has found a link between anxiety and depression and phantom tooth pain, but the association remains unclear. Phantom tooth pain is a dysfunction or short-circuiting of the nerves that carry sensations from the teeth and jaw to the brain. Molecular or biochemical changes have been observed in areas of the brain that process pain, which could be the cause of the phantom pain.

Treatment

Dental treatment usually does not alleviate phantom tooth pain. It may lessen the severity, but it often returns. This is because the pain is a result of a dysfunction of the brain and nerves that process pain.

Phantom tooth pain is treated using a variety of medications, most commonly tricyclic antidepressants, such as amitriptyline, which in this case are prescribed for their pain-relieving properties, rather than their antidepressant benefits. Medicines prescribed for chronic pain conditions, such as gabapentin, baclofen, and duloxetine, are also often prescribed. This treatment reduces the pain but may not eliminate it completely.

Phantom tooth pain may or may not be a permanent condition, but in some cases, the symptoms disappear after a length of time or with prolonged treatment. Sometimes the pain persists and may require lifelong medication.

Phantom tooth pain is a rare condition, and some dentists may not be familiar with its diagnosis and treatment. It is best to consult a dentist with an advanced specialization, such as oral medicine or orofacial pain.

References

1. "Sensitive Teeth: Causes and Treatment," American Dental Association (ADA), December 2003.

2. Carr, Alan. "What Causes Sensitive Teeth, and How Can I Treat Them?" Mayo Clinic, December 6, 2014.

3. "What Causes a Toothache?" Delta Dental, June 2010.

4. "Tooth Abscess," Mayo Clinic, February 16, 2016.

5. Falace, D. "Atypical Odontalgia," American Academy of Oral Medicine (AAOM), January 22, 2015.

6. "Cracked Teeth," American Association of Endodontists (AAE),, n.d.

Chapter 13

Medications Used in Dentistry

Dentists may prescribe several different types of medications as part of a patient's treatment plan. Medications are commonly used in oral care to help relieve pain and anxiety, prevent tooth decay, or control plaque and gingivitis, infections, and dry mouth. To ensure the effectiveness and reduce the risk of dental medications, it is important for patients to keep their dentist informed of any changes in symptoms, any health conditions they may have, and any other medications they may be taking.

Managing Pain and Anxiety

Many patients worry about the pain involved in dental procedures. As a result, pain management and anxiety control are important facets of dental care. At the dentist's office, patients may receive topical, local, or general anesthetics to help them deal with this common complication. They may also use prescription or over-the-counter (OTC) analgesics at home to relieve discomfort following dental procedures.

- **Topical anesthetics.** Many dentists apply topical anesthetics to numb the gums prior to injecting local anesthetics. In addition, they may prescribe topical anesthetics to provide patients with temporary relief from pain or irritation caused

"Medications Used in Dentistry," © 2017 Omnigraphics. Reviewed July 2019.

by cold sores, canker sores, fever blisters, teething, braces, or dentures. These medications are available in many forms, including gels, ointments, pastes, lozenges, and aerosol sprays. Some of the common brand name dental anesthetics include Anbesol, Chloraseptic®, Orajel®, and Xylocaine. It is important to note that topical anesthetics are generally intended to provide temporary pain relief, and patients should seek dental treatment if the discomfort lasts more than a few days.

- **Local anesthetics.** Dentists typically inject local anesthetics—such as lidocaine and mepivacaine—into the gum tissues of the mouth prior to dental procedures that involve drilling or cutting. These medications reduce pain by inhibiting the impulses from pain-sensing nerves.

- **General anesthetics.** Oral surgeons may administer intravenous anesthetic medications to enable patients to sleep through complex dental procedures.

- **Analgesics.** Analgesics are pain-relieving medications that are often recommended for patients who have undergone dental procedures. Narcotic analgesics, such as codeine or hydrocodone (brand names Tylenol #3 or Vicodin) may be prescribed to manage severe pain conditions. To relieve minor pain and inflammation associated with toothaches or dental appliances, a number of OTC nonnarcotic analgesics are available including ibuprofen (Advil®, Nuprin®, Motrin®) and acetaminophen (Tylenol®).

- **Anti-inflammatory medications.** Corticosteroids are anti-inflammatory medications that may help relieve discomfort from tooth and gum problems. They usually take the form of topical pastes and are sold under such brand names as Orabase-HCA, Oracort, and Oralone®. It is important to note that corticosteroids should not be used for teething due to the potential for dangerous side effects in infants and young children.

- **Sedatives.** Dentists may also use medications to help patients relax during dental procedures. Inhaled antianxiety agents, such as nitrous oxide, may be used along with local anesthetics. Benzodiazepines, such as diazepam (Valium), may also be prescribed to help relieve the symptoms of anxiety. Finally, muscle relaxants may be prescribed to reduce stress in patients who grind their teeth or experience headaches or jaw pain from temporomandibular joint disorders (TMJ).

Controlling Plaque and Gingivitis

Plaque is a sticky, bacteria-containing film that coats the teeth and other surfaces in the mouth. Gingivitis is a mild form of gum disease that is caused by the buildup of plaque. Symptoms of gingivitis include redness, swelling, and irritation of the gums. Both plaque and gingivitis can usually be controlled through good oral hygiene, including brushing the teeth at least twice per day and flossing between teeth regularly. In addition, many different antiseptic mouth rinses are available OTC to help reduce plaque and gingivitis and kill bacteria in the mouth that cause bad breath.

Chlorhexidine is an antibiotic used to control plaque and gingivitis in the mouth. Dentists may also prescribe chlorhexidine in conjunction with certain dental procedures, such as scaling or root planing, or to reduce the depth of periodontal pockets (the space between the teeth and gums). The medication is available as a mouth rinse or in a chip form under the brand names Peridex®, PerioChip®, and PerioGuard®. Although chlorhexidine can help control bacteria in the mouth, it may also cause unwanted side effects, such as an increase in tartar on the teeth or staining of the teeth, dentures, or other mouth appliances.

Tetracyclines are a category of antibiotics (including demeclocycline, doxycycline, minocycline, oxytetracycline, and tetracycline) that may be used to treat gingivitis and eliminate bacteria associated with more advanced periodontal disease. Tetracyclines are available as gels, mouth rinses, fibers, and particles for use as dental antibiotics. Tetracyclines should not be used by pregnant women or children under age eight, however, because they may cause permanent discoloration of developing teeth.

Preventing Tooth Decay

Fluoride is a medication that helps prevent tooth decay by strengthening teeth and making them better able to resist damage from acids and bacteria. Fluoride is added to many municipal water supplies, and it is also available in nonprescription form in many toothpastes and mouth rinses. Prescription-strength fluoride is also available in liquid, tablet, and chewable form for young children who do not have access to a fluoridated water supply.

Alleviating Dry Mouth

Dry mouth can occur as a complication of autoimmune disorders, certain medications, and some other conditions. The symptoms can often be alleviated through the use of saliva substitute medications, such as Moi-Stir, Mouth Kote, Optimoist, Salivar, Salix, and Xero-Lube. Most dry mouth treatments take the form of sprays that the patient can apply as needed. Pilocarpine, sold under the brand name Salagan, is a prescription medication that helps relieve dry mouth by stimulating saliva production.

Treating Dental Infections

In addition to helping control bacteria in the mouth that cause periodontal disease, antibiotics are also used in dentistry to prevent and treat infections and abscesses. Antibiotics are often used to treat infections that develop in the bone and soft tissue following dental procedures. In some cases, antibiotics are also prescribed prior to dental procedures to prevent bacteria in the mouth from entering the bloodstream. People with medical conditions that put them at high risk of infection—such as a compromised immune system, artificial heart valves, or liver disease—may need to take antibiotics both before and after undergoing dental procedures.

Penicillin and amoxicillin are among the antibiotics most commonly prescribed to treat infections that result from dental procedures. Patients who are allergic to penicillin are usually prescribed erythromycin instead. Clindamycin may be prescribed to treat infections that do not respond to other antibiotics. These medications may be administered orally, intramuscularly, or intravenously.

Antifungal medications such as nystatin are used to treat candidiasis (oral thrush), an infection caused by the Candida albicans fungus. Antifungal medications are available in lozenges or liquid suspensions that the patient holds in the mouth and swishes around before swallowing.

References

1. "Drugs Used in Dentistry," WebMD, 2016.

2. "Medications Used in Dentistry," Cleveland Clinic, 2010.

3. Ogbru, Annette. "Medications Used in Dentistry," WebMD, 2016.

Chapter 14

Sedation Techniques Used by Dentists

Sedation in dentistry involves administering medication to reduce patients' level of awareness and make them feel more relaxed and comfortable. Although sedation does not control pain, it can help decrease patients' level of anxiety about undergoing dental procedures. Studies have shown that up to 20 percent of people experience some form of anxiety or phobia with regard to dental treatment. Depending on its severity, dental anxiety can cause patients to postpone or avoid necessary dental care, resulting in poor oral health. People with poor oral health, in turn, generally require more extensive and complicated dental procedures, which serves to further increase their anxiety levels.

Fear and apprehension create physiological responses that can make dental treatment more difficult for patients and dentists alike. These emotions trigger the release of stress chemicals in the brain that put bodily systems on alert. Muscles become tense, nerves become hypersensitive to stimuli, and pain tolerance becomes lower. Management of patients' pain and anxiety is thus a major concern for successful dental practices. Various sedation techniques are available that suppress the central nervous system, allowing patients to feel relaxed, peaceful, and comfortable while still remaining conscious

"Sedation Techniques Used by Dentists," © 2017 Omnigraphics. Reviewed July 2019.

and in control. By helping patients overcome anxiety, sedation dentistry also enables the dental team to work more efficiently and confidently.

Levels of Sedation

There are several different levels of sedation available to meet patients' needs. The level of sedation is determined by the degree to which the medication suppresses the patient's central nervous system and awareness of their surroundings.

- Conscious or minimal sensation, also known as "anxiolysis," induces a mildly depressed level of consciousness. The patient remains conscious and able to respond to verbal commands or physical stimuli. Although the patient's thought processes may be slightly impaired, this level of sedation should not affect breathing or heart function.

- Moderate sedation is similar to minimal sedation but involves a more depressed level of consciousness. Patients can generally respond to verbal commands, such as "open your mouth," that are accompanied by light tactile stimuli. Ventilation and cardiovascular function are usually unaffected.

- Deep sedation induces a loss of consciousness in the patient. Although the patient may respond to repeated stimulation, it may be difficult to arouse them. In addition, positive-pressure ventilation may be required and cardiovascular function may be impaired.

- General anesthesia is the deepest level of sedation. Patients cannot be aroused even by painful stimuli. Ventilation assistance is often required, and cardiovascular function may be impaired.

Sedation Techniques

Medications used for sedation in dentistry are typically administered orally, through inhalation, or intravenously. In some cases, different routes of drug administration are used in combination to induce the desired level of sedation.

- Oral (enteral) sedation is commonly used to help alleviate mild to moderate anxiety in dental patients. Patients take the medication by mouth, either by swallowing it or allowing it to dissolve under the tongue. Many people find the oral administration easy and convenient and appreciate the fact that injections are not required. Some of the oral sedatives often used in dentistry include benzodiazepines such as diazepam (Valium), lorazepam (Ativan), triazolam (Halcion), and midazolam (Versed), and nonbenzodiazepines such as zolpidem (Ambien) and zaleplon (Sonata). These medications help patients relax and feel more comfortable during dental procedures. In some cases, they also produce an amnesia effect that dampens patients' memory of what happened in the dental chair. Even though the sedation effect is mild, patients should always be accompanied by a responsible person to drive them home from the dentist's office.

- Inhalation sedation involves the administration of nitrous oxide mixed with oxygen to the lungs. Patients inhale the gases through a nasal hood, which looks like a small plastic cup that fits over the nose. It produces a light-headed, euphoric feeling in patients that helps reduce pain and apprehension during dental treatment. Bodily functions remain unaffected, however, and the effects wear off quickly once the gas is turned off.

- Intravenous (IV) sedation involves the administration of sedatives directly into the bloodstream through the veins. The drugs most commonly used include a benzodiazepine in combination with an opioid, such as fentanyl or demerol. Since IV sedation requires specialized training, it is mainly used by oral surgeons and periodontists. Although IV sedation works quickly and allows the level of sedation to be adjusted easily, bodily functions like heart rate, blood pressure, and breathing must be monitored carefully. Due to the higher level of risk involved, IV sedation is typically considered when other sedation methods are ineffective.

Safety and Effectiveness

The sedative medications used in dentistry have been tested extensively and have proven safe and effective in most situations. To minimize the risk of adverse reactions, it is important for patients to provide their dentists with information about any underlying medical conditions they may have, such as diabetes; any prescription medications, over-the-counter (OTC) drugs, or natural or herbal supplements they may be taking; and any lifestyle choices, such as smoking or excessive alcohol consumption, that may affect sedation. Patients should also follow the dentist's instructions about not eating or drinking for at least six hours before their appointment and bring a responsible person to drive them home following any dental procedure that involves sedation.

References

1. Assaf, Hussein M., and Negrelli, Marna L. "Sedation in the Dental Office: An Overview," DentalCare.com, January 5, 2015.

2. Silverman, Michael D. "Oral Sedation Dentistry," Dear Doctor: Dentistry and Oral Health, February 1, 2009.

Chapter 15

Alternatives to Dental Drills

Many patients dread going to the dentist because of the dental drill. Whether they object most to the noise, vibration, heat, or smell, many people find having their teeth drilled to be an unpleasant experience. In addition, procedures that require drilling usually involve the use of local anesthesia, which can entail several hours of discomfort due to numb lips, tongue, and cheeks. Recognizing the negative associations many patients have toward the dental drill, some dentists have adopted alternative methods of preparing and treating teeth, such as air abrasion and dental lasers.

Air Abrasion

Air abrasion, also known as "micro-abrasion," is a technique that uses compressed air to propel a tiny stream of aluminum oxide particles onto the tooth. It has been compared to the process of sandblasting. Dentists can use air abrasion in place of a standard dental drill to fix minor cracks and discolorations or to remove decay from the tooth's surface and prepare it for fillings, sealants, or restoration placement.

Air abrasion offers several advantages over a traditional dental drill. It is very quiet and virtually painless, so patients do not require an anesthetic. It also allows the dentist to operate with greater precision, which helps to safeguard soft tissue, preserve more tooth structure, and reduce the risk of micro-fractures in tooth enamel. In addition, there is no odor or vibration associated with the air abrasion technique. Although patients may have some dust residue in their mouth, it can easily be removed by rinsing with water. The main disadvantage of air abrasion is that it cannot be used on restorations, such as crowns and bridges.

Dental Lasers

Dental lasers offer another alternative to dental drills. Lasers use targeted pulses of infrared light energy to perform many of the typical functions of drills. Lasers can be used to remove decayed areas from a tooth to prepare it for filling and to strengthen the bond between the filling and the tooth. They can also be used in tooth-whitening procedures to enhance the action of bleaching chemicals applied to the tooth surface. Finally, lasers can be used to cut into gums and soft tissue during root canal procedures.

There are many different types of dental lasers available that use different wavelengths of light to vaporize water molecules or minerals like hydroxyapatite within teeth. A computer usually determines the pattern of laser pulses, although the dentist still controls the instrument. Most types of lasers do not produce heat or vibration, and many patients do not experience pain and thus avoid the need for anesthesia. In addition, dental lasers offer precision that can help preserve tooth structure and protect soft tissue from damage.

Dental lasers do have a few disadvantages, however. They cannot be used on teeth that already contain fillings, for instance, and they cannot be used to remove crowns or prepare teeth for bridgework. Even in situations when lasers can be used, traditional dental drills are sometimes needed to shape and polish fillings following laser treatment. Dental laser systems also tend to be an extremely costly investment for dental practices as compared to standard drills. Finally, although dental lasers have been approved for use by the U.S. Food and Drug Administration (FDA), as of 2015 they had not yet met the American Dental Association's (ADA) standards for safety and effectiveness. However, the ADA did express optimism about future applications of dental lasers as an alternative to more traditional treatment.

References

1. "Dental Alternative to the Drill: Drilless Dentistry," Drakeshire Dental, 2016.

2. Gwynne, Peter. "Laser Offers Alternative to the Dental Drill," Inside Science, June 4, 2014.

3. "Laser Use in Dentistry," WebMD, 2016.

Chapter 16

Dental Fillings

Chapter Contents

Section 16.1

Dental Amalgam Fillings

This section includes text excerpted from "About Dental Amalgam Fillings," U.S. Food and Drug Administration (FDA), December 5, 2017.

What Is Dental Amalgam?

Dental amalgam is a dental filling material used to fill cavities caused by tooth decay. It has been used for more than 150 years in hundreds of millions of patients around the world.

Dental amalgam is a mixture of metals, consisting of liquid (elemental) mercury and a powdered alloy composed of silver, tin, and copper. Approximately 50 percent of dental amalgam is elemental mercury by weight. The chemical properties of elemental mercury allow it to react with and bind together the silver/copper/tin alloy particles to form an amalgam.

Dental amalgam fillings are also known as "silver fillings" because of their silver-like appearance. Despite the name, "silver fillings" do contain elemental mercury.

When placing dental amalgam, the dentist first drills the tooth to remove the decay and then shapes the tooth cavity for placement of the amalgam filling. Next, under appropriate safety conditions, the dentist mixes the powdered alloy with the liquid mercury to form an amalgam putty. This softened amalgam putty is placed and shaped in the prepared cavity, where it rapidly hardens into a solid filling.

What Should I Know before Getting a Dental Amalgam Filling?

Deciding what filling material to use to treat dental decay is a choice that must be made by you and your dentist.

The U.S. Food and Drug Administration (FDA) continues to evaluate the available information on dental amalgam and will update the information on this webpage as necessary. As you consider your options, you should keep in mind the following information.

Benefits

Dental amalgam fillings are strong and long-lasting, so they are less likely to break than some other types of fillings.

Dental amalgam is the least expensive type of filling material.

Potential Risks

Dental amalgam contains elemental mercury. It releases low levels of mercury in the form of a vapor that can be inhaled and absorbed by the lungs. High levels of mercury vapor exposure are associated with adverse effects in the brain and the kidneys.

The U.S. Food and Drug Administration has reviewed the best available scientific evidence to determine whether the low levels of mercury vapor associated with dental amalgam fillings are a cause for concern. Based on this evidence, FDA considers dental amalgam fillings safe for adults and children ages 6 and above. The weight of credible scientific evidence reviewed by the FDA does not establish an association between dental amalgam use and adverse health effects in the general population. Clinical studies in adults and children ages six and above have found no link between dental amalgam fillings and health problems.

The developing neurological systems in fetuses and young children may be more sensitive to the neurotoxic effects of mercury vapor. Very limited to no clinical data is available regarding long-term health outcomes in pregnant women and their developing fetuses, and children under the age of six, including infants who are breastfed. Pregnant women and parents with children under six who are concerned about the absence of clinical data as to long-term health outcomes should talk to their dentist.

However, the estimated amount of mercury in breast milk attributable to dental amalgam is low and falls well below the general levels for oral intake that the U.S. Environmental Protection Agency (EPA) considers safe. Despite the limited clinical information, the FDA concludes that the existing risk information supports a finding that infants are not at risk for adverse health effects from the mercury in the breast milk of women exposed to mercury vapor from dental amalgam. Some individuals have an allergy or sensitivity to mercury or the other components of dental amalgam (such as silver, copper, or tin). Dental amalgam might cause these individuals to develop oral lesions or other contact reactions. If you are allergic to any of the metals in dental amalgam, you should not get amalgam fillings. You can discuss other treatment options with your dentist.

Why Is Mercury Used in Dental Amalgam?

Approximately half of a dental amalgam filling is liquid mercury and the other half is a powdered alloy of silver, tin, and copper.

Mercury is used to bind the alloy particles together into a strong, durable, and solid filling. Mercury's unique properties (it is a liquid at room temperature and that bonds well with the alloy powder) make it an important component of dental amalgam that contributes to its durability.

What Is Bioaccumulation?

Bioaccumulation refers to the buildup or steadily increasing concentration of a chemical in organs or tissues in the body. Mercury from dental amalgam and other sources (e.g., fish) is bioaccumulative. Studies of healthy subjects with amalgam fillings have shown that mercury from exposure to mercury vapor bioaccumulates in certain tissues of the body, including kidneys and brain. Studies have not shown that bioaccumulation of mercury from dental amalgam results in damage to target organs.

Is the Mercury in Dental Amalgam the Same as the Mercury in Some Types of Fish?

No. There are several different chemical forms of mercury: elemental mercury, inorganic mercury, and methylmercury. The form of mercury associated with dental amalgam is elemental mercury, which releases mercury vapor. The form of mercury found in fish is methylmercury, a type of organic mercury. Mercury vapor is mainly absorbed by the lungs. Methylmercury is mainly absorbed through the digestive tract. The body processes these forms of mercury differently and has different levels of tolerance for mercury vapor and methylmercury.

If I Am Concerned about the Mercury in Dental Amalgam, Should I Have My Fillings Removed?

If your fillings are in good condition and there is no decay beneath the filling, the FDA does not recommend that you have your amalgam fillings removed or replaced. Removing sound amalgam fillings results in unnecessary loss of healthy tooth structure, and exposes you to additional mercury vapor released during the removal process.

However, if you believe you have an allergy or sensitivity to mercury or any of the other metals in dental amalgam (such as silver, tin, or copper), you should discuss treatment options with your dentist.

Section 16.2

Mercury in Dental Amalgam

This section includes text excerpted from "Mercury in Dental Amalgam," U.S. Environmental Protection Agency (EPA), February 7, 2018.

What Are Dental Amalgam Fillings?

Sometimes referred to as "silver filling," dental amalgam is a silver-colored material used to fill (restore) teeth that have cavities. Dental amalgam is made of two nearly equal parts:

1. Liquid mercury

2. A powder containing silver, tin, copper, zinc, and other metals

Amalgam is one of the most commonly used tooth fillings and is considered a safe, sound, and effective treatment for tooth decay.

Are Dental Amalgam Fillings Safe?

When amalgam fillings are placed in or removed from teeth, they can release a small amount of mercury vapor. Amalgam can also release small amounts of mercury vapor during chewing. People can absorb these vapors by inhaling or ingesting them. However, the U.S. Food and Drug Administration (FDA) considers dental amalgam fillings safe for adults and children over the age of six.

The U.S. Food and Drug Administration regulates dental amalgam as a medical device and FDA is responsible for ensuring that dental amalgam is reasonably safe and effective. Among other things, the FDA also makes sure the product labeling for dentists has adequate directions for use and includes applicable warnings.

Background: Since the 1990s, the FDA, the Centers for Disease Control and Prevention (CDC), and other government agencies have reviewed the scientific literature looking for links between dental amalgams and health problems. The CDC reported in 2001 that there is little evidence:

• That the health of the vast majority of people with dental amalgam is compromised, or

• That removing amalgam fillings has a beneficial effect on health.

In 2002, the FDA published a proposed rule to classify dental amalgam as a class II medical device with special controls. In 2008, the FDA reopened the comment period for that proposed rule. After reviewing all comments, the FDA issued a rule in 2009.

Are There Alternatives to Using Dental Amalgam Fillings?

Presently, there are five other types of restorative materials for tooth decay:

1. Resin composite
2. Glass ionomer
3. Resin ionomer
4. Porcelain
5. Gold alloys

The choice of dental treatment rests with dental professionals and their patients, so talk with your dentist about available dental treatment options.

How Does Amalgam Waste Affect the Environment?

If improperly managed by dental offices, dental amalgam waste can be released into the environment. Although most dental offices currently use some type of basic filtration system to reduce the amount of mercury solids passing into the sewer system, dental offices are the single largest source of mercury at sewage treatment plants.

The installation of amalgam separators, which catch and hold the excess amalgam waste coming from office spittoons, can further reduce discharges to wastewater. Without these separators, the excess amalgam waste will be released to the sewers.

From sewers, amalgam waste goes to publicly-owned treatment works (POTWs) (sewage treatment plants). POTWs have around a 90 percent efficiency rate of removing amalgam from wastewaters. Once removed, the amalgam waste becomes part of the POTW's sewage sludge, which is then disposed of:

- **In landfills.** If the amalgam waste is sent to a landfill, the mercury may be released into the groundwater or air.

- **Through incineration.** If the mercury is incinerated, mercury may be emitted to the air from the incinerator stacks.

- **By applying the sludge to agricultural land as fertilizer.**
  If mercury-contaminated sludge is used as an agricultural
  fertilizer, some of the mercury used as fertilizer may also
  evaporate to the atmosphere.

Through precipitation, this airborne mercury eventually gets deposited onto bodies of water, land, and vegetation. Some dentists throw
their excess amalgam into special medical waste containers, believing
this to be an environmentally safe disposal practice. If waste amalgam
is improperly disposed of in medical waste bags, however, the amalgam
waste may be incinerated and mercury may be emitted to the air from
the incinerator stacks. This airborne mercury is eventually deposited
into bodies of water and onto land.

Section 16.3

Amalgam Filling Alternatives

This section includes text excerpted from "Alternatives to
Dental Amalgam," U.S. Food and Drug Administration (FDA),
December 5, 2017.

Other materials can also be used to fill cavities caused by dental
decay. Like dental amalgam, these direct filling materials are used to
restore the biting surface of a tooth that has been damaged by decay.
Your dentist can discuss treatment options based on the location of
cavities in your mouth and the amount of tooth decay.
The primary alternatives to dental amalgam are as follows:

- Composite resin fillings

- Glass ionomer cement fillings

Every restorative material has advantages and disadvantages.

Composite Resin Fillings

Composite resin fillings are the most common alternative to dental
amalgam. They are sometimes called "tooth-colored" or "white" fillings

because of their color. Composite resin fillings are made of a type of plastic (an acrylic resin) and reinforced with a powdered glass filler. The color (shade) of composite resins can be customized to closely match surrounding teeth. Composite resin fillings are often light cured by a "blue-light" in layers to build up the final restoration.

Advantages of composite resin fillings include:

- Blends in with surrounding teeth

- High strength

- Requires minimal removal of healthy tooth structure for placement

Disadvantages of composite resin fillings include:

- More difficult to place than dental amalgam

- May be less durable than dental amalgam and may need to be replaced more frequently

- Higher cost of placement

Glass Ionomer Cement Fillings

Glass ionomer cement contain organic acids, such as eugenol, and bases, such as zinc oxide, and may include acrylic resins. Like some composite resins, glass ionomer cement includes a component of a glass filler that releases fluoride over time. Also, like composite fillings, glass ionomer cement is tooth-colored. The composition and properties of glass ionomer cement are best suited for very small restorations. Unlike composite resin fillings, glass ionomer cement is self-curing and usually does not need a "blue light" to set (harden). The advantages of glass ionomer cement are ease of use and appearance. Their chief disadvantage is that they are limited to use in small restorations.

Chapter 17

Rebuilding and Reshaping Teeth

Crowns and Bridges
What Is a Dental Crown?

A dental crown is a cap that covers a tooth that is cracked, broken, or discolored, or one in which fillings have deteriorated or been lost. The purpose of a dental crown is to restore the shape, size, and strength of the tooth, as well as to improve its appearance.

Numerous options are available for dental crown material. Depending on its location, the dentist may suggest permanent crowns made of resin, ceramic, stainless steel, metal (gold or other alloy), or porcelain that is fused to metal. A dental crown should last between 5 and 15 years, depending on how much wear and tear it receives and how good the oral hygiene is, as well as on other individual habits, such as grinding or clenching teeth, biting fingernails, and chewing ice.

When Is a Crown Needed?

A person may require a dental crown to:

• Prevent cracking or breaking of a weak tooth

• Hold together or restore an already broken tooth

"Rebuilding and Reshaping Teeth," © 2017 Omnigraphics. Reviewed July 2019.

- Act as an anchor for a dental bridge

- Cover worn out or discolored teeth

- Provide the tooth with cover and support for a large filling

- Cover a dental implant or a root canal
  A crown may be required for children on primary (baby) teeth to:

- Save a tooth severely damaged by decay

- Protect teeth when the child is at high risk of tooth decay, especially when there is difficulty in maintaining proper dental hygiene

- Decrease use of general anesthesia in children unable to sit through proper dental care requirements (due to age, behavior, or medical history)

How Is a Tooth Prepared for a Crown?

Usually, two visits to the dentist are required to prepare the tooth for a crown. In the first visit, the dentist examines the tooth by taking x-rays to check its root and the surrounding bone. A root canal may be required if there is either extensive tooth decay or the risk of injury or infection to the pulp of the tooth. The tooth will then be reshaped to accommodate the crown, and a paste or putty impressions will be made of the tooth that will receive the crown, along with those above or below it.

These impressions will then be sent to a dental lab, and the crown will arrive at the dentist's office in about two or three weeks. In the interim, the patient will be fitted with a temporary crown made of acrylic, which will protect the prepared tooth. The dentist will usually suggest a few special precautions to take care of this temporary crown. In the second visit, the dentist will inspect the fit and color of the permanent crown, and if they are satisfactory, it will be cemented in place.

What Is a Dental Bridge?

A dental bridge is a ceramic structure that fills the gap created by a missing or extracted tooth. It is used for a number of purposes, including to restore the ability to speak or chew properly, to prevent teeth from moving out of position, to restore the person's smile, and to maintain the shape of the face.

To create a bridge, an artificial tooth (called a "pontic"), commonly made of ceramic, is fused with two or more crowns on the teeth on either side of the gap. These crowns become the anchors for the pontic, and are known as "abutment teeth." Porcelain, gold, alloys, or a combination of these materials can be used to make a bridge, which can last from 5 to 15 years, depending on good oral hygiene and regular dental checkups.

How Is a Bridge Prepared?

Preparing a bridge generally requires at least two dental visits. In the first, the abutment teeth are reshaped to make room for the crowns to be placed over them. The impressions of these teeth are then made and will be used as the model in the dental lab to prepare the pontic, crowns, and bridge. The shape and color of both the crowns and the pontic will be made to match those of the patient's natural teeth. As with crowns, the dentist will make a temporary bridge to help protect the exposed teeth and gums between visits.

In the second visit, the fit and appearance of the bridge will be checked. Adjustments will be made if required, and when the bridge fits properly, it will be installed permanently. This fitting process sometimes requires more than one visit, and in some cases the dentist may cement it only temporarily for a few weeks to ensure that it fits properly before the final placement.

Is Special Care Required for Dental Crowns and Bridges?

Special care is not generally needed for a crowned tooth or a bridge, however, it is important to maintain good oral hygiene. In addition to brushing at least twice daily and flossing (especially where the gum meets the tooth), using an antibacterial mouthwash to rinse at least once per day is recommended. In the case of a bridge, strong and healthy adjoining teeth are needed to provide sturdy support, so practicing good oral hygiene is crucial to prevent tooth loss due to decay or gum disease. And a regular cleaning schedule and visits to the dentist will help identify complications at an early stage.

Dental Veneers

A dental veneer, sometimes called a "porcelain veneer" or a "dental porcelain laminate," is a thin shell used to cover the front surface of a tooth. It is made from either porcelain or resin composite material to provide strength to the tooth and improve its appearance. The veneer is custom-made to match the person's natural teeth and is typically used to correct teeth that are slightly out of position, discolored, fractured or chipped, unevenly shaped, or have gaps between them. It functions as an intermediate option between bonding (the application of resin directly to the tooth) and a crown for individuals who want only a slight change in the appearance of the tooth. Veneers usually last from five to ten years, after which they need to be replaced.

How Is a Veneer Prepared?

Preparing a veneer might require multiple visits to the dentist's office. The first visit will be a consultation with the dentist to determine if a veneer is the right option for the patient. The dentist will examine the teeth, discuss the procedure, outline the plusses and minuses, and suggest alternatives, if there are any.

To prepare for a veneer, the dentist will remove about half a millimeter of enamel from the surface of the tooth. This is roughly equal to the thickness of the veneer that will be bonded to that tooth's surface. An impression of the tooth will then be made and sent to the dental lab that will make the veneer. It can take up to two weeks for the dentist to receive the veneer from the lab, and in the interim, the patient may opt for a temporary veneer, usually at additional cost.

In the next visit, the veneer will be placed temporarily on the tooth to test its fit and color. Small adjustments will be made to the fit if needed, and the color can be fine-tuned with different shades of cement. The tooth will then be prepared to receive the veneer by cleaning, polishing, and then etching the surface to roughen it for a stronger bond. Once the veneer is cemented into position, the excess cement is removed, the bite is evaluated, and final adjustments are made, if needed. A follow-up visit might be required after a couple of weeks for the dentist to see how the gums respond to the veneer and to examine its placement once again. Regular professional visits to the dentist will also be required to polish the veneer with a special nonabrasive paste.

Is Special Care Required for a Veneer?

Maintaining a porcelain veneer does not generally demand special care, other than normal oral hygiene, including brushing twice daily, flossing, and rinsing daily with an antiseptic mouthwash. But the dentist might recommend a nighttime bite guard if the patient grinds or clenches her or his teeth often. Though veneers are stain resistant, the dentist might also recommend avoiding food and beverages, such as coffee, tea, and red wine, which strain teeth.

References

1. "Crowns and Bridges," National Dental Care (NDC), n.d.

2. Wyatt Jr., Alfred D. "Dental Crowns," WebMD, September 29, 2014.

3. Friedman, Michael. "Dental Health and Bridges," WebMD, May 24, 2016.

4. Wyatt Jr., Alfred D. "Dental Health and Veneers," WebMD, January 30, 2015.

5. "Porcelain Veneers," American Academy of Cosmetic Dentistry (AACD), n.d.

Chapter 18

Having a Tooth Pulled

Tooth extraction, or having a tooth pulled, is a dental procedure that involves removing a tooth from its socket in the jawbone. Simple extractions are typically performed by a general dentist using a local anesthetic. Surgical extractions, on the other hand, are usually performed by an oral surgeon and often require an intravenous (IV) or general anesthetic.

Reasons for Tooth Extraction

People have teeth extracted for a number of different reasons. One or more teeth may need to be pulled in cases where they:

- Become damaged by trauma or decay and cannot be repaired with a filling, crown, or other dental treatment

- Become loose due to periodontal (gum) disease affecting the bones and tissues of the mouth

- Are too crowded for permanent teeth to come in properly or for orthodontic treatment to align teeth properly

- Become impacted (stuck in the jaw), especially wisdom teeth

- Develop an infection that cannot be successfully treated with antibiotics or root canal therapy

- Create a high risk of infection in people with weakened immune systems due to chemotherapy, organ transplant, or other medical conditions, or

- Get in the way of radiation treatment to the head or neck

Before Having a Tooth Pulled

When a dentist diagnoses a problem that requires the removal of a tooth, the first step in the process involves assessing the patient's medical condition and history. Although tooth extraction is generally considered to be a very safe procedure, it can allow bacteria from the mouth to enter the bloodstream. As a result, people with medical conditions that put them at high risk of infection—such as a compromised immune system, heart disease, or liver disease—may need to take antibiotics before and after having a tooth pulled.

Patients should also provide a list of all medications they take, including prescriptions, over-the-counter (OTC) drugs, vitamins, and dietary supplements. Some medications, such as bisphosphonates (which are commonly prescribed to treat osteoporosis and other forms of bone loss), can increase the risk of complications from oral surgery.

After taking a medical history, the dentist or oral surgeon will usually take a series of x-rays or a panoramic x-ray to help them plan the extraction. X-rays can provide important information about the relationship between upper teeth and sinuses, or between lower teeth and the inferior alveolar nerve in the jawbone. In addition, x-rays can help identify infections, tumors, or bone diseases that may be affecting the teeth.

The Tooth Extraction Process

Prior to the tooth extraction, the patient usually receives some form of anesthesia. For a simple extraction where the tooth is fully exposed or already loose, the dentist may inject a local anesthetic to numb the area of the mouth near the tooth. For more complex procedures involving an impacted tooth or multiple teeth, an oral surgeon may administer a general anesthetic. Depending on the type of anesthetic used, the patient may remain conscious but feel very calm and sedated, or the patient may sleep through the entire procedure. It is important for patients to follow preoperative instructions and avoid eating, drinking, or smoking if they will receive general anesthesia.

For a simple extraction, the dentist will typically use an instrument called an "elevator" to loosen the tooth, then grasp it with forceps and wiggle it gently to remove it. In a surgical extraction, the oral surgeon will usually make a small incision in the gum to expose the tooth and then cut away the bone and tissue holding it in place. Finally, the oral surgeon will grasp the tooth with forceps and rock it gently to loosen and remove it. Teeth that are impacted or difficult to pull out sometimes must be broken and removed in pieces.

Once the extraction has been completed, the dentist will pack the tooth socket with gauze and ask the patient to bite down to put pressure on the wound for 20 to 30 minutes. Since cuts in the mouth cannot dry out and form a scab, they tend to bleed for a longer period of time than cuts on the skin. In some cases, minor bleeding may continue for 24 hours. Eventually, however, a blood clot should form in the socket. The dentist may use a few stitches to close the edges of the gum over the extraction site. The stitches may dissolve on their own, or they may need to be removed by the dentist at a follow-up appointment.

After Having a Tooth Pulled

Most people who have a tooth extracted are able to return home a few hours after the procedure is completed. In most cases, patients are encouraged to have a responsible person accompany them and drive them home. The initial recovery from a tooth extraction typically takes a few days. During that time, the following suggestions can help patients minimize pain and discomfort, reduce the risk of infection, and promote a quick and full recovery:

- Keep a gauze pad in place for three to four hours to control bleeding and allow a blood clot to form in the tooth socket. Change the pad whenever it becomes soaked with blood or saliva.

- Avoid spitting, rinsing, or drinking from a straw for 24 hours after the extraction to prevent the clot from being dislodged.

- Take nonsteroidal anti-inflammatory drugs (NSAIDs), such as ibuprofen, as directed by the dentist to help manage pain and reduce swelling. Stronger painkillers may be prescribed for the first few days following a surgical tooth extraction.

- Apply an icepack to the face in 15-minute increments to help control inflammation.

- Limit physical activity for one to two days after the procedure.

- When lying down, prop the head up on pillows to inhibit bleeding.

- Brush the teeth and tongue gently to reduce the risk of infection, being careful to avoid the extraction site.

- After 24 hours, rinse the mouth gently with a warm saltwater solution (1/2 teaspoon salt dissolved in 8 ounces of warm water) to keep the extraction area clean.

- Eat foods that are soft and cool—such as yogurt, pudding, or applesauce—for the first 24 hours, reintroducing solid foods gradually as the wound heals.

- Do not smoke, which can delay healing.

Risks of Tooth Extraction

Although tooth extraction is generally viewed as a very safe procedure, there are a few risks associated with it. Some of the complications the patient may experience after having a tooth pulled include the following:

- Infection of the extraction site

- Accidental damage to nearby teeth or fillings

- Fracture of the jaw

- Puncture of the sinus cavity

- Injury to the inferior alveolar nerve in the jaw, causing temporary or permanent numbness of the chin and lower lip

- Dry socket, a painful condition in which the blood clot in the socket breaks off, exposing the underlying bone to air and food

Some pain, discomfort, swelling, and soreness of the jaw is normal after a tooth extraction. Patients are advised to seek medical attention, however, if they experience the following symptoms:

- Severe pain or bleeding that continues for more than 4 hours after the procedure

- Redness, oozing, or excessive discharge that occurs after the first 24 hours

- Swelling that becomes worse over time rather than better

- Fever, chills, or other signs of infection

- Trouble swallowing

- Nausea or vomiting

- Pain in the extraction site that begins 3 days after the procedure, which may indicate dry socket

Most people who have a tooth pulled will fully recover within one to two weeks, although it may take several months for new bone and gum tissue to fill the gap where the tooth used to be. In many cases, the dentist may recommend a second procedure to replace the missing tooth with an implant, bridge, or denture.

References

1. "Pulling a Tooth," WebMD, 2014.

2. "Tooth Extraction," Colgate Oral Care Center, May 2, 2014.

Chapter 19

Dentures

Chapter Contents

Section 19.1

What Are Dentures?

"What Are Dentures?" © 2017 Omnigraphics. Reviewed July 2019.

Dentures, also called "false teeth," are prosthetic devices that replace two or more natural teeth that have been lost as a result of decay, periodontal disease, or developmental defects. They are held in place by the hard and soft tissues of the mouth and can, to a large extent, take over the functions of natural teeth, such as chewing and speech. In addition to functional benefits, dentures also help maintain facial structure and improve appearance.

The Process

Dentures are made in commercial laboratories by technicians called "denturists." Today, many dentures are made from acrylic resins and have better functionality and aesthetic appeal than their forerunners. They are very resilient and generally have a life span of about eight years. Porcelain may also be used, but this material is not generally recommended for some applications, as it can wear away the natural teeth that come in contact with them. The teeth in dentures are mounted on a saddle-shaped plastic or metal frame whose form is designed to conform to the user's gums and palate. Plastic frames are becoming more common, because they are highly wear-resistant and can easily be reshaped at the dentist's office.

The manufacturing process begins with the creation of a diagnostic cast. This involves making a preliminary wax impression of the patient's maxillary and mandibular arches (upper and lower sets of dentition). The preliminary cast is adjusted by applying pressure to the soft tissues to simulate a biting effect. This helps ensure proper alignment of the dentures and gums. The preliminary cast is used as a template for the permanent cast, which is made of gypsum. Acrylic resin is filled in the final mold to manufacture the denture. The packed mold is then heated to enable the resin to harden. Finally, the hardened acrylic denture is removed by breaking the mold.

Types of Dentures

Depending on whether they replace all or some of the teeth, dentures are classified as full or partial. A full denture replaces the complete set of teeth and requires the removal of any remaining natural teeth prior to its placement. The denture is typically not fixed immediately following tooth removal, as the gums and jawbones take a while to heal and reshape. The dentist may, in fact, wait several months after tooth removal to order a full denture. This helps avoid the need for alterations or relining of the denture to accommodate structural changes in the gums and bones, a process which inevitably follows tooth removal.

A partial denture, on the other hand, is designed to replace one, or a few, missing teeth. It is usually anchored to the natural teeth using metal clasps and can be easily removed. The clips may occasionally be made from material that closely resembles gum or tooth, although this type is generally not as strong as those made from metal.

Dentures, whether full or partial, may be permanent or removable. Removable dentures depend on the underlying bone for support and are low in cost and less invasive to fit. In many cases, however, removable dentures might not be the ideal solution, since bone loss may result in the lack of a suitable anchoring point. Permanent dentures may be the only option in such cases. This type of denture is permanently fixed in the mouth and is supported by dental implants. More invasive and more expensive than removable dentures, permanent dentures replace both visible structures and the root structures of the teeth.

Disadvantage of Dentures

Although dentures have helped many people regain the ability to eat normally, enunciate better, enhance their appearance, and boost their self-esteem, they are not without problems. While some of the issues associated with dentures may subside after a break-in period, during which the patient becomes accustomed to the prosthesis, others may persist and often require additional visits to the dentist or orthodontist.

Common Problems with Dentures

Before considering being fitted with dentures, it is important to be aware of some of the problems associated with them, including:

Awkwardness

One of the most common issues experienced by denture-wearers is getting used to having a foreign object in their mouths. And the dentures may slip out frequently. When this happens, especially with the lower denture, the user will in time learn to bite down softly and push the denture back into position. Pronunciation of certain sounds may also take some practice. But, usually, these issues tend to lessen after a brief period of adjustment.

Irritation

Pain, swelling, and increased salivation are other common problems following denture placement. However, these issues usually subside as healing takes place and the wearer adapts to the dentures. The dentist may recommend a special adhesive to help keep the denture in place, however, it is best not to overuse denture adhesives and to avoid those containing zinc. If pain and irritation persist, the dentist may recommend pain-relieving gels, as well as antiseptics to prevent possible infection.

Difficulty Chewing

Chewing feels different with dentures, and this may take some getting used to. Unlike natural teeth, prostheses lack nerve sensations, and the wearer may not become aware of food textures and changes in temperature. While dentures help you eat most foods, there are some sticky or crunchy foods that pose problems for the denture wearer. For example, nut butters and crunchy fruits and vegetables may not be denture-friendly, and you may need to substitute these with nonsticky protein-rich spreads, cooked vegetables, stewed fruit, or smoothies.

Resorption

Bone resorption is a process that normally accompanies tooth removal. When there are no teeth to support, the bony ridges that once held the natural teeth begin to reduce in mass and density. As the body recognizes the loss of function in the supporting bones, the nutrients that normally aid bone growth are rerouted elsewhere. This resorption can be accelerated as the dentures exert pressure on the gums and underlying bony tissues. As a result, dentures may begin to lose their fit after some time and might need to be remodeled or relined on occasion.

Care and Hygiene

Caring for your dentures is as important as caring for your natural teeth. Your dentist or orthodontist will recommend how long you need to wear your dentures and how to care for them properly. Clean dentures contribute to good oral health and hygiene and can prevent problems, such as gum disease, bad breath, and oral infections.

Some tips for denture care include:

- Soak dentures overnight in warm water and cleansing solution to prevent drying or warping.

- Brush dentures at least once per day, ideally after every meal, to remove food remnants and prevent the buildup of tartar.

- Brush with a soft-bristled brush and soapy water or a commercial denture cleaner.

- Never use housecleaning liquids or abrasive chemicals.

- Massage and clean the roof of the mouth, tongue, and gums each day before putting on your dentures.

- Never sleep with your dentures in place.

References

1. "Dental Health and Dentures," WebMD, 2005–2016.

2. Horne, Steven B., DDS. "Dentures," MedicineNet, Inc., 2016.

3. "Denture," MadeHow.com, 2016.

Section 19.2

Denture Adhesives

This section includes text excerpted from "Denture Adhesives," U.S. Food and Drug Administration(FDA), September 4, 2018.

Denture adhesives are pastes, powders, or adhesive pads that may be placed in or on dentures to help them stay in place. Sometimes denture adhesives contain zinc to enhance adhesion.

In most cases, properly fitted and maintained dentures should not require the use of denture adhesives. Over time, shrinkage in the bone structure in the mouth causes dentures to gradually become loose. When this occurs, the dentures should be relined or new dentures made that fit the mouth properly. Denture adhesives fill gaps caused by shrinking bone and give temporary relief from loosening dentures.

Zinc and Potential Risk

Zinc is a mineral that is an essential ingredient for good health. It is found in protein-rich foods, such as shellfish, beef, chicken, and nuts, as well as in some dietary supplements.

However, an excess of zinc in the body can lead to health problems, such as nerve damage, especially in the hands and feet. This damage appears slowly, over an extended period of time.

The overuse of zinc-containing denture adhesives, especially when combined with dietary supplements that contain zinc and other sources of zinc, can contribute to an excess of zinc in your body.

Reports of Problems

The U.S. Food and Drug Administration (FDA) is aware of case reports in the medical literature linking negative reactions, such as nerve damage, numbness, or tingling sensations from denture adhesives that contain zinc to chronic overuse of the products. The subjects of these case reports used at least two tubes of zinc-containing denture adhesive each week. Some product instructions indicate that one tube should last seven to eight weeks.

The FDA has also received reports of adverse events linked to the use of denture adhesives. However, the FDA's adverse event reporting system is not designed to establish injury rates and individual reports vary in the amount and reliability of data included.

Neither published data nor FDA adverse event surveillance data are adequate to associate injuries with specific device types or brands.

The FDA has not found conclusive evidence that these problems result from using zinc-containing denture adhesive as instructed in the product labeling.

To help address the potential risk that overuse of zinc-containing denture adhesives may pose, the FDA asked makers of zinc-containing denture adhesives to consider:

- Including directions that will prevent overuse if zinc is an ingredient. (Some companies include graphics of the amount of adhesive to use or the amount of time that a tube should last under correct usage.)

- Modifying the labeling to specify that the product contains zinc as an ingredient, if appropriate, and replacing zinc with an ingredient that presents fewer health risks in situations of overuse.

Manufacturers, importers, and distributors of denture adhesives are required by the FDA to register their facilities, list their products, and report adverse events. In addition, they are required to adhere to other general regulatory controls, such as good manufacturing practice and adequate directions for use or a clear definition of an unsafe dosage or methods or duration of application.

Advice for Denture Wearers

Denture wearers may have difficulty determining the proper amount of denture adhesive to use if the instructions are not clear. If a denture wearer is uncertain about how much to use, she or he should contact a dental-health professional to help determine the correct amount.

Denture wearers should know that a large amount of denture adhesive will not necessarily address problems with ill-fitting dentures, and prolonged use of ill-fitting dentures may lead to an increase in bone loss.

The FDA recommends that consumers of denture adhesive products:

- Follow the instructions provided with the denture adhesive. If the product does not come with instructions or the instructions are unclear, consult with a dental professional.

- Do not use more adhesive than recommended.

- Understand that some denture adhesives contain zinc and that although they are safe to use in moderation as directed, if overused, they could have harmful effects.

- Know that manufacturers may not always list their product ingredients.

- Know that there are zinc-free denture adhesives products.

- Stop using the denture adhesive and consult your physician if you experience symptoms, such as numbness or tingling sensations in the extremities.

- Start with a small amount of adhesive—if the adhesive oozes off the denture into your mouth, you are likely using too much adhesive.

- Know that a 2.4-ounce tube of denture adhesive used by a consumer with upper and lower dentures should last seven to eight weeks.

- Track how much denture adhesive you use by marking on a calendar when you started a new tube, and when the tube is empty.

- Consider speaking to your dentist to see that your dentures fit properly. Dentures can become ill-fitting as a person's gums change over time.

Part Three

Dental Care for Infants and Children

Chapter 20

Oral Health for Infants

Chapter Contents

Section 20.1

A Healthy Mouth for Your Baby

This section includes text excerpted from "A Healthy Mouth for Your Baby," National Institute of Dental and Craniofacial Research (NIDCR), August 2017.

Healthy teeth are important—even baby teeth. Children need healthy teeth to help them chew and to speak clearly, and baby teeth hold space for adult teeth. This can help you keep your baby's mouth healthy and give your baby a healthy start.

Protect Your Baby's Teeth with Fluoride

Fluoride protects teeth from tooth decay. It can even heal early decay. Fluoride is in the drinking water of many towns and cities. Ask a dentist or doctor if your water has fluoride in it. If it does not, ask about other kinds of fluoride (such as fluoride varnish or drops) that can help keep your baby's teeth healthy.

Check and Clean Your Baby's Teeth

Check Your Baby's Teeth

Healthy teeth should be all one color. If you see spots or stains on the teeth, take your baby to a dentist.

Clean Your Baby's Teeth

Clean them as soon as they come in with a clean, soft cloth or a baby's toothbrush. Clean the teeth at least once a day. It is best to clean them right before bedtime. At about age two (or sooner if a dentist or doctor suggests it) you should start putting fluoride toothpaste on your child's toothbrush. Use only a pea-sized drop of toothpaste. Young children cannot get their teeth clean by themselves. Until they are seven or eight years old, you will need to help them brush. Try brushing their teeth first and then letting them finish.

Feed Your Baby Healthy Food

- Choose foods without a lot of sugar in them.

- Give your child fruits and vegetables for snacks.

- Save cookies and other treats for special occasions.

Do Not Put Your Baby to Bed with a Bottle

Milk, formula, juice, and other drinks such as soda all have sugar in them. If sugary liquids stay on your baby's teeth too long, it can lead to tooth decay. (And decayed teeth can cause pain for your baby.)

What Is One of the Most Important Things You Can Do to Keep Your Baby from Getting Cavities?

Avoid putting your baby to bed with a bottle—at night or at nap time. (If you do put your baby to bed with a bottle, fill it only with water.)

Here Are Some Other Things You Can Do

- Between feedings, do not give your baby a bottle or sippy cup filled with sweet drinks to carry around.

- Near your baby's first birthday, teach your baby to drink from an open cup.

- If your baby uses a pacifier, do not dip it in anything sweet like sugar or honey.

Take Your Child to the Dentist

Your child should have a dental visit by the first birthday. At this visit, the dentist will:

- Check your child's teeth

- Show you the best way to clean your child's teeth

- Talk to you about other things, such as a healthy diet and fluoride that can keep your child's mouth healthy

Section 20.2

Teething

This section includes text excerpted from "Brush Up on
Oral Health—Babies Who Are Teething," Early Childhood
Learning and Knowledge Center (ECLKC), March 2019.

Babies Who Are Teething

Teething happens when a baby's primary teeth push through the
gums into the baby's mouth. For some babies, teething is uncomfortable. Head Start* staff support parents whose baby is teething by providing information on teething and other tips to parents for comforting
their baby who has teething pain.

** Head Start programs support children's growth and development in a positive learn-
ing environment through a variety of services.*

Teething Basics

Most babies begin teething around the age of 6 months. But,
teething can start at any time between ages 3 and 12 months. As the
primary teeth come into the mouth, babies may feel pain from the
tooth pushing through the gum. Babies who are teething may become
cranky, drool more, have red and swollen spots on their gums, and
chew on things more frequently.

Tips for Parents to Ease Baby's Teething Pain

- **Keep it safe.** Here are some ideas for choosing safe teething toys.

  - Avoid liquid-filled teething toys. The baby may chew a hole
    into them.

  - Find teething toys that are made of a single piece of durable
    material. Otherwise, loose pieces could break off in the baby's
    mouth and cause choking.

  - Do not hang teething toys on a cord around a baby's neck
    or attach them to clothes. They could get tangled around
    the baby's neck and cause choking. These toys include chew
    beads, chew necklaces, or pacifiers.

- **Clean it.** Many strategies for comforting a teething baby include
  putting something in the baby's mouth. Everything that goes in

the mouth should be cleaned first to keep the baby healthy. Read the package for directions on how to clean the item. Some items are dishwasher safe and some are not.

- **Massage it.** Gently rub the baby's gums with a clean finger for about two minutes. Many babies find the pressure soothing. For babies who already have some teeth, be careful the baby does not bite you!

- **Cool it.** Cold helps ease the pain of sore gums. Give the baby a cool clean wet washcloth, spoon, pacifier, or teething ring to chew on. Teething rings can be put in the refrigerator but not the freezer. Chewing frozen teething rings can make a baby's cheeks or chin become bumpy and turn reddish-purple. Note: To prevent injuries to the mouth, do not let a baby walk while holding a spoon.

- **Freeze it.** Some frozen foods can help ease teething pain.

- **Do not use it.** Over-the-counter (OTC) teething gels and liquids on babies' gums are not recommended because they offer little to no benefit for treating oral pain. They all contain benzocaine, which, if used incorrectly, can cause serious health problems, including blood disorders and death. If nothing works to ease a baby's teething pain, ask the baby's doctor or dentist for directions on what pain medications can be used and how to use them safely.

It is important to remember that once a tooth comes into the mouth, the tooth is at risk for developing tooth decay. Encourage parents to brush their child's teeth using an infant-sized toothbrush with soft bristles with a smear (rice-sized amount) of fluoride in the morning and before bedtime.

Section 20.3

Soothing Teething Pain and Sensory Needs in Babies

This section includes text excerpted from "Safely Soothing Teething Pain and Sensory Needs in Babies and Older Children," U.S. Food and Drug Administration (FDA), May 23, 2018.

Teething is normal but may be a painful experience for infants and toddlers. Too often, well-meaning parents and caregivers who want to ease a child's pain turn to medications and products that could be harmful.

Soothing children's gums with prescription or over-the-counter (OTC) drugs, homeopathic drugs, or teething jewelry marketed for relieving teething pain may seem like good options. But, those products can be dangerous and lead to serious injury or even death. This also applies to older children with special needs who may use teething jewelry for sensory stimulation.

The American Academy of Pediatrics (AAP) recommends alternative ways for treating teething pain, including rubbing infants' gums with a clean finger or providing a teething ring made of firm rubber to chew on. For children with sensory stimulation needs, parents and caregivers should talk to their child's healthcare provider about safer options.

On average, children begin teething around 4 to 7 months and have a total of 20 "baby teeth" by age 3. According to the AAP, occasional symptoms of teething include mild irritability, a low-level fever, drooling, and an urge to chew something hard.

The Risks of Teething Bracelets, Necklaces, and Other Jewelry

Teething jewelry includes necklaces, bracelets, and other jewelry worn by either an adult or child, used by parents and caregivers, and is marketed to relieve an infant's teething pain. It may also be marketed for use by people with special needs, such as autism or attention deficit hyperactivity disorder, to provide sensory stimulation or redirect chewing on clothes or body parts.

The beads of the jewelry may be made with various materials, such as amber, wood, marble, or silicone. Jewelry marketed for teething is not the same as teething rings or teethers, which are made of hard plastic or rubber and not wearable by an adult or child.

Serious risks are associated with using jewelry marketed for relieving teething pain. Choking, strangulation, injury to the mouth, and infection, other concerns include potential injury to the mouth or infection if a piece of the jewelry irritates or pierces the child's gums.

Teething Creams and Gels Also Have Risks

Parents and caregivers might also look to relieve a teething baby by rubbing numbing medications on the child's gums. But, the U.S. Food and Drug Administration (FDA) warns against using any sort of topical medication to treat teething pain in children, including prescription or OTC creams and gels, or homeopathic teething tablets. They offer little to no benefit and are associated with serious risk.

Benzocaine—a local anesthetic—is the active ingredient in several OTC oral healthcare products, such as Anbesol®, Baby Orajel, Cepacol®, Chloraseptic®, Hurricaine®, Orabase®, Orajel®, and Topex. These products should not be used for teething because they can be dangerous and are not useful because they wash out of a baby's mouth within minutes.

The use of benzocaine gels, sprays, ointments, solutions, and lozenges for mouth and gum pain can lead to a serious—and sometimes fatal—condition called "methemoglobinemia,' in which the oxygen-carrying capacity of your baby's red blood cells is greatly reduced.

Prescription and OTC benzocaine oral healthcare drug products are also widely used in adults. Doctors and dentists often use sprays containing benzocaine to numb the mucous membranes of the mouth and throat or to suppress the gag reflex during medical and surgical procedures, such as transesophageal echocardiograms, endoscopy, intubation, and feeding tube replacements. But, benzocaine sprays are not FDA-approved for these uses.

Talk to your healthcare professional about using benzocaine and other local anesthetics, especially if you have heart disease, are elderly, are a smoker, or have breathing problems, such as asthma, bronchitis, or emphysema. Those conditions put you at greater risk for complications relating to methemoglobinemia.

What You Can Do to Ease Teething Pain

If your child's gums are swollen and tender, gently rub or massage the gums with your finger, or give your child a teething ring made of firm rubber to chew. Make sure the teething ring is not frozen. If the object is too hard, it can hurt your child's gums. Parents should supervise their children so they do not accidentally choke on the teething ring.

Parents and caregivers of children with special needs who may require sensory stimulation should talk to their child's healthcare provider about safer options and treatment. Jewelry marketed for relieving teething pain and to provide sensory stimulation can lead to serious injuries, including strangulation and choking.

The FDA continues to closely monitor the use of teething jewelry and other teething pain relief products and is evaluating whether other actions are necessary to address the risks associated with these products, as part of its commitment to protecting public health—especially when it comes to the health and safety of children.

Consumers and healthcare professionals should notify the FDA of any adverse side effects when using drugs and devices the agency regulates, by reporting them online to MedWatch, the FDA's safety information and adverse event reporting program, or by telephone at 800-FDA-1088 (800-332-1088).

Section 20.4

Benzocaine and Teething

This section includes text excerpted from "Benzocaine and Babies: Not a Good Mix," U.S. Food and Drug Administration (FDA), November 6, 2017.

When a baby is teething, many a mom or dad reaches for a pain remedy containing benzocaine to help soothe sore gums. Benzocaine is a local anesthetic and can be found in such over-the-counter (OTC) products as Anbesol®, Hurricaine®, Orajel, Baby Orajel, and Orabase®.

But, the use of benzocaine gels and liquids for mouth and gum pain can lead to a rare but serious—and sometimes fatal—condition called "methemoglobinemia," a disorder in which the amount of oxygen carried through the bloodstream is greatly reduced. In the most severe cases, says pharmacist Mary Ghods, R.Ph., of the U.S. Food and Drug Administration (FDA), methemoglobinemia can result in death.

And children under two years old appear to be at particular risk.

Since the FDA first warned about potential dangers in 2006, the agency has received 29 reports of benzocaine gel-related cases of methemoglobinemia. Nineteen of those cases occurred in children, and 15 of the 19 cases occurred in children under 2 years of age, says FDA pharmacist Kellie Taylor, Pharm.D., MPH.

The agency repeated the warning in April 2011 and remains particularly concerned about the use of OTC benzocaine products in children for relief of pain from teething, says Taylor. This concern is fueled by the serious potential outcomes and the difficulty parents may have to recognize the signs and symptoms of methemoglobinemia when using these products at home. These symptoms may not always be evident or attributed to the condition.

For these reasons, the FDA recommends that parents and caregivers not use benzocaine products for children younger than two years, except under the advice and supervision of a healthcare professional.

Danger Signs

Symptoms of methemoglobinemia include:

- Pale, gray, or blue-colored skin, lips, and nail beds
- Shortness of breath
- Fatigue
- Confusion
- Headache
- Light-headedness
- Rapid heart rate

"Symptoms can occur within minutes to hours after benzocaine use," Ghods says. "They can occur after using the drug for the first time, as well as after several uses."

If your child has any of these symptoms after using benzocaine, she adds, stop using the product and seek medical help immediately by calling 911.

Methemoglobinemia caused by benzocaine may require treatment with medications and admission to a hospital. Serious cases should be treated right away. If left untreated or if treatment is delayed, methemoglobinemia may cause permanent injury to the brain and body tissues, and even death, from the insufficient amount of oxygen in the blood.

Teething: What Parents Can Do

As for the crying baby, what is a mom or dad to do? The American Academy of Pediatrics offers some alternatives for treating teething pain:

- Give the child a teething ring chilled in the refrigerator.
- Gently rub or massage the child's gums with your finger.

If these remedies do not provide relief, contact your healthcare professional for advice on other treatments.

Adults Can Be Affected, Too

Benzocaine products—which are sold as gels, liquids, sprays, and lozenges—are also widely used by adults. Doctors and dentists often use sprays containing benzocaine to numb the mucous membranes of the mouth and throat during such procedures as transesophageal echocardiograms, endoscopy, intubation, and feeding tube replacements.

Even though children are more at risk, it is still a good idea to talk to your healthcare professional about using benzocaine, especially if you have heart disease, are a smoker, or have breathing problems, such as asthma, bronchitis, or emphysema. These conditions put you at greater risk for complications relating to methemoglobinemia, says Taylor.

The FDA advises consumers to:

- Store any products containing benzocaine out of the reach of children
- Use benzocaine gels and liquids sparingly and only when needed. Do not use them more than four times a day.
- Read the label to see if benzocaine is an active ingredient when buying OTC products. Labels on OTC products containing benzocaine are not currently required to carry warnings about the risk of methemoglobinemia. If you have any concerns, talk to your healthcare professional before using them.

Section 20.5

Using a Pacifier

This section includes text excerpted from "Brush Up on
Oral Health—Babies and Pacifier Use," Early Childhood
Learning and Knowledge Center (ECLKC), June 2018.

Babies and Pacifier Use

Most babies have a natural need to suck, and most find it calming.
This type of sucking is also called "nonnutritive sucking" because the
baby is not being fed. Giving a baby a pacifier can satisfy a baby's
need to suck.

Between ages two and four, most children stop using a pacifier on
their own. If a child continues to use a pacifier after age five, it can
affect the way their teeth bite together. For example, it can cause an
overbite. It can also affect the growth of jaws and bones that support
the child's teeth.

Tips for Parents about Pacifier Use

If parents choose to give their baby a pacifier, here are some tips
for using it safely:

- **Wait until breastfeeding is going well (usually after about
  three to four weeks).** If a pacifier is given to a baby before
  then, nipple confusion may occur and make breastfeeding hard
  to establish. After a pacifier is introduced, it should never be
  used to delay or replace regular feedings.

- **Let a baby decide whether to use a pacifier.** If a baby shows
  no interest in using a pacifier, do not force it.

- **Offer a pacifier at naptime and bedtime.** If a baby uses a
  pacifier, the best times to offer it are at naptime and bedtime.
  Using a pacifier at these times may help lower a baby's risk for
  sudden infant death syndrome (SIDS).

- **Do not coat pacifiers.** Sucking on a pacifier coated with
  anything, especially sugar, honey, or jam, increases a baby's risk
  for tooth decay.

- **Attach pacifiers with clips that have short ribbons to
  keep from falling.** Never tie a pacifier to a baby's wrist or neck

or to a baby's crib. The string can get tangled around the baby's neck and make the baby choke.

- **Clean pacifiers and replace them regularly.** Wash a pacifier that has fallen on the ground or floor with soap and warm water before giving it back to a baby. Parents who clean pacifiers with their mouths pass bacteria that cause tooth decay to the baby. Carrying extra pacifiers is a good idea.

- **Check pacifiers for wear and tear.** Over time, pacifiers can break down. Look at the rubber every now and then to see if it is discolored, cracked, or torn. If it is, replace it.

- **Do not share pacifiers.** Each baby should have their own pacifier(s). Letting babies share a pacifier can pass bacteria that cause tooth decay and increases a baby's risk for tooth decay.

Tips to Help Parents Wean Their Child from a Pacifier

If a child shows no interest in self-weaning from the pacifier by age four, parents need to help. Here are some ideas to share with parents.

- **Take it away gradually.** Limit pacifier use to certain times (such as naptime or bedtime) or to certain places (such as in bed). In most cases, when a child uses a pacifier in bed, it falls out of the child's mouth during sleep. Parents can gradually increase the amount of time the child is not using a pacifier until the child completely stops using it.

- **Throw it away.** Encourage the child to throw their pacifier away. If the child asks for a pacifier, parents can remind them that the child threw it away, that the child is a big kid, and that big kids do not use pacifiers.

- **Trade it.** Encourage the child to put pacifiers under the pillow for the "pacifier fairy" (or another positive cultural character) who will trade them for a gift, like a toy or something soothing. If the child keeps asking for a pacifier, remind the child that all the pacifiers were given to the pacifier fairy (or other character), who gave the child a gift.

- **Poke holes in it.** This alters the pacifier so it is no longer satisfying to suck on. It is best to use a clean pin to poke two to three holes in the tip.

Chapter 21

Weaning a Child from a Bottle

For children who drink infant formula or breast milk from a bottle, at some point, parents will wonder if it is time to start weaning their child. As children begin to eat more solid foods and drink from a cup, parents can wean their child from a bottle.

The American Academy of Pediatrics (AAP) and the American Academy of Pediatric Dentistry (AAPD) recommend that children be weaned from a bottle by age 12 to 14 months. The longer parents wait, the harder the process can be.

This chapter explains why weaning from a bottle is important and offers tips that Head Start* staff can share with parents to help. It also provides a recipe for a healthy snack that can be made in a Head Start classroom or at home.

* Head Start programs support children's growth and development in a positive learn- ing environment through a variety of services.

Why Weaning a Child from a Bottle Is Important

Children who keep drinking from a bottle after age 14 months are more likely to develop tooth decay than children the same age who

This chapter includes text excerpted from "Brush Up on Oral Health—Weaning a Child from a Bottle," Early Childhood Learning and Knowledge Center (ECLKC), April 2016.

have been weaned. This is especially true if a child is allowed to drink throughout the day and/or at bedtime from a bottle filled with anything other than water.

Drinking from a bottle after age 14 months can also prevent the top and bottom front teeth from meeting and create an "open bite" when the child bites down. Like long-term thumbsucking, this behavior can affect appearance, interfere with the ability to bite food and speak clearly, and cause crowding of permanent teeth. In addition, children who keep drinking from a bottle after age 14 months tend to drink more milk than recommended. This can reduce their appetite for solid foods, which can cause nutritional deficiencies, such as an iron deficiency. Also, children who keep drinking from a bottle after age 14 months may not develop the eating skills they need to stay healthy.

Weaning Tips for Head Start Staff to Share with Parents
Preparing for Weaning

Some preparation may help make weaning easier.

- Do not introduce a bottle if the child is breastfed solely until age 9 to 12 months and never fed breast milk from a bottle. Serve breast milk, infant formula, or cow's milk (starting at age 1) in a cup.

- Starting at age 4 to 6 months, let the child drink water from a cup. This helps the child get used to drinking from a cup. A sippy cup can be used. However, sippy cups are meant to be used for a short time only to help a child move from a bottle to a cup.

Note: The AAP recommends that no fruit juice should be served to children under age 1. If fruit juice is served to children after age 1, it should be served in a cup at mealtimes and limited to 4 to 6 ounces per day.

Using a Gradual Approach

- Introduce a cup in place of a bottle when a child is least interested in feeding or at mealtimes when other people are drinking from cups.

- Feed small amounts of breast milk or infant formula in a cup. Feed the liquid slowly, tilting the cup so that only a small amount leaves the cup, so the child can swallow without hurrying.

- Let the child pick out a special new cup.

- Decrease the number of bottles you offer the child every day, and replace them, one at a time, with a cup of breast milk, infant formula, or cow's milk (starting at age 1).

- Stop giving the least important bottle first, such as one in the middle of the day.

Going Cold Turkey

- For about a week before taking bottles away, talk to the child about giving up the bottle. Remind the child often that soon she or he is no longer going to have a bottle. Then, remove all the bottles from the house. Show the child they are gone.

- Offer a reward, such as an activity that the child enjoys, for making it through a day or night without a bottle.

- Serve a snack at the time of day when the child asks for a bottle most.

- Give the child a soothing object, such as a blanket or favorite toy, whenever she or he misses a bottle.

Deciding on which weaning approach to use depends on many things, including the child's age and ability to cooperate. Most parents find a gradual approach works well. However, this approach may not work for children who are very attached to a bottle. Taking a bottle away suddenly can be difficult for the child and the parents for a short time, but it may work best.

Chapter 22

Routine Care of Children's Teeth

Chapter Contents

153

Section 22.1

Finding and Visiting a Dental Clinic with Your Child

This section contains text excerpted from the following sources: Text under the heading "Finding a Dental Clinic" is excerpted from "Finding a Dental Clinic for Your Child," Early Childhood Learning and Knowledge Center (ECLKC), August 14, 2018; Text under the heading "Visiting the Dental Clinic with Your Child" is excerpted from "Visiting the Dental Clinic with Your Child," Early Childhood Learning and Knowledge Center (ECLKC), September 11, 2018.

Finding a Dental Clinic

Children need to visit the dental clinic to keep their teeth and mouth healthy. If children have regular dental visits, the dentist and dental hygienist can take care of their teeth and find oral health problems early. Here are tips for finding a dental clinic that is best for you and your child.

Tips for finding a dental clinic:

- Ask your child's Head Start* teacher or other parents for suggestions.

- Ask your child's doctor for a referral.

* Head Start programs support children's growth and development in a positive learning environment through a variety of services

Questions to ask when choosing a dental clinic:

- Is your clinic taking new patients?

- Does your clinic take my child's insurance (for example, Medicaid or Children's Health Insurance Program (CHIP))?

- Do any of your staff speak my language? Can they translate so I can understand?

- Does clinic staff have training or experience treating young children?

- When is the next appointment for a new patient?

- What happens during a new patient visit?

- Is your clinic close to public transportation?

- When is your clinic open? Is it open evenings or on weekends?

- What information or forms do I need to bring to fill out your paperwork (for example, my child's insurance card or a Head Start oral health form)?

- Are there books, toys, or other things for children in your waiting room?

Visiting the Dental Clinic with Your Child

Children need to visit the dental clinic to keep their teeth and mouth healthy. If children have regular dental visits, the dentist and dental hygienist can take care of their teeth and find oral health problems early. Having regular dental visits also teaches children to value good oral health.

At the dental clinic, the dental team will:

- Check your child's teeth and mouth

- Talk to you about the best way to take care of your child's teeth. For example, brushing your child's teeth with fluoride toothpaste after breakfast and before bed.

- Share other ways to help prevent tooth decay (cavities). For example, putting fluoride varnish on children's teeth.

Tips for visiting the dental clinic:

- If your child asks what will happen at the dental clinic, give a simple answer. For example, say:

  - "They may count how many teeth you have."

  - "They may clean your teeth to make them shiny and bright!"

- If you do not like going to the dental clinic, do not tell your child. That might make your child worry about going, too.

- Set up a pretend dental chair. Pretend to be the dentist or dental hygienist. Look in your child's mouth and count the teeth; then talk to your child about brushing the teeth.

- Read books or watch videos with your child about visiting the dental clinic. Do not use books or videos that have words, such as hurt, pain, shot, drill, afraid, or any other words that might scare your child.

- Let your child bring a favorite toy or blanket to the clinic.

- If you find out that your child will receive a small toy or new toothbrush at the end of the visit, remind your child of this reward.

- Plan a fun activity for after the clinic visit.

Section 22.2

Primary Teeth

This section includes text excerpted from "Brush Up on Oral Health—Primary (Baby) Teeth," Early Childhood Learning and Knowledge Center (ECLKC), June 2015. Reviewed July 2019.

Many parents believe that primary (baby) teeth are less important than permanent teeth because primary teeth are going to "fall out anyway." However, primary teeth are key to a child's growth and development. Head Start* staff play a vital role in helping parents better understand the importance of primary teeth and offers publications that explain why primary teeth are important, as well as information about primary teeth.

* Head Start programs support children's growth and development in a positive learning environment through a variety of services.

Facts about Primary Teeth: Information for Head Start Staff to Share with Parents

- **Primary teeth are important.** Primary teeth are key to young children's health and development in five very important ways. These include:

  - **Maintaining good health.** The health of primary teeth affects children's overall health and well-being. Untreated tooth decay in primary teeth can lead to infections that can cause fever and discomfort. Infection from an abscessed primary tooth can spread to other areas in the head and neck and lead to pain, severe swelling, and, in rare cases, death. Using antibiotics to treat dental infections may work temporarily. However, the infection will always return if the decay is not treated.

- **Maintaining good nutrition with proper chewing.** To grow and be strong, children need to eat healthy food every day. Children with decay in their primary teeth are less likely to eat crunchy foods, such as fresh fruits and vegetables, that promote good nutrition and a healthy weight. These children are also at risk for developing dietary deficiencies and becoming malnourished.

- **Helping with the development of speech.** Missing teeth can interfere with the development of a young child's speech. Young children with missing teeth have difficulty making "th," "la," and other sounds. This can make it hard for others to understand the child. In some cases, the child may need speech therapy to change speech patterns she or he developed because of missing teeth.

- **Maintaining space for permanent teeth.** Primary teeth hold space for permanent teeth developing underneath them in the jaw. If primary teeth are lost too early, teeth in the mouth move into space and block the space for the incoming permanent teeth. This can cause crowding of the permanent teeth.

- **Promoting self-esteem and confidence.** Young children can be quick to point out other children with teeth that are decayed, chipped, or discolored. Children with tooth decay tend to avoid smiling, cover their mouth with their hands when they speak, or minimize interaction with others. A healthy smile gives children the self-confidence they need to have positive social experiences.

- **Tooth decay in primary teeth matters.** Children with pain from tooth decay do more poorly in school and have more behavior problems. Untreated tooth decay can also spread from one tooth to another. Children with severe tooth decay may need to be put to sleep and receive treatment in a hospital operating room.

- **Brushing primary teeth with a fluoride toothpaste every day promotes good oral health.** Parents should begin brushing a baby's teeth with a smear (rice-sized amount) of fluoride toothpaste twice a day as soon as the first tooth appears in the mouth. Making this a daily habit lowers the number of bacteria in the mouth, helps prevent tooth decay, and starts a lifetime of good oral health habits.

- **Having a dental visit by age one promotes good oral health.** The American Academy of Pediatric Dentistry (AAPD) recommends that a child have her or his first dental visit by age one. A young child's dental visit is simple and quick. The oral health professional examines the child's mouth, identifies potential problems, and explains what changes to expect in the child's mouth as she or he develops and grows. The oral health professional also shows parents how to take care of their child's teeth and applies fluoride varnish to the child's teeth.

Section 22.3

Keeping Children's Teeth Healthy

This section includes text excerpted from "Chew on This," *NIH News in Health*, National Institutes of Health (NIH), February 2013. Reviewed July 2019.

Teeth help us bite, chew, speak clearly, and smile. Even babies need healthy teeth. But, teeth need proper care to stay healthy and strong. It is never too early to start kids on the path to good dental health.

Diet plays a role in tooth decay. When you eat or drink foods that contain sugar, germs in your mouth use the sugar to make acids. Over time, the acids can cause tooth decay or cavities. Tooth decay is the most common chronic disease in children, yet it is mostly preventable.

Although baby teeth eventually fall out, it is still important to take care of them. They play an important role in the mouth. "Baby teeth, of course, are used to chew, but they also guide the growth of the jawbones and create room for permanent teeth to come in," says Dr. Tim Iafolla, a dental-health expert at the National Institutes of Health (NIH).

"Start cleaning your baby's mouth even before the first teeth come in, so your baby gets used to having her or his mouth cleaned. Wipe gums with a clean, soft cloth," says Iafolla. "When teeth come in, clean them twice a day with a cloth or soft brush, as they are immediately susceptible to tooth decay and plaque."

One important way to protect baby teeth is not putting your baby to bed with a bottle. Milk, formula, and juice all contain sugar. If sugary liquids stay on your baby's teeth too long, it can lead to tooth decay. If you give your baby a bottle to keep at bedtime or to carry around between feedings, fill it only with water.

"It's important to catch tooth decay early," Iafolla says. He recommends taking your child to the dentist by age one. The dentist can tell if teeth are coming in properly, detect early signs of decay, and give you tips on caring for your child's teeth.

The best defense against tooth decay is fluoride, a mineral found in most tap water. If your water does not have fluoride, ask a dentist about fluoride drops, gel or varnish.

Start using fluoride toothpaste at about age two. Iafolla recommends using just a pea-sized drop of fluoridated toothpaste until kids have the ability to spit and rinse.

Young kids need help brushing their teeth properly. Try brushing their teeth first and letting them finish. You might try using a timer or a favorite song so your child learns to brush for two minutes. Continue to supervise brushing until your child is seven or eight years old.

Have kids brush their teeth at least twice daily: in the morning, at bedtime, and preferably after meals.

Offer healthy foods and snacks to children. If kids do eat sugary or sticky foods, they should brush their teeth afterward.

Also, ask your child's dentist about sealants—a simple, pain-free way to prevent tooth decay. These thin plastic coatings are painted on the chewing surfaces of permanent back teeth. They quickly harden to form a protective shield against germs and food. If a small cavity is accidentally covered by a sealant, the decay would not spread because germs trapped inside are sealed off from their food supply.

Section 22.4

Brushing Your Child's Teeth

This section includes text excerpted from "Brushing Your Child's Teeth," Early Childhood Learning and Knowledge Center (ECLKC), August 9, 2018.

Brushing is one of the main ways you can keep your child's teeth healthy. You should brush your child's teeth with fluoride toothpaste twice each day to help prevent tooth decay (cavities). Begin brushing as soon as your child's first tooth begins to show.

Tips for brushing your child's teeth:

- Brush your child's teeth after breakfast and before bed.

- Use a child-sized toothbrush with soft bristles and fluoride toothpaste.

- For children under age three, use a small smear of fluoride toothpaste.

- For children ages three to six, use fluoride toothpaste the size of a pea.

Young children like to do things by themselves. It is good to let children brush their teeth while an adult watches. But, children under age seven or eight cannot brush their teeth well yet. An adult needs to brush the child's teeth too.

- Find a position where your child is comfortable and you can see your child's teeth while you brush. For example, sit on the floor with your baby's or young child's head in your lap. Or stand behind your child in front of the mirror.

- Gently brush your child's teeth using small circles. Brush all surfaces of the teeth, including the insides and outsides.

- After brushing, have your child spit out the remaining toothpaste but not rinse. The small amount of toothpaste that stays in your child's mouth is good for the teeth.

- If you are having trouble brushing your child's teeth, use a timer, a counting game, or a song while brushing. You can also ask the staff at your child's dental clinic for help.

Chapter 23

Fluoride Consumption during Tooth Development

Chapter Contents

Section 23.1

Dental Fluorosis

This section includes text excerpted from "Fluorosis," Centers for
Disease Control and Prevention (CDC), March 8, 2019.

The proper amount of fluoride helps prevent and control tooth decay
in children and adults. Fluoride works both while the teeth are developing and every day after the teeth have emerged through the gums.
Fluoride consumed during tooth development can also result in a range
of visible changes to the enamel surface of the tooth. These changes
have been broadly termed "dental fluorosis."

What Is Dental Fluorosis?

Dental fluorosis is a condition that causes changes in the appearance of tooth enamel. It may result when children regularly consume
fluoride during the teeth-forming years, age 8 and younger. Most dental fluorosis in the United States is very mild to mild, appearing as
white spots on the tooth surface that may be barely noticeable and do
not affect dental function. Moderate and severe forms of dental fluorosis, which are far less common, cause more extensive enamel changes.
In the rare, severe form, pits may form in the teeth. The severe form
hardly ever occurs in communities where the level of fluoride in water
is less than two milligrams per liter.

What Causes Dental Fluorosis

Dental fluorosis is caused by taking in too much fluoride over a long
period of time as the teeth are forming under the gums. Only children
age eight and younger are at risk because this is when permanent
teeth are developing; children older than eight years, adolescents, and
adults cannot develop dental fluorosis. The severity of the condition
depends on the dose (how much), duration (how long), and timing
(when consumed) of fluoride intake.

Increases in the occurrence of mostly mild dental fluorosis were recognized as more sources of fluoride became available to prevent tooth
decay. These sources include drinking water with fluoride, fluoride
toothpaste—especially if swallowed by young children—and dietary
prescription supplements in tablets or drops (particularly if prescribed
to children already drinking fluoridated water).

Forms of Dental Fluorosis

- **Very mild and mild forms of dental fluorosis**—Teeth have scattered white flecks, occasional white spots, frosty edges, or fine, lacy chalk-like lines. These changes are barely noticeable and difficult to see except by a dental healthcare professional.

- **Moderate and severe forms of dental fluorosis**—Teeth have larger white spots and, in the rare, severe form, rough, pitted surfaces.

What Can Parents and Caregivers Do to Reduce the Occurrence of Dental Fluorosis?
Know the Fluoride Concentration of Your Drinking Water

You should know the fluoride concentration in your primary source of drinking water, especially if you have young children. This information should help with decisions about using other fluoride products, particularly fluoride tablets or drops that your physician or dentist may prescribe for your young child. Fluoride tablets or drops should not be used at all if your drinking water has the recommended fluoride concentration of 0.7 mg/L or higher.

If you live in a state that participates in the Centers for Disease Control and Prevention's (CDC) My Water's Fluoride, you can find out your water system's fluoridation status online. If you are on a public water system, you can call the water utility company and request a copy of the utility's most recent Consumer Confidence Report.

For children younger than two, consult first with your doctor or dentist regarding the use of fluoride toothpaste. You should clean your child's teeth as soon as the first tooth appears by brushing without toothpaste with a small, soft-bristled toothbrush and plain water.

For children aged two to six years, apply no more than a pea-sized amount of fluoride toothpaste to the brush and supervise their tooth brushing, encouraging the child to spit out the toothpaste rather than swallow it. Until about age six, children have poor control of their swallowing reflex and frequently swallow most of the toothpaste placed on their brush.

Use an Alternative Source of Water for Children Eight Years of Age and Younger If Your Primary Drinking Water Contains Greater Than 2 mg / L of Fluoride

In some regions of the United States, public water systems and private wells contain a natural fluoride concentration of more than 2 mg/L; at this concentration, children eight years and younger have a greater chance for developing dental fluorosis, including the moderate and severe forms. These children should have an alternative source of drinking water that contains fluoride at the recommended level.

What Can Healthcare and Public Health Professionals Do to Reduce the Occurrence of Dental Fluorosis?

Counsel Parents and Caregivers Regarding Use of Fluoride Toothpaste by Young Children

Parents or caregivers should be counseled on the use of fluoride toothpaste by young children, especially those younger than two years. There is an increased chance for dental fluorosis for children younger than six years, and especially for those younger than two years, because they are more likely to swallow the toothpaste than older children.

For children younger than two years, you should consider the fluoride level in the community drinking water, other sources of fluoride, and factors likely to affect susceptibility to tooth decay when weighing the risk and benefits of using fluoride toothpaste. When assessing the risks and benefits, determine if the child may be at high risk for tooth decay because of factors, such as poor hygiene, poor diet, or history of decay in the child, and in their siblings or parents.

Target Mouth Rinses to Children at High Risk for Developing Tooth Decay

Because fluoride mouth rinses have resulted in only limited reductions in tooth decay among children, especially as their exposure to other sources of fluoride has increased, their use should be targeted to individuals and groups at high risk for decay.

Children younger than six years should not use a fluoride mouth rinse without parents first consulting a dentist or physician because there is a possibility for dental fluorosis if these rinses are repeatedly swallowed.

Prescribe Fluoride Supplements Judiciously

Fluoride supplements can be prescribed for children at high risk for tooth decay and whose primary source of drinking water has a low fluoride level. If the children are younger than 6 years, however, then the dentist or physician should weigh the risks for developing decay without supplements with the possibility of developing dental fluorosis. Access to other sources of fluoride, especially drinking water, should be considered when determining this balance. Parents and caregivers should be informed of both the benefits and risks of fluoride supplements.

Fluoride supplements can be prescribed for persons as appropriate or used in school-based programs. When practical, supplements should be prescribed as chewable tablets or lozenges to maximize the topical effects of fluoride.

Is My Child at Increased Risk of Fluorosis If They Are Being Fed Infant Formula?

Three types of infant formula are available in the United States: powdered formula, which comes in bulk or single-serve packets, concentrated liquid, and ready-to-feed formula. Ready-to-feed formula contains little fluoride and does not cause dental fluorosis. The kinds of formula that must be mixed with water—powdered or liquid concentrates—may increase the chance of dental fluorosis if they are the child's main source food and if the water is fluoridated.

Section 23.2

Infant Formula and Fluorosis

This section contains text excerpted from the following sources: Text
in this section begins with excerpts from "Infant Formula," Centers
for Disease Control and Prevention (CDC), November 3, 2015.
Reviewed July 2019; Text under the heading "How Can I Prevent
Dental Fluorosis in My Children?" is excerpted from
"How Can I Prevent Dental Fluorosis in My Children?"
U.S. Department of Health and Human Services (HHS),
August 11, 2014. Reviewed July 2019.

Breastfeeding is ideal for infants. Breast milk is easy to digest and contains antibodies that can protect infants from bacterial and viral infections.

If breastfeeding is not possible, formula can be used. Parents should speak with their pediatrician about what type of infant formula is best for their child.

Does Using Infant Formula Increase Risk for Dental Fluorosis?

Because most infant formulas contain low levels of fluoride, regularly mixing powdered or liquid infant formula concentrate with fluoridated water may increase the chance of a child developing the faint white markings of mild fluorosis.

Does the Type of Infant Formula I Use Affect My Child's Chance of Getting Dental Fluorosis?

Three types of infant formula are available in the United States: powdered formula, which comes in bulk or single-serve packets, concentrated liquid, and ready-to-feed formula. Ready-to-feed formula contains little fluoride and does not cause dental fluorosis. The kinds of formula that must be mixed with water—powdered or liquid concentrates—may increase the chance of dental fluorosis if they are the child's main source food and if the water is fluoridated.

Can I Use Fluoridated Tap Water to Mix Infant Formula?

Yes, you can use fluoridated water for preparing infant formula. However, if your child is only consuming infant formula mixed with fluoridated water, there may be an increased chance for mild dental fluorosis. To lessen this chance, parents can use low-fluoride bottled water some of the time to mix infant formula; these bottled waters are labeled as de-ionized, purified, demineralized, or distilled, and without any fluoride added after purification treatment. The U.S. Food and Drug Administration (FDA) requires the label to indicate when fluoride is added.

Can I Use Bottled Water to Mix Infant Formula?

Yes, you can use bottled water to reconstitute (mix) powdered or liquid concentrate infant formulas, but be aware that the fluoride content in bottled water varies. If your child is exclusively consuming infant formula reconstituted with water that contains fluoride, there may be an increased chance for mild dental fluorosis (a change in the appearance of tooth enamel creating barely visible lacy white markings). To lessen this chance, parents may choose to use low-fluoride bottled water some of the time to mix infant formula. These bottled waters are labeled as de-ionized, purified, demineralized, or distilled and are without any fluoride added after purification treatment (the FDA requires the label to indicate when fluoride is added). Some water companies make available bottled waters marketed for infants and for the purpose of mixing with formula. When water is labeled as intended for infants, the water must meet tap water standards established by the U.S. Environmental Protection Agency (EPA) and indicate that the water is not sterile.

How Can I Prevent Dental Fluorosis in My Children?

There is some potential for developing dental fluorosis when young children consume fluoride during the time when teeth are forming under the gums (birth through age 8). To help prevent both tooth decay and dental fluorosis, the Centers for Disease Control and Prevention (CDC) recommends the following:

Children younger than six years have a poor swallowing reflex and tend to swallow much of the toothpaste on their brush. Toothpaste that is swallowed (but not toothpaste that is spit out) contributes to a child's total fluoride intake.

As soon as the first tooth appears, begin cleaning by brushing without toothpaste with a small, soft-bristled toothbrush and plain water after each feeding. Begin using toothpaste with fluoride when the child is two years old. Use toothpaste with fluoride earlier if your child's doctor or dentist recommends it.

- Do not brush your child's teeth more than two times a day with a fluoride toothpaste,

- Apply no more than a pea-sized amount of toothpaste to the toothbrush, and

- Supervise your child's tooth brushing, encouraging the child to spit out toothpaste rather than swallow it.

- If your child's pediatrician or dentist prescribes a fluoride supplement (or vitamin supplement that contains fluoride), ask her or him about any risk factors your child has for decay and the potential for dental fluorosis. If you live in an area with fluoridated water, fluoride supplements are not recommended.

Chapter 24

Preventing Tooth Decay in Children

Chapter Contents

Section 24.1

Prevalence of Dental Caries (Cavities) in Children in the United States

This section includes text excerpted from "Dental Caries and Sealant Prevalence in Children and Adolescents in the United States, 2011–2012," Centers for Disease Control and Prevention (CDC), November 6, 2015. Reviewed July 2019.

- Approximately 23 percent of children aged 2 to 5 years had dental caries in primary teeth.

- Untreated tooth decay in primary teeth among children aged 2 to 8 was twice as high for Hispanic and non-Hispanic Black children compared with non-Hispanic White children.

- Among those aged 6 to 11, 27 percent of Hispanic children had any dental caries in permanent teeth compared with nearly 18 percent of non-Hispanic White and Asian children.

- Dental sealants were more prevalent for non-Hispanic White children (44%) compared with non-Hispanic Black and Asian children (31% each) aged 6 to 11.

Although dental caries has been declining in permanent teeth for many children since the 1960s, previous findings showed caries in primary teeth for preschool children increasing from 24 to 28 percent between 1988 and 2004. Disparities in caries continue to persist for some race and ethnic groups in the United States. Prevalence of dental sealants—applied to the tooth chewing surfaces to help prevent caries—has also varied among sociodemographic groups. This section describes U.S. youth dental caries and sealant prevalence by race and Hispanic origin for 2011 to 2012.

How Prevalent Was Any Caries in Children's Primary Teeth?

Approximately 37 percent of children aged 2 to 8 years had experienced dental caries in primary teeth in 2011 to 2012 (Figure 24.1). Dental caries among children aged 2 to 5 was nearly 23 percent compared with 56 percent among those aged 6 to 8. Caries prevalence was higher for Hispanic (46%) and non-Hispanic Black (44%)

children compared with non-Hispanic White children (31%) aged 2 to 8. Non-Hispanic Asian children were less likely to have experienced dental caries (36%) compared with Hispanic children (46%) aged 2 to 8, but were not different from non-Hispanic White or non-Hispanic Black children.

In 2011 to 2012, 14 percent of children aged 2 to 8 had untreated tooth decay in primary teeth. Untreated caries in primary teeth was twice as high for children aged 6 to 8 (20%) compared with children aged 2 to 5 (10%). Tooth decay was significantly higher for both non-Hispanic Black (21%) and Hispanic (19%) children compared with non-Hispanic White children aged 2 to 8 (10%). The prevalence of untreated dental caries in primary teeth in non-Hispanic Asian children did not significantly differ from that in any of the other race and Hispanic origin groups.

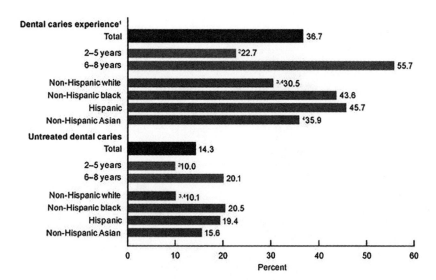

Figure 24.1. *Prevalence of Dental Caries in Primary Teeth, by Age and Race and Hispanic Origin among Children Aged 2 to 8 Years: United States, 2011 to 2012* (Source: Centers for Disease Control and Prevention (CDC)/National Center for Health Statistics (NCHS), National Health and Nutrition Examination Survey (NHANES), 2011–2012.)
[1] Includes untreated and treated (restored) dental caries.
[2] Significantly different from those aged 6 to 8 years, p < 0.05.
[3] Significantly different from non-Hispanic Black children, p < 0.05.
[4] Significantly different from Hispanic children, p < 0.05.

What Percentage of Children Had Any Dental Caries in Permanent Teeth?

In 2011 to 2012, 21 percent of children aged 6 to 11 had experienced dental caries in permanent teeth (Figure 24.2). Dental caries among children aged 6 to 8 was nearly 14 percent and was twice as high for children aged 9 to 11 (29%). Caries prevalence was higher among Hispanic children aged 6 to 11 (27%) compared with non-Hispanic White children (19%) or non-Hispanic Asian children (18%).

Approximately 6 percent of children aged 6 to 11 had untreated tooth decay in permanent teeth. Untreated caries in permanent teeth was twice as high for children aged 9 to 11 (8%) compared with children aged 6 to 8 years (3%). Prevalence of untreated caries was higher for Hispanic children (9%) compared with non-Hispanic White children (4%) aged 6 to 11 years.

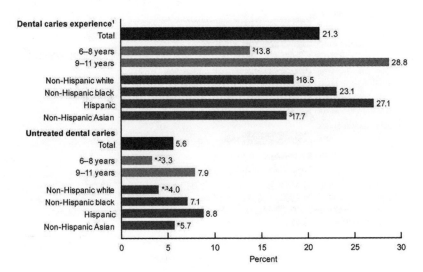

Figure 24.2. *Prevalence of Dental Caries in Permanent Teeth, by Age and Race and Hispanic Origin among Children Aged 6 to 11 Years: United States, 2011 to 2012* (Source: Centers for Disease Control and Prevention (CDC)/National Center for Health Statistics (NCHS), National Health and Nutrition Examination Survey (NHANES), 2011–2012.)

* *Does not meet standards of statistical reliability and precision (relative standard error of ≥ 30% but < 40%).*
[1] *Includes untreated and treated (restored) dental caries.*
[2] *Significantly different from those aged 9 to 11 years, p < 0.05.*
[3] *Significantly different from Hispanic children, p < 0.05.*

How Prevalent Were Dental Sealants among Children?

Nearly one-half of children aged 9 to 11 had at least one dental sealant on a permanent tooth, whereas 31 percent of children aged 6 to 8 had a dental sealant (Figure 24.3). Non-Hispanic Black and non-Hispanic Asian children aged 6 to 11 (31%) had lower dental sealant prevalence compared with non-Hispanic White children (44%). Hispanic children (40%) had higher dental sealant prevalence compared with non-Hispanic Black children aged 6 to 11 (31%).

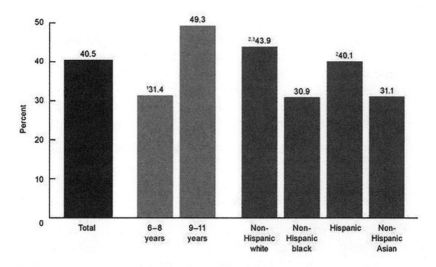

Figure 24.3. *Prevalence of Dental Sealants in Permanent Teeth, by Age and Race and Hispanic Origin among Children Aged 6 to 11 Years: United States, 2011 to 2012* (Source: Centers for Disease Control and Prevention (CDC)/National Center for Health Statistics (NCHS), National Health and Nutrition Examination Survey (NHANES), 2011–2012.)

[1] *Significantly different from those aged 9 to 11 years, p < 0.05.*
[2] *Significantly different from non-Hispanic Black children, p < 0.05.*
[3] *Significantly different from non-Hispanic Asian children, p < 0.05.*

Section 24.2

Tooth Decay and Children

This section includes text excerpted from "Brush Up on Oral
Health—Risky Business: Tooth Decay and Children," Early
Childhood Learning and Knowledge Center (ECLKC), May 2016.

Tooth decay is caused by bacteria in the mouth that use sugar in
food to make acid. Acid removes minerals from the outer tooth surface
(enamel). Over time, acid breaks the tooth surface down and creates
a cavity (hole) in the tooth.

Many factors can increase a child's risk for developing tooth decay.
Likewise, many factors can lower a child's risk for developing tooth
decay. This issue explains why it is important to lower the factors that
cause tooth decay and increase the factors that protect teeth from tooth
decay. Head Start* staff can share this information with parents. This
issue also includes a recipe for a healthy snack that can be made in a
Head Start classroom or at home.

** Head Start programs support children's growth and development in
a positive learning environment through a variety of services.*

Factors That Increase a Child's Risk for Tooth Decay

- **Parent has untreated tooth decay.** Parents with untreated
  tooth decay have high levels of the bacteria that cause tooth
  decay in their mouths. Parents can pass these bacteria to their
  child through saliva-sharing activities. Examples of these
  activities are cleaning a pacifier by mouth and giving it to a child
  and sharing forks or spoons.

- **Child enrolled in a public insurance plan.** Children who
  are enrolled in their state Medicaid or Child's Health Insurance
  Program may have a difficult time accessing oral healthcare
  because some oral health providers refuse to take public insurance.

- **Child has frequent between-meal snacks or drinks that
  contain sugar.** When children snack and/or drink foods or
  beverages containing natural or added sugar frequently, their
  teeth are bathed in acid for long periods of time. The acid has
  time to break tooth surfaces down and cause tooth decay.

- **Child is put to bed with a bottle with liquids that contain
  natural or added sugar.** When children are put to bed with

174

a bottle or sippy cup containing breast milk, infant formula, or any liquid with natural or added sugar, their teeth are bathed in acid for long periods of time. The acid has time to break tooth surfaces down and cause tooth decay.

- **Child has dental plaque on teeth.** Dental plaque is a film on the surface of a tooth that is a mix of saliva, bacteria, and food. If dental plaque is not removed by brushing with fluoride toothpaste twice a day, it increases the child's risk for developing tooth decay.

- **Child has a medical condition or a disability.** Children with medical conditions, such as asthma, may take medicines that contain sugar or make their mouths dry. Children with disabilities may have oral habits that can wear or break teeth, or they may have soft diets that can lead to more dental plaque on teeth. Having one or more of these issues increases the child's risk for developing tooth decay.

- **Child has had tooth decay in the past.** Once children have had tooth decay, their risk for developing more tooth decay increases. This is true even for children who have fillings to treat earlier tooth decay.

- **Child has early signs of tooth decay.** Chalky white spots along the gum line of the upper front teeth are the beginning of tooth decay.

Factors That Lower a Child's Risk for Tooth Decay

- **Child receives fluoride.** Fluoride puts minerals back into teeth that acid has removed. It also destroys bacteria that cause tooth decay and keeps the bacteria from growing. The three main ways children can receive fluoride are:

  - **Fluoridated water.** Fluoride is added to many community water supplies to protect teeth from tooth decay.

  - **Fluoride toothpaste.** As soon as the first tooth comes in, brushing with the right amount of fluoride toothpaste twice a day helps to protect teeth from tooth decay.

  - **Fluoride treatments.** Health staff in medical and dental offices or clinics can put fluoride varnish on a child's teeth as soon as the first tooth comes into the mouth and then every few months afterward.

- **Child has a dental home, a regular source of oral healthcare.** The teeth of children with a dental home are checked regularly for early signs of tooth decay. These children also receive services to protect teeth from tooth decay and repair early stages of tooth decay.

Section 24.3

Sugar and Tooth Decay

This section includes text excerpted from "Brush Up on Oral Health—Sugar and Children's Oral Health," Early Childhood Learning and Knowledge Center (ECLKC), July 2018.

Sugar and Children's Oral Health

Children who consume foods and drinks containing natural and/or added sugar frequently (for example, every hour) during the day are more likely to develop tooth decay than those who consume them less often. Parents and Head Start* staff may not know that many of the foods and drinks they give children contain sugar.

It is important to educate yourself about sugar and to understand how consuming foods and drinks containing sugar often during the day increases the risk of developing tooth decay. Learn to read food labels to identify hidden sugars in the product. Head Start staff can share with parents other tips about limiting their child's sugar intake.

* Head Start programs support children's growth and development in a positive learning environment through a variety of services.

How Often Children Consume Foods and Drinks with Sugar during the Day Matters

Sugar plays a key role in tooth decay. Most foods, such as milk and milk products, fruit, vegetables, grains, and processed and prepared foods contain sugar.

Bacteria that cause tooth decay breakdown foods and drinks that contain sugar to form acid. Each time a person consumes foods or drinks containing sugar, acid is in the mouth for 20 to 40 minutes. Children who are fed meals and snacks at scheduled times are at lower risk for developing tooth decay than children who are fed often during the day.

If a child consumes foods and drinks containing sugar often, over time the child is more likely to develop tooth decay.

Finding Hidden Sugar

Many foods and drinks contain added sugar. Sugar in foods can be listed by many different names. The best place to check for sugar is in the ingredients list on the food label. Look for words like:

- Beet sugar
- Brown sugar
- Cane sugar
- Corn sweeteners
- Corn syrup
- Cane juice
- High fructose corn syrup
- Honey
- Malt syrup
- Maple syrup
- Molasses
- Raw sugar
- White sugar

Tips to Help Parents Limit Their Child's Sugar Intake

Head Start staff can help prevent tooth decay by teaching parents about hidden sugar in foods and drinks and about feeding and eating habits that can reduce their child's risk for developing tooth decay.

- Explain to parents the role sugar plays in the tooth decay process and that how often a child consumes foods and drinks containing sugar can make a big difference.

- Show parents how to identify sugars listed on ingredient labels.

- Work with parents to set up a schedule for serving meals and snacks. Encourage parents not to feed their child or graze on foods and drinks often through the day, especially those containing natural and/or added sugar.

Section 24.4

Dental Sealant FAQs

This section includes text excerpted from "Dental Sealant FAQs," Centers for Disease Control and Prevention (CDC), March 8, 2019.

What Are Dental Sealants?

Dental sealants are thin coatings that when painted on the chewing surfaces of the back teeth (molars) can prevent cavities (tooth decay) for many years. Sealants protect the chewing surfaces from cavities by covering them with a protective shield that blocks out germs and food. Once applied, sealants protect against 80 percent of cavities for two years and continue to protect against 50 percent of cavities for up to four years.

What Is a Cavity?

A cavity is a permanent hole in a tooth. If it is not treated, it will get bigger; it can hurt and get infected. The most common place for cavities is in the grooves of the back teeth.

Is Sealing a Tooth Better than Filling the Cavity?

Sealants are a quick, easy, and painless way to prevent cavities. A tooth without a cavity is stronger and healthier than a tooth with a filling or untreated decay. Sealants are also less expensive and easier to apply than fillings.

Should I Ask the Dentist to Put Sealants on My Child's Teeth?

Yes. Dental cavities are one of the most common chronic conditions among children and teens. Left untreated, cavities can cause pain and infection and problems in eating, speaking, and learning. Sealants are an extremely effective yet underutilized shield that protects children's teeth from cavities.

When Can My Child Get Sealants?

Sealants prevent the most cavities when applied soon after permanent molars come into the mouth (around age 6 for 1st molars and age 12 for 2nd molars).

Will It Hurt to Get a Sealant?

Getting a sealant is easy and does not hurt. The tooth is cleaned and a gel may be placed on the chewing surface for a few seconds. The tooth is then rinsed and dried. Next, the sealant is painted on the tooth. The dentist or dental hygienist also may shine a light on the tooth to help harden the sealant to form a protective shield.

Will Sealants Make Teeth Feel Different?

Sealants are very thin and fill the pits and grooves of the teeth. Sometimes children can feel the sealant with their tongues for a short while after the sealant is placed.

What Do Sealants Look Like?

Sealants can be clear, white, or slightly tinted. Usually, you cannot see a sealant when a child talks or smiles.

How Long Will Sealants Last?

Sealants have shown to still work nine years after placement. However, sometimes they do fall off, so they should be checked at regular dental appointments. If a tooth loses a sealant, the protective shield is gone and the tooth can get a cavity. Missing sealants are easy to replace.

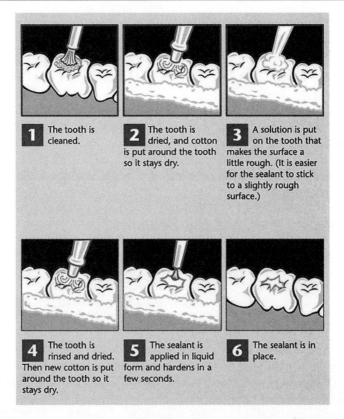

Figure 24.4. *How Sealants Are Put On* (Source: "Seal Out Tooth Decay," National Institute of Dental and Craniofacial Research (NIDCR).)

If My Water Has Fluoride, Should My Child Still Get Sealants?

Yes. Sealants and fluoride both prevent tooth decay, but in different ways. Sealants keep germs and food out of the grooves in the back teeth by covering them with a safe protective shield. Fluoride in drinking water and dental products, such as toothpaste, protects against cavities by making teeth stronger.

Where Can My Child Get Sealants?

- Ask your child's dentist to apply sealants when appropriate.

- Some schools offer sealants as part of a community public health program. Ask if your school has a sealant program. If they do, sign your child up to participate. If they do not, ask them to start one.

- If you need to find a dentist, use the Insure Kids Now Dentist Locator (www.insurekidsnow.gov).

If My Child Has Dental Sealants, Is There Anything Else I Need to Do to Protect Their Teeth?

Sealants are one part of a child's total preventive dental care.

Chapter 25

Mouth Injuries in Children

Chapter Contents

Section 25.1

Children and Oral Injuries

This section includes text excerpted from "Brush Up on Oral Health—Oral Injuries," Early Childhood Learning and Knowledge Center (ECLKC), February 2019.

Oral Injuries

Injuries to the head, face, and mouth are common in young children. Parents and Head Start* staff play an important role in preventing oral injuries. However, even when parents and staff do their best to keep children safe, oral injuries can happen. This chapter identifies supplies to include in a first aid kit for treating oral injuries. It also explains how to give first aid for the five most common oral injuries that happen to young children with primary (baby) teeth.

* Head Start programs support children's growth and development in a positive learning environment through a variety of services.

First Aid Supplies for Responding to Oral Injuries

It is important that first aid kits have supplies for responding to oral injuries, such as these supplies included in all Head Start kits:

- Instructions on how to assess and provide first aid for oral injuries

- Nonlatex gloves to wear while inspecting or cleaning the injured area

- Clean gauze and cotton swabs to stop bleeding and clean the injured area

- Floss to remove anything stuck between teeth to relieve pain

- Clean clothes to wrap ice or instant cold ice packs to put on the injured area to reduce swelling

- Plastic bags to dispose of biohazard waste, such as blood-soaked gauze or gloves

- Phone number for the child's dentist in case of a dental emergency, like a tooth knocked loose or pushed into the gum

- Emergency medical service (EMS) phone numbers (911 or 9-911) for a medical emergency, like a child who is unconscious or has trouble breathing or has bleeding that cannot be stopped

Giving First Aid for Oral Injuries

If a child has an oral injury, keep the child as calm as you can and assess the type of injury:

- **Tongue or lip injured.** Injured tongues or lips often bleed a lot. Clean the injured area and press a clean piece of gauze or a cotton swab on it to stop the bleeding. Also, keep the child's head up and facing forward to prevent choking. Put ice, wrapped in a clean cloth, on the area to reduce swelling. If bleeding does not stop after 30 minutes, take the child to the dentist, doctor, or nearest urgent care center immediately

- **Tooth chipped or cracked.** If a child's tooth is chipped or cracked, contact the dentist and, if needed, the child's parents immediately. Quick action can prevent infection and reduce the amount of treatment needed to fix the tooth. Clean the injured area. If the child can rinse, have the child rinse with water. Press a clean piece of gauze or a cotton swab on the gum around the tooth to stop any bleeding. If there are other injuries around the mouth, put ice, wrapped in a clean cloth, on the area to reduce swelling.

- **Tooth knocked out.** If a tooth is knocked out, check the child's health record, if possible, to determine if it is a primary tooth or a permanent tooth. Permanent teeth usually appear between ages 6 and 8. If it is a primary tooth, contact the and dentist and, if needed, the child's parents immediately. Do not try to put the tooth back into the mouth. Doing this may damage the permanent tooth underneath. Clean the injured area. If there is bleeding, have the child bite on a clean piece of gauze on the area for 15 to 30 minutes to stop it. If there are other injuries around the mouth, put ice, wrapped in a clean cloth, on the area to reduce swelling.

- **Tooth knocked loose, moved, or pushed into the gum.** If a child's tooth has been knocked loose, moved forward or backward, or pushed into the gum, contact the dentist and, if needed, the child's parents immediately. Ask the dentist if the child needs to be seen. If the child can rinse, have the child rinse with water. Press a clean piece of gauze or a cotton swab on the gum around the tooth to stop bleeding. If there are other injuries around the mouth, put ice, wrapped in a clean cloth, on the area to reduce swelling.

• **Toothache.** If a child has a toothache, it is likely that the tooth is decayed. An appointment should be made as soon as possible for a dentist to assess the problem and treat it.

Section 25.2

Preventing Oral Injuries

This section includes text excerpted from "Brush Up on Oral Health—Preventing Oral Injuries," Early Childhood Learning and Knowledge Center (ECLKC), April 2017.

Oral injuries to the face and mouth happen often among young children. Because oral injuries can affect children for the rest of their lives, it is important to try to prevent these injuries.

The following strategies can be used to help prevent these injuries.

Causes and Types of Oral Injuries

Most oral injuries happen when children fall. Children may stumble as they are learning to walk and when they are physically active. Injuries may happen when children trip on things, are pushed by another child, climb on stairs and furniture, or run with items in their mouths. Children's top front teeth are injured most often. They can be chipped, pushed into the gum, pushed forward or back in the mouth, or knocked out. Bruises or cuts in or near the mouth are also common oral injuries. Some children receive burns from chewing on electrical cords that are plugged into a socket.

Impact of Oral Injuries

Preventing oral injuries is important for many reasons. Injured primary teeth can turn brown or black, be painful, become infected, or have to be removed. Any one of these outcomes can affect the child's self-esteem, ability to learn, and/or ability to eat healthy foods. Early loss of primary teeth as a result of an oral injury or tooth decay can affect the condition of the child's permanent teeth as well. Primary teeth keep space open for permanent teeth forming underneath. When primary teeth are lost too early, there may not be enough space for permanent teeth. Injuries to a child's primary teeth can also damage the permanent teeth that are forming under the primary teeth. If a primary tooth is pushed into the gum, it can disturb the cells that are building the permanent tooth. This can cause discolored or deformed permanent teeth or permanent teeth that decay quickly. Injuries to primary and permanent teeth can affect a child's speech, nutrition, self-confidence, and overall health.

What Head Start Staff Can Do

Adults can protect children from oral injuries by making the center and play areas safe. Here are some steps to take to help prevent oral injuries:

- **Do health and safety sweeps.** Tour areas where children spend time. Use safety gates and cover sharp corners on furniture. Remove hazards or obstacles that might make a child fall. Make sure that toys and other things are picked up off the floor to help prevent children from tripping. Check that there is enough uncluttered space for children to move and play. Look over playground equipment to make sure it is age-appropriate.

- **Set and enforce policies and procedures.** Work with Head Start Health Services Advisory Committee (HSAC) members, parent committees, home visitors, child-safety experts, and others to identify behaviors that could cause oral injuries, and develop policies and procedures to help prevent oral injuries. Some examples include using child safety straps on high chairs, having children wear helmets when riding wheeled toys, and keeping toys picked up from the floor, playground, and yard. The policies and procedures should also address how to handle oral injuries.

- **Record, track, and analyze oral injuries.** Document all injuries and, as needed, inform parents if their child is injured. Keep a log of all injuries, and review the log quarterly to identify patterns about where and when injuries happen. This information can be used to determine what changes are needed to help prevent injuries.

- **Educate staff, parents, and children.** Use staff training and coaching opportunities, parent meetings, newsletters, and social media to teach Head Start staff, parents, and children how to avoid oral injuries. Invite oral health professionals, safety experts, and others to talk about how to prevent injuries.

Chapter 26

Bruxism

Bruxism is a disorder characterized by grinding, gnashing, and clenching of the teeth. Although it can have many different causes, it is often related to stress. Bruxism is widely prevalent, affecting an estimated 30 to 40 million people in the United States. People with bruxism may unconsciously clench their jaws during the day or grind their teeth while they are asleep at night. In most cases, bruxism is treatable with proper care and attention.

Symptoms and Diagnosis of Bruxism

Bruxism is usually diagnosed through a visit to a dentist. During a regular dental checkup, a dentist will look for and inquire about the following symptoms:

- Damaged teeth
- Unusual teeth sensitivity
- Swelling and pain in the jaw or facial muscles around the mouth
- Tongue indentations
- Headaches or earaches
- Frequent awakening or poor quality of sleep

"Bruxism," © 2015 Omnigraphics. Reviewed July 2019.

If the patient shows signs of bruxism, the dentist may prescribe a splint or mouthguard to prevent the teeth from grinding together. If the problem seems to be stress-related, the patient may be referred to a therapist or a counselor who will suggest methods for modifying the patient's behavior and sleep patterns.

Causes of Bruxism

Although various factors may contribute to bruxism, it is often related to the patient's emotional and psychological state. Nearly 70 percent of cases of bruxism can be traced to stress and anxiety. For children, the stress may be due to such causes as school exams, bullying by classmates, scolding from parents, or moving to a new neighborhood. Some small children may grind their teeth as part of the teething process or due to frequent earaches. Among children, bruxism often appears between the ages of three and ten years and then disappears on its own at puberty.

For adults, common sources of stress may include workplace tensions, family problems, relationship issues, or anxiety about health conditions. Certain personality types tend to be more vulnerable to stress-related bruxism, including those who are highly aggressive, competitive, or hyperactive.

Certain lifestyle factors can increase the risk of developing bruxism, such as smoking, alcohol consumption, and drug use. Some dental disorders, such as improper teeth alignment or jaw movement, can also aggravate bruxism. Bruxism may also develop as a side effect of certain medications or as a symptom of neurological disorders, such as Huntington disease and Parkinson disease. Finally, bruxism is often related to sleep disorders, such as excessive snoring, pauses in breathing, or obstructive sleep apnea.

Treatments of Bruxism

Treatments for bruxism should be selected to best fit the individual patient and the underlying cause of the disorder. When a dental problem is determined to be the cause of bruxism, a dental appliance such as a splint or mouthguard might alleviate the condition. These devices help prevent the teeth from grinding together and also help protect the tooth enamel from further damage. Various dental procedures can also be performed to correct misalignment of the teeth and jaw or address damage to the teeth from clenching and grinding.

Behavioral therapy can also help patients deal with improper mouth and jaw alignment. Correcting the position and placement of the tongue, teeth, and lips can bring about a significant improvement in the condition. Biofeedback is another treatment method used to assess and alter the movement of the muscles around the mouth and jaw. The doctor may use monitoring equipment to help guide the patient toward overcoming the habit of clenching the jaw or grinding the teeth.

If the primary cause of bruxism is determined to be psychological in nature, a number of behavioral and related therapies may help alleviate the condition. Stress management is the foremost issue to be addressed in people with bruxism. Counseling sessions with experts can help patients develop coping strategies. Other popular means of reducing stress include meditation, relaxation, exercise, and music. Hypnosis is a proven method of treatment for people who tend to grind their teeth at night. Most people with bruxism respond well with the proper treatment.

References

1. "Causes of Bruxism," Bruxism Association, n.d.
2. "Bruxism," The Nemours Foundation/KidsHealth®, 2015.

Chapter 27

Oral Conditions in Children with Special Needs

Oral Development

Tooth eruption may be delayed, accelerated, or inconsistent in children with growth disturbances. Gums may appear red or bluish-purple before erupting teeth break through into the mouth. Eruption depends on genetics, growth of the jaw, muscular action, and other factors. Children with Down syndrome may show delays of up to two years.

Malocclusion, a poor fit between the upper and lower teeth, and crowding of teeth occur frequently in people with developmental disabilities. Muscle dysfunction contributes to malocclusion, particularly in people with cerebral palsy. Teeth that are crowded or out of alignment are more difficult to keep clean, contributing to periodontal disease and dental caries.

Tooth anomalies are variations in the number, size, and shape of teeth. People with Down syndrome, oral clefts, ectodermal dysplasias, or other conditions may experience congenitally missing, extra, or malformed teeth.

Developmental defects appear as pits, lines, or discoloration in the teeth. Very high fever or certain medications can disturb tooth

This chapter includes text excerpted from "Oral Conditions in Children with Special Needs—A Guide for Healthcare Providers," National Institute of Dental and Craniofacial Research (NIDCR), August 2016.

formation and defects may result. Many teeth with defects are prone to dental caries, are difficult to keep clean, and may compromise appearance.

Oral Trauma

Trauma to the face and mouth occur more frequently in people who have intellectual disability, seizures, abnormal protective reflexes, or muscle incoordination. People receiving restorative dental care should be observed closely to prevent chewing on anesthetized areas.

Bruxism

Bruxism, the habitual grinding of teeth, is a common occurrence in people with cerebral palsy or severe intellectual disability. In extreme cases, bruxism leads to tooth abrasion and flat biting surfaces.

Oral Infections

Dental caries, or tooth decay, may be linked to frequent vomiting or gastroesophageal reflux, less than normal amounts of saliva, medications containing sugar, or special diets that require prolonged bottle-feeding or snacking. When oral hygiene is poor, the teeth are at increased risk for caries. It is important that on daily oral hygiene include frequent rinsing with plain water and use of a fluoride-containing toothpaste or mouth rinse.

Viral infections are usually due to the herpes simplex virus. Children rarely get herpetic gingivostomatitis or herpes labialis before six months of age. Herpetic gingivostomatitis is most common in young children, but may occur in adolescents and young adults. Viral infections can be painful and are usually accompanied by a fever. These lesions are infectious and patients need frequent fluids to prevent dehydration.

Early, severe periodontal (gum) disease can occur in children with impaired immune systems or connective tissue disorders and inadequate oral hygiene. Simple gingivitis results from an accumulation of bacterial plaque and presents as red, swollen gums that bleed easily. Periodontitis is more severe and leads to tooth loss if not treated. Professional cleaning by an oral healthcare provider, systemic antibiotics, and instructions on home care may be needed to stop the infection.

Gingival Overgrowth

Gingival overgrowth may be a side effect from medications, such as calcium channel blockers, phenytoin sodium, and cyclosporine. Poor oral hygiene aggravates the condition and can lead to superimposed infections. Severe overgrowth can impair tooth eruption, chewing, and appearance.

Part Four

Orthodontic, Endodontic, Periodontic, and Orofacial Conditions and Procedures

Chapter 28

Orthodontia

Not everyone is gifted with naturally perfect teeth. There are some people who find it very hard getting used to the way their teeth are arranged. People who have spacing problems between their teeth and difficulties while biting their food may need orthodontic care. The term "orthodontia" is a branch of dentistry that deals with jaw and teeth abnormalities.

Why Do People Need Braces?

Why do people need braces?—The answer is easily stated: when the upper and the lower jaws are not aligned correctly, people need professional teeth braces, which help correct dental abnormalities. When it comes to alignment of the jaws, some people's upper jaws are bigger than the lower jaws, and vice versa. The condition wherein a larger upper jaw is left hanging with the mouth closed is called "overbite" while a bigger lower jaw left hanging is called "underbite."

The other disorder in the process of tooth growth is that not everyone has correctly angled and spaced teeth; some teeth may overlap or be crooked while others may even grow rotated or twisted. The medical term for such disorders is "malocclusion." These dental anomalies are not anyone's fault; they are generally inherited traits similar to how people have brown eyes and big feet.

"Orthodontia," © 2019 Omnigraphics. Reviewed July 2019.

In rare cases, early injuries to permanent or baby teeth, thumb-sucking, accidents, or certain medical conditions may result in teeth disorder.

This medical condition, called "malocclusion," may interfere with chewing. Proper chewing of food is important for eating and digestion. Improper tooth alignment could make it difficult for chewing and, in turn, result in indigestion. These dental conditions could be rectified with the use of braces. Proper alignment of the teeth will not only enhance your appearance but will also help you maintain a healthy mouth.

Braces

Braces are wire-based equipment that is used for orthodontic treatment. Use of dental braces will help in the correction of misaligned teeth and jaws. To optimally align teeth, braces are worn even as early as during the teenage years. An adult may have to wear braces a little longer than a young person as the facial bones have stopped growing, but the result produced will be similar. The main aim of using braces for dental treatment is to align the teeth and jaws to provide even biting. If the dentist finds that a patient requires braces, the patient is referred to an orthodontist who is specialized in treating misaligned teeth and jaws.

Diagnosis of Dental Alignment Problems

Orthodontists diagnose problems before prescribing appropriate measures to correct abnormalities. The diagnosis involves various methods that include:

- **Oral exam:** This includes a complete examination of jaws, teeth, and mouth.

- **X-rays:** X-rays help in determining the position of the teeth. There are three types of x-rays: panoramic, head x-rays, and 3D x-rays. A panoramic x-ray is common and helps in determining the biting position of the upper and lower teeth. This type of x-ray also helps in determining the developing of teeth within the jaw.

- **Plaster models:** An impression of the patient's teeth and jaw is taken in a soft material that serves as the exact model of the teeth and jaw. This helps the orthodontist to evaluate the biting position of the teeth.

- **Potential tooth extraction:** There may be limited or no space in the jaw for the existing teeth if a patient's mouth is overcrowded. In such cases, an orthodontist might suggest removal of one or more permanent teeth to create room for the other teeth to fit in comfortably.

Treatment

Once the diagnosis is completed the orthodontist will decide the optimal treatment for the patient based on the particular complications she or he has. If there are no complications, then a removable retainer is all that will be needed. However, if there are complications, such as an extreme overbite or underbite, then surgery is needed. Braces will be the solution in most of the cases. Treatment time may vary, but generally, it might take about 12 to 30 months and a little longer for adults.

Types of Braces

Dental braces are categorized into two types:

- **Fixed type:** The fixed type is called "brackets" or "braces."

- **Removable type:** This type is the traditional method of treating bad bites.

These dental braces are made of different materials, such as metals, ceramic, plastic, or a combination of these materials.

Based on the materials used, the braces are further categorized into four types:

- **Metal braces:** Metal braces are otherwise called "traditional braces." They are made of metal and are the most notable among all types of braces. They are the least expensive too.

- **Ceramic braces:** These braces are of the same size and shape as of the metal braces but the color of the ceramic braces is tooth-colored and comparatively less notable than metal braces.

- **Lingual braces:** These braces are made of metal but they are placed from the inside and hence not visible. Lingual braces, however, are uncomfortable and difficult to clean. The time consumed for regular adjustments is not long when compared to that of metal braces.

- **Invisalign braces:** These are a set of 18 to 30 custom-made mouth-guardlike plastic aligners. These aligners are removable and almost invisible. These will not be suitable for serious dental problems. These are removable and can be replaced every two weeks.

Risks of Braces

Dental braces are safe and offer various benefits. However, there are also certain risks in dental treatment.

Short-Term Risks

Dental braces create tiny spaces between the teeth. Food particles can settle in these tiny spaces and pave the way for plaque if not cleaned properly. These deposits of uncleaned food particles and plaque can lead to loss of minerals in the outer enamel of the teeth, thereby causing permanent whitish stains on your teeth. This also leads to gum diseases and tooth decay.

Long-Term Risks

In the course of moving a tooth, some tooth bones in the path of the moving tooth also get dissolved (but new bone is behind it). In such cases, permanent loss of tooth root length may occur and cause less stable teeth. However, this typically does not cause any problems.

If you do not follow the instructions of your orthodontist once the braces are removed, there are chances for loss of correction, in which some of the corrections gained made during the treatment will be lost.

Retainers

A retainer is a device that your orthodontist will want you to use once you remove your braces; it prevents the teeth from shifting back to their original position, even if the braces are removed. This stage is called the "retention period." There are two types of retainers:

- Bonded or fixed retainers
- Removable retainers

Roughly half of the orthodontic patients use bonded retainers and the other half wear the removable retainer. Your orthodontist will help you choose the type of retainer that will best suit you based on your teeth's condition.

References

1. "Braces—Orthodontics," 32dentalcare, December 11, 2008.

2. "Dental Braces," Mayo Foundation for Medical Education and Research (MFMER), May 21, 2019.

3. "All about Orthodontia," TeensHealth, February 1, 2001.

Chapter 29

Endodontic Conditions and Treatment

Endodontics

Endodontics is a dental specialty that studies and treats the pulp of teeth. The word "endodontic" is derived from the Greek words "endo," which means "inside," and "odont," which translates as "tooth."

To understand endodontic treatment, it helps know a bit about dental anatomy. The tooth is covered by a hard layer of enamel. Another hard layer, called "dentin," lies under the enamel and covers soft tissue known as the "pulp," a collection of blood vessels, nerves, and connective tissue that is responsible for nourishing the tooth. The pulp is located in the center of the tooth and extends from under the crown down to the tissue under the root. Pulp is especially important during tooth growth and development, but once the tooth is fully grown, it can survive without the pulp because the surrounding tissues are able to provide nourishment.

Almost all teeth can be treated endodontically. However, in some cases treatment may not be possible. For example, this might be the case if the chambers that contain the root (called "root canals") are not accessible, if the tooth is badly fractured, or if there is inadequate bone support. Endodontics has advanced so much that teeth that would have been considered lost a few years ago can be saved today.

Root Canal Treatment

The most common type of endodontic procedure is a root canal treatment, often called simply a "root canal." It is a routine procedure that relieves pain, saves millions of teeth every year, and can help improve appearance.

This procedure becomes necessary when a tooth's pulp becomes inflamed or infected. The infection may arise as a result conditions, such as tooth decay, repeated dental work, or a crack in the tooth. If left untreated, the infection may lead to an abscess, a more serious infection that can be life threating.

In root canal treatment, the pulp is fully removed from the tooth. The pulp chamber is cleaned and shaped, and the empty space is filled and sealed with an inert material. In subsequent visits, the dentist generally fixes a crown on the tooth or performs some other type of restorative work to return the tooth to its full function and appearance.

Symptoms Indicating That a Root Canal May Be Necessary

Signs that root canal treatment may be needed include tooth pain, sensitivity to heat and cold, and tenderness to touch and chewing. You should also look for tooth discoloration and tenderness of lymph nodes, gum tissue, and bone. But sometimes infection requiring a root canal can be present with virtually no symptoms at all.

The Procedure

Root canal treatment generally consists of the following steps:

- The endodontist examines the tooth and x-rays it. A local anesthetic is then administered, and a sheet known as a "dental dam" may be placed in the mouth to isolate the tooth and keep it free of saliva.

- The endodontist drills through the crown of the tooth and uses various tools to remove the pulp.

- The space is then shaped and cleaned before it is filled with a biocompatible material, such as a rubber-like substance called "gutta-percha." It is placed with adhesive cement, completely sealing the chamber. The tooth is then covered with a temporary filling, which remains in place until the next office visit.

- In the next step, the dentist or endodontist will prepare the tooth for a crown or will perform other restorative work to provide normal tooth function.

- If the tooth is incapable of holding the restoration on its own, the endodontist will fix a post inside the tooth, which will serve as an anchor.

Root Canal Treatment and Pain

Modern anesthetics and techniques are generally able to ensure that little pain is felt during a root canal procedure. But after a root canal, the tooth and surrounding area may be sensitive. This can be treated by prescription medication or by over-the-counter (OTC) pain relievers. However, if pain persists for more than a few days after the treatment, consult your endodontist immediately.

Cost of Root Canal Treatment

As with any medical treatment, the cost of a root canal can depend on the complexity of the procedure. For example, molars tend to be more difficult to treat than other teeth and thus might cost more. But most dental insurance policies cover endodontic procedures, and in any case, endodontic treatment and tooth restoration is likely to be less expensive than tooth extraction, because the latter involves the additional cost of fixing an implant or bridge at the site of the extraction to restore chewing function and prevent teeth from shifting.

After Root Canal Treatment

To avoid fracture or other damage, you must not bite or chew on food with the tooth that has undergone endodontic treatment until the restoration work has been done. After the procedure is complete, it is important to practice good basic dental hygiene, like brushing, flossing, dental checkups, and cleaning.

The restored tooth should last for a long time. But in some cases, the treated tooth might not heal and could become infected again in the future. In some cases, new trauma, decay, or a crack may result in an infection in the treated tooth. Or the endodontist may discover that complicating factors caused the tooth to be treated improperly to begin with. In such cases, a second endodontic procedure may be able to save the tooth.

Endodontic Surgery

In cases where root canal treatment will not suffice, an endodontist may recommend surgery, which can often save a tooth by providing better access for treatment. Surgery can also help the endodontist make a diagnosis that might otherwise not be possible, since some conditions do not show up in diagnostics, such as x-rays. And in some cases, a tiny fracture or canal may remain undetected in nonsurgical treatment. With surgery, the endodontist will be able to make a more thorough inspection of the area and provide the required treatment.

In addition, it can become difficult to reach the end of the root with instruments in a root canal procedure if there is calcification in the canal. With endodontic surgery, a dentist will be able to reach the end of the root to clean and seal it properly. Or, after a root canal, the tooth might not heal fully and become infected. This could occur sometime after successful treatment. Endodontic surgery is often required to save the tooth in such cases.

Finally, endodontic surgery is often performed to treat damage to the root surface or the surrounding bone when no other type of treatment would be effective.

Apicoectomy

An apicoectomy, also called a "root-end resection" or "root-end filling," is the most common type of oral surgery. It generally involves the following steps:

- The gum tissue around the tooth is opened and the underlying bone is exposed.

- Any inflamed or infected tissue is then removed, along with the end of the root.

- The end of the root canal is often sealed with a filling, and the gum tissue is sutured.

- The gum tissue generally heals in a few weeks, while it may take a few months for the bone to heal fully.

Other Types of Endodontic Surgery

Other endodontic surgical procedures include dividing a tooth in half, repairing injured roots, and removing the root. Another type of endodontic surgery, intentional replantation, involves extracting the tooth, then replacing it in the socket after an endodontic procedure has been completed.

Endodontic Surgery and Pain

Endodontic surgeries are usually done under local anesthesia and are generally not painful during the procedure. However, pain is typically felt during the healing process. The endodontist will likely prescribe medication to alleviate the pain. You will also be given postoperative instructions to follow. Talk to your endodontist if you have any questions after surgery or if the pain does not respond to medication.

After Endodontic Surgery

In many cases, patients are able to drive themselves home after endodontic surgery. But if your surgeon suggests otherwise, be sure that you make suitable arrangements for transportation.

Most patients find that they are able return to work the next day, however recovery time and postoperative effects vary from individual to individual. The endodontist will discuss recovery time with you during your consultation.

Although successful healing and full recovery are typical, there are, of course, no guarantees with any type of medical or dental treatment, including surgery. A particular procedure is recommended by an endodontist because she or he believes it offers the best possible treatment option for saving your natural tooth. An endodontist will discuss the chances of success so that you are able to make an informed decision.

Cost of Endodontic Surgery

As with root canal treatment, the cost of endodontic surgery varies with the complexity of the procedure and a number of other factors. Some insurance plans cover certain types of treatment, while others do not. Talk to your employer or insurance company to learn if your particular surgery is covered under your plan.

Endodontic Retreatment

A tooth that has undergone endodontic treatment can last a lifetime with proper care. But when a treated tooth does not heal properly, becomes infected, and causes pain, a second procedure may be needed to save the tooth. If you experience pain or discomfort in a tooth that was previously treated, talk to your endodontist about retreatment.

Retreatment Procedure

The endodontist will first discuss the procedure with you. If retreatment is required, the endodontist will generally follow these steps:

- Reopen the tooth to get access to the filling in the root canals by disassembling the crown, post, and filling material.

- Once the filling has been removed, the endodontist will examine the canals with magnification and illumination to assess their condition.

- Clean and seal the canals with a temporary filling. If the canals are very narrow or blocked, the endodontist may suggest endodontic surgery.

Once the retreatment is complete, you will need to make additional visits for restoration procedures in order to regain full tooth function and appearance.

Why Endodontic Retreatment May Be Required

The best possible option always is to save your natural teeth. So even if initial treatment fails, retreatment may be able to allow teeth to function properly for many years. Technological improvements are always being made in endodontics, and it is possible that retreatment may be able to employ tools and techniques that did not even exist just a few years ago.

If nonsurgical retreatment will be ineffective, then surgical retreatment may be necessary. This will entail a process similar to that of an initial endodontic surgery, including incision, assessment, cleaning, and stitches. Your endodontist will discuss the options and necessary treatment with you.

Cost of Endodontic Retreatment

Understandably, the cost of retreatment depends on the complexity of the condition. The endodontist will need to remove the filling, assess the previous work and the underlying structures, and then redo the procedure, or use an entirely different procedure. Therefore, retreatment will likely cost more than the initial procedure, especially if surgical retreatment is necessary.

Dental insurance may cover the expenses for all or part of retreatment, but some plans cover just the initial endodontic procedure. Your employer or insurance company can help clarify this.

Alternatives to Endodontic Treatment

Tooth extraction is generally the only alternative to endodontic treatment. Once a tooth has been extracted, it must be replaced with a bridge, implant, or a partially removable denture to restore chewing function and to prevent adjacent teeth from shifting. Since extraction involves additional procedures to maintain tooth function, endodontic treatment is usually the best option, from a cost perspective, as well as for utility and appearance. Although, artificial teeth can be very effective, nothing is better than having natural teeth, and an endodontic procedure can help you retain those teeth for a long time.

References

1. "Endodontic Surgery Explained," American Association of Endodontists (AAE), n.d.

2. "Root Canals Explained," American Association of Endodontists (AAE), n.d.

3. "Endodontic Retreatment Explained," American Association of Endodontists (AAE), n.d.

4. "An Overview of Root Canals," WebMD, June 10, 2016.

5. Horne, Steven B., DDS. "Root Canal," MedicineNet, n.d.

6. "Oral Surgery," WebMD, July 28, 2016.

Chapter 30

Periodontal (Gum) Disease

Chapter Contents

Section 30.1

Understanding Periodontal Disease

This section includes text excerpted from documents published by two public domain sources. Text under the headings marked 1 are excerpted from excerpted from "Gum Disease," National Institute of Dental and Craniofacial Research (NIDCR), July 2018; Text under the heading marked 2 is excerpted from "Periodontal (Gum) Disease," National Institute of Dental and Craniofacial Research (NIDCR), September 15, 2013. Reviewed July 2019.

What Is Periodontal Disease?[1]

Periodontal (gum) disease is an infection of the tissues that hold your teeth in place. It is typically caused by poor brushing and flossing habits that allow plaque—a sticky film of bacteria—to build up on the teeth and harden. In advanced stages, periodontal disease can lead to sore, bleeding gums, painful chewing problems, and even tooth loss.

Who Gets Gum Disease[2]

People usually do not show signs of gum disease until they are in their 30s or 40s. Men are more likely to have gum disease than women. Although teenagers rarely develop periodontitis, they can develop gingivitis, the milder form of gum disease. Most commonly, gum disease develops when plaque is allowed to build up along and under the gum line.

Causes of Periodontal Disease[1]

Our mouths are full of bacteria. These bacteria, along with mucus and other particles, constantly form a sticky, colorless "plaque" on teeth. Brushing and flossing help get rid of plaque. Plaque that is not removed can harden and form "tartar" that brushing does not clean. Only a professional cleaning by a dentist or dental hygienist can remove tartar.

There are a number of risk factors for gum disease, but smoking is the most significant. Smoking also can make treatment for gum disease less successful. Other risk factors include diabetes; hormonal changes in girls and women; medications that lessen the flow of saliva; certain illnesses, such as acquired immunodeficiency syndrome (AIDS), and their medications; and genetic susceptibility.

Symptoms of Periodontal Disease[1]

Symptoms of gum disease include:

- Bad breath that would not go away
- Red or swollen gums
- Tender or bleeding gums
- Painful chewing
- Loose teeth
- Sensitive teeth
- Receding gums or longer appearing teeth

Diagnosis of Periodontal Disease[1]

At a dental visit, a dentist or dental hygienist will:

- Examine your gums and note any signs of inflammation
- Use a tiny ruler called a "probe" to check for and measure any pockets around the teeth. In a healthy mouth, the depth of these pockets is usually between one and three millimeters. This test for pocket depth is usually painless.
- Ask about your medical history to identify conditions or risk factors (such as smoking or diabetes) that may contribute to gum disease

The dental professional may also:

- Take an x-ray to see whether there is any bone loss
- Refer you to a periodontist. Periodontists are experts in the diagnosis and treatment of gum disease and may provide you with treatment options that are not offered by your dentist.

Treatment of Periodontal Disease[1]

The main goal of treatment is to control the infection. The number and types of treatment will vary, depending on the extent of the gum disease. Any type of treatment requires that the patient keep up good daily care at home. The dentist may also suggest changing certain behaviors, such as quitting smoking, as a way to improve your treatment results.

Helpful Tips

You can keep your gums and teeth healthy by:

- Brushing your teeth twice a day with a fluoride toothpaste

- Flossing regularly to remove plaque from between teeth. Or, you can use a device, such as a special brush, wooden or plastic pick, or a "water flosser" recommended by a dental professional.

- Visiting the dentist routinely for a checkup and professional cleaning

- Quitting smoking

Section 30.2

Causes and Risk Factors of Gum Disease

This section includes text excerpted from "Periodontal (Gum) Disease," National Institute of Dental and Craniofacial Research (NIDCR), September 15, 2013. Reviewed July 2019.

What Causes Gum Disease

Our mouths are full of bacteria. These bacteria, along with mucus and other particles, constantly form a sticky, colorless "plaque" on teeth. Brushing and flossing help get rid of plaque. Plaque that is not removed can harden and form "tartar" that brushing does not clean. Only a professional cleaning by a dentist or dental hygienist can remove tartar.

Gingivitis

The longer plaque and tartar are on teeth, the more harmful they become. The bacteria cause inflammation of the gums that is called "gingivitis." In gingivitis, the gums become red, swollen and can bleed easily. Gingivitis is a mild form of gum disease that can usually be reversed with daily brushing and flossing, and regular cleaning by a dentist or dental hygienist. This form of gum disease does not include any loss of bone and tissue that hold teeth in place.

Periodontitis

When gingivitis is not treated, it can advance to "periodontitis" (which means "inflammation around the tooth"). In periodontitis, gums pull away from the teeth and form spaces (called "pockets") that become infected. The body's immune system fights the bacteria as the plaque spreads and grows below the gum line. Bacterial toxins and the body's natural response to infection start to break down the bone and connective tissue that hold teeth in place. If not treated, the bones, gums, and tissue that support the teeth are destroyed. The teeth may eventually become loose and have to be removed.

Risk Factors

- **Smoking.** Need another reason to quit smoking? Smoking is one of the most significant risk factors associated with the development of gum disease. Additionally, smoking can lower the chances for successful treatment.

- **Hormonal changes in girls/women.** These changes can make gums more sensitive and make it easier for gingivitis to develop.

- **Diabetes.** People with diabetes are at higher risk for developing infections, including gum disease.

- **Other illnesses and their treatments.** Diseases such as acquired immunodeficiency syndrome (AIDS) and its treatments can negatively affect the health of gums, as can treatments for cancer.

- **Medications.** There are hundreds of prescription and over-the-counter (OTC) medications that can reduce the flow of saliva, which has a protective effect on the mouth. Without enough saliva, the mouth is vulnerable to infections such as gum disease. And some medicines can cause abnormal overgrowth of the gum tissue; this can make it difficult to keep teeth and gums clean.

- **Genetic susceptibility.** Some people are more prone to severe gum disease than others.

Section 30.3

Chronic Periodontal Infections

This section includes text excerpted from "Public
Health Implications of Chronic Periodontal Infections in
Adults," Centers for Disease Control and Prevention (CDC),
July 10, 2013. Reviewed July 2019.

Periodontitis is a chronic infectious disease that affects approximately 34 percent of the U.S. population over age 30 (about 36 million persons), and it is a major cause of tooth loss in about 13 percent of adults. The disease begins as an acute inflammation of the gingival tissue known as "gingivitis," manifested by bleeding, especially during tooth brushing. In susceptible individuals, gingivitis progresses to periodontitis, in which the destructive inflammatory process extends into the deeper periodontal tissues. Clinical signs of periodontitis are gingival bleeding, loss of periodontal attachment as detected by increasing probing depth around the necks of the teeth, and radiographic loss of alveolar bone. As the disease advances, the teeth may become loose, periodontal abscesses may form, and the affected teeth may be lost.

Periodontitis is caused by a small group of predominantly gram-negative anaerobic bacteria among which Porphyromonas gingivalis is especially important. Biofilms containing these pathogenic bacteria form on the tooth surfaces and extend apically between the surface of the tooth root and gingiva to cause a destructive inflammation that destroys the attachment of gingival tissue to the tooth. Consequently, periodontal pockets form and collagenous fibers of the periodontal ligament and the bony housing of the tooth roots are destroyed.

Lipopolysaccharide, antigenic bacterial components, and intact bacteria have ready access through the ulcerated pocket wall into the inflamed tissue, where they may enter the circulation and become systemically disseminated. Bacteria and their components stimulate a dense infiltrate of inflammatory cells including neutrophilic granulocytes, macrophages, and lymphoid cells. Bacterial substances activate macrophages and neutrophilic granulocytes to produce and release large quantities of proinflammatory cytokines and prostanoids especially interleukin-1 (IL-1), tumor necrosis factor-alpha (TNF-alpha), prostaglandin E2 (PGE2) and matrix metalloproteinases. Resident connective tissue fibroblasts also are involved in this process. Binding of the C1 component of complement and cytokines, such as IL-1 and TNF-alpha causes the fibroblasts to contribute to the growing concentrations of proinflammatory cytokines, prostaglandins, and matrix metalloproteinases. PGE2 mediates alveolar bone destruction, and the matrix metalloproteinases destroy the collagens and other connective tissue components of the gingiva and periodontal ligament.

A growing body of evidence suggests that periodontitis, in addition to being a major cause of tooth loss in adults, also enhances the risk for several potentially deadly systemic diseases and conditions. This enhanced risk may be related to the systemic dissemination of gram-negative anaerobic bacteria and their components present in subgingival biofilms as well as inflammatory mediators that reach very high levels in the diseased periodontal tissues.

Periodontitis is a chronic infectious disease that affects approximately 34 percent of the U.S. population over age 30 (about 36 million persons), and it is a major cause of tooth loss in about 13 percent of adults. The disease begins as an acute inflammation of the gingival tissue known as "gingivitis," manifested by bleeding, especially during tooth brushing. In susceptible individuals, gingivitis progresses to periodontitis, in which the destructive inflammatory process extends into the deeper periodontal tissues. Clinical signs of periodontitis are gingival bleeding, loss of periodontal attachment as detected by increasing probing depth around the necks of the teeth, and radiographic loss of alveolar bone. As the disease advances, the teeth may become loose, periodontal abscesses may form, and the affected teeth may be lost.

Periodontitis is caused by a small group of predominantly gram-negative anaerobic bacteria among which Porphyromonas gingivalis is especially important. Biofilms containing these pathogenic bacteria form on the tooth surfaces and extend apically between the surface of the tooth root and gingiva to cause a destructive inflammation that destroys the attachment of gingival tissue to the tooth. Consequently, periodontal pockets form and collagenous fibers of the periodontal ligament and the bony housing of the tooth roots are destroyed.

Lipopolysaccharide, antigenic bacterial components, and intact bacteria have ready access through the ulcerated pocket wall into the inflamed tissue, where they may enter the circulation and become systemically disseminated. Bacteria and their components stimulate a dense infiltrate of inflammatory cells including neutrophilic granulocytes, macrophages, and lymphoid cells. Bacterial substances activate macrophages and neutrophilic granulocytes to produce and release large quantities of proinflammatory cytokines and prostanoids especially interleukin-1 (IL-1), tumor necrosis factor-alpha (TNF-alpha), prostaglandin E2 (PGE2) and matrix metalloproteinases. Resident connective tissue fibroblasts also are involved in this process. Binding of the C1 component of complement and cytokines, such as IL-1 and TNF-alpha causes the fibroblasts to contribute to the growing concentrations of proinflammatory cytokines, prostaglandins, and matrix metalloproteinases. PGE2 mediates alveolar bone destruction, and the matrix metalloproteinases destroy the collagens and other connective tissue components of the gingiva and periodontal ligament.

A growing body of evidence suggests that periodontitis, in addition to being a major cause of tooth loss in adults, also enhances the risk for several potentially deadly systemic diseases and conditions. This enhanced risk may be related to the systemic dissemination of gram-negative anaerobic bacteria and their components present in subgingival biofilms as well as inflammatory mediators that reach very high levels in the diseased periodontal tissues.

Section 30.4

Treatment of Gum Disease

This section includes text excerpted from
"Periodontal (Gum) Disease," National Institute of
Dental and Craniofacial Research (NIDCR),
September 15, 2013. Reviewed July 2019.

The main goal of treatment is to control the infection. The number and types of treatment will vary, depending on the extent of the gum disease. Any type of treatment requires that the patient keep up good daily care at home. The doctor may also suggest changing certain behaviors, such as quitting smoking, as a way to improve treatment outcome.

Deep Cleaning (Scaling and Root Planing)

The dentist, periodontist, or dental hygienist removes the plaque through a deep-cleaning method called "scaling and root planing." Scaling means scraping off the tartar from above and below the gum line. Root planing gets rid of rough spots on the tooth root where the germs gather, and helps remove bacteria that contribute to the disease.

In some cases a laser may be used to remove plaque and tartar. This procedure can result in less bleeding, swelling, and discomfort compared to traditional deep cleaning methods.

Medications

Medications may be used with treatment that includes scaling and root planning, but they cannot always take the place of surgery. Depending on how far the disease has progressed, the dentist or periodontist may still suggest surgical treatment. Long-term studies are needed to find out if using medications reduces the need for surgery and whether they are effective over a long period of time. Listed on the next page are some medications that are currently used.

Surgical Treatments
Flap Surgery

Surgery might be necessary if inflammation and deep pockets remain following treatment with deep cleaning and medications. A dentist or periodontist may perform flap surgery to remove tartar deposits in deep pockets or to reduce the periodontal pocket and make it easier for the patient, dentist, and hygienist to keep the area clean. This common surgery involves lifting back the gums and removing the tartar. The gums are then sutured back in place so that the tissue fits snugly around the tooth again. After surgery the gums will heal and fit more tightly around the tooth. This sometimes results in the teeth appearing longer.

Bone and Tissue Grafts

In addition to flap surgery, your periodontist or dentist may suggest procedures to help regenerate any bone or gum tissue lost to periodontitis. Bone grafting, in which natural or synthetic bone is placed in the area of bone loss, can help promote bone growth. A technique that can be used with bone grafting is called "guided tissue regeneration." In this procedure, a small piece of mesh-like material is inserted between the bone and gum tissue. This keeps the gum tissue from growing into the area where the bone should be, allowing the bone and connective tissue to regrow. Growth factors—proteins that can help your body naturally regrow bone—may also be used. In cases where gum tissue has been lost, your dentist or periodontist may suggest a soft tissue graft, in which synthetic material or tissue taken from another area of your mouth is used to cover exposed tooth roots.

Table 30.1. Medications for Gum Disease

Medications	What Is It?	Why Is It Used?	How Is It Used?
Prescription antimicrobial mouthrinse	A prescription mouthrinse containing an antimicrobial called "chlorhexidine"	To control bacteria when treating gingivitis and after gum surgery	It is used like a regular mouthwash.
Antiseptic chip	A tiny piece of gelatin filled with the medicine chlorhexidine	To control bacteria and reduce the size of periodontal pockets	After root planing, it is placed in the pockets where the medicine is slowly released over time.
Antibiotic gel	A gel that contains the antibiotic doxycycline	To control bacteria and reduce the size of periodontal pockets	The periodontist puts it in the pockets after scaling and root planing. The antibiotic is released slowly over a period of about seven days.
Antibiotic microspheres	Tiny, round particles that contain the antibiotic minocycline	To control bacteria and reduce the size of periodontal pockets	The periodontist puts the microspheres into the pockets after scaling and root planing. The particles release minocycline slowly over time.
Enzyme suppressant	A low dose of the medication doxycycline that keeps destructive enzymes in check	To hold back the body's enzyme response—If not controlled, certain enzymes can break down gum tissue	This medication is in tablet form. It is used in combination with scaling and root planing.
Oral antibiotics	Antibiotic tablets or capsules	For the short-term treatment of an acute or locally persistent periodontal infection	These come as tablets or capsules and are taken by mouth.

Since each case is different, it is not possible to predict with certainty which grafts will be successful over the long term. Treatment results depend on many things, including how far the disease has progressed, how well the patient keeps up with oral care at home, and certain risk factors, such as smoking, which may lower the chances of success. Ask your periodontist what the level of success might be in your particular case.

How Can I Keep My Teeth and Gums Healthy?

- Brush your teeth twice a day (with a fluoride toothpaste).

- Floss regularly to remove plaque from between teeth. Or use a device such as a special brush or wooden or plastic pick recommended by a dental professional.

- Visit the dentist routinely for a checkup and professional cleaning.

- Do not smoke.

Can Gum Disease Cause Health Problems beyond the Mouth?

In some studies, researchers have observed that people with gum disease (when compared to people without gum disease) were more likely to develop heart disease or have difficulty controlling blood sugar. Other studies showed that women with gum disease were more likely than those with healthy gums to deliver preterm, low birthweight babies. But, so far, it has not been determined whether gum disease is the cause of these conditions.

There may be other reasons people with gum disease sometimes develop additional health problems.

For example, something else may be causing both the gum disease and the other condition, or it could be a coincidence that gum disease and other health problems are present together.

More research is needed to clarify whether gum disease actually causes health problems beyond the mouth, and whether treating gum disease can keep other health conditions from developing.

In the meantime, it is a fact that controlling gum disease can save your teeth—a very good reason to take care of your teeth and gums.

Section 30.5

Preventing Gum Diseases

This section includes text excerpted from "Mind Your Mouth—
Preventing Gum Disease," *NIH News in Health*, National Institutes
of Health (NIH), July 2010. Reviewed July 2019.

If you have it, you are not alone. Many adults nationwide have some form of gum disease. It can simply cause swollen gums or give you bad breath. It can also ruin your smile or even make you lose your teeth. The good news is that gum disease can be prevented with daily dental care.

The problem begins with bacteria. Our mouths are packed with these tiny microbes. They combine with mucus and other particles to form a sticky, colorless film—called "plaque"—on our teeth. Brushing and flossing can get rid of some plaque. But any that remains can harden and form tartar, a yellowish deposit that can become rock-hard.

Plaque and tartar buildup can lead to gum disease—technically known as "periodontal disease." The most common and mild type of gum disease is called "gingivitis." The gums become red and swollen, and they can bleed easily. Daily brushing and flossing and regular cleanings by dental professionals can usually clear up gingivitis.

If gingivitis is not treated, it can become a more severe type of gum disease called "periodontitis." Symptoms of periodontitis include bad breath that would not go away; gums that are red, swollen, tender, or bleeding; painful chewing; and loose or sensitive teeth.

In periodontitis, the gums pull away from the teeth and form "pockets" that become infected. Bacterial toxins and your body's natural response to infection start to break down the bone and soft tissues that hold teeth in place. If not treated, the tissues will be destroyed. Your teeth may eventually become loose and have to be removed. If you have periodontitis, your dentist may recommend a deep-cleaning method called "scaling and root planing." In more severe cases, you may need surgery.

Most people do not show signs of gum disease until they are in their 30s or 40s. But, getting older does not necessarily mean you will get gum disease. Daily dental care and regular visits to your dentist can reduce your risk of gum disease.

Smoking greatly increases your risk for periodontitis—another reason not to smoke. Other factors that boost your risk include hormonal changes in women, certain medications and some illnesses, such as diabetes, cancer, and acquired immunodeficiency syndrome (AIDS).

National Institutes of Health (NIH)-supported researchers are working to learn about preventing and treating gum problems. Some are exploring whether stem cells might help to restore damaged tissues that support the teeth. Others are searching for genes and proteins produced by our bodies and by the bacteria in our mouths to see how they interact to affect gum health.

Some studies suggest that gum disease may increase the risk of heart attack or stroke or cause other health problems. But, so far, it has not been confirmed that gum disease contributes to these conditions.

Although many aspects of gum disease are still being investigated, one thing is clear: controlling gum disease can save your teeth. That alone is an excellent reason to take good care of your teeth and gums every day.

Section 30.6

Periodontal Disease in Seniors (Age 65 and Over)

This section includes text excerpted from "Periodontal Disease in Seniors (Age 65 and Over)," National Institute of Dental and Craniofacial Research (NIDCR), July 2018.

Overall, the prevalence of periodontal (gum) disease in seniors has decreased from the early 1970s until the latest (1999–2004) National Health and Nutrition Examination Survey. In spite of this improvement, significant disparities remain in some population groups.

The research definitions of periodontal disease are not necessarily the same as the common definition of gum disease, which may include both gingivitis (inflammation of the gums without any loss of bone and tissue) and periodontitis (as defined below):

For the purposes of epidemiological research, periodontal disease is defined very specifically. For a person to have periodontal disease, she or he must have at least one periodontal site with three millimeters or more of attachment loss and four millimeters or more of pocket depth. Moderate periodontal disease is defined as having at least two teeth with interproximal attachment loss of four millimeters or more OR at least two teeth with five millimeters or more of pocket depth at interproximal sites. Severe periodontal disease is defined as having at least two teeth with interproximal attachment loss of six millimeters or more AND at least one tooth with five millimeters or more of pocket depth at interproximal sites.

Prevalence of Periodontal Disease

- 17.20 percent of seniors age 65 and over have periodontal disease.

- Older seniors, Black and Hispanic seniors, current smokers, and those with lower incomes and less education are more likely to have periodontal disease.

Prevalence of periodontal disease among seniors with teeth, age 65 and over years of age, by selected characteristics: United States, National Health and Nutrition Examination Survey, 1999–2004

Table 30.2. Seniors, Prevalence of Periodontal Disease

Characteristic	Percent with periodontal disease*
Age	
65 to 74 years	10.2
75 years and over	11.03
Sex	
Male	12.97
Female	8.56
Race and Ethnicity	
White, non-Hispanic	8.99
Black, non-Hispanic	23.92
Mexican American	17.23
Poverty Status (Income compared to Federal Poverty Level)	
Less than 100%	17.49
100% to 199%	11.59
Greater than 200%	8.62

Table 30.2. Continued

Characteristic	Percent with periodontal disease*
Education	
Less than High School	16.56
High School	8.3
More than High School	8.9
Smoking History	
Current Smoker	13.8
Former Smoker	9.2
Never Smoked	11.12
Overall	10.58

Data Source: The National Health and Nutrition Examination Survey (NHANES) has been an important source of information on oral health and dental care in the United States since the early 1970s. Table presents the latest NHANES data regarding periodontal disease in seniors.

Chapter 31

Dental Implants

Dental implants are metal posts or frames that are surgically implanted in the gums. They fuse to the jawbone and serve as permanent anchors or roots for dental prosthetics—including crowns, bridges, and dentures—that replace missing natural teeth.

Dental implants offer many advantages over conventional tooth-replacement techniques. Most patients find that bridges and dentures placed on implants fit securely, feel comfortable and natural, and do not shift while eating or speaking. Ordinary dentures that rest on top of the gums, in contrast, often affect speech, create problems while eating, or cause sore gums by moving around. An advantage over ordinary bridges is that dental implants do not require adjacent teeth to be ground down in order to provide an attachment point to hold the replacement teeth in place.

Dental implants also play an important role in stabilizing and preserving the alveolar bone in the jaw. When teeth are missing, the underlying bone that once connected and supported them breaks down as part of a natural process called "resorption." Studies have shown that the bone width can decrease by 25 percent in the first year after a tooth is lost. As the bone loss progresses, it can lead to aesthetic and functional problems in the mouth. Dental implants fuse to the bone and provide stimulation that helps to keep the bone healthy and strong.

The main disadvantage of dental implants is their cost, which is generally higher than other methods of tooth replacement and not as

"Dental Implants," © 2017 Omnigraphics. Reviewed July 2019.

likely to be covered by insurance. In addition, to be eligible to receive dental implants, a patient must be in good health and have adequate bone to support the implants. Medical conditions such as uncontrolled gum disease, diabetes, or cancer—as well as lifestyle factors such as smoking or alcoholism—can prevent dental implants from fusing to the bone. Finally, patients who receive dental implants must commit to practicing good oral hygiene and making regular dental visits to keep the structures healthy.

Getting Dental Implants

Getting dental implants is a multistep process that involves a team of specialists. The implant dentistry team is likely to include a periodontist, oral surgeon, or general dentist with training in implant surgery; a dental laboratory technician with training in fabrication of crowns, bridgework, and dentures that attach to implants; and a restorative dentist with training in planning and placing tooth restorations. The team works together to assess and plan the placement of the dental implants and the design of the tooth restorations.

To begin the process, the team will typically conduct a detailed assessment of the patient's teeth, jaws, and bite to determine the exact positioning of the dental implants. This assessment will likely involve specialized x-rays and computerized tomography (CT) scans to create a three-dimensional model of the patient's mouth. Once the assessment is complete, the periodontist uses the information to guide the precise surgical placement of the implants. Channels are created in the jawbone, and metal posts are fitted into the sites. In cases where resorption of the bone has occurred, additional surgery may be needed to graft bone into tooth sockets or regenerate bone that has been lost in order to provide a sufficient base for anchoring the implants.

The bone will generally fuse with the implants within two to six months of the surgery. Temporary healing caps may be placed on the implants until they are fully fused. At that point, tooth restorations are fabricated in a dental laboratory to match the patient's existing teeth. Finally, the artificial teeth are screwed or cemented onto the implants. Once the restorations are attached, they are virtually indistinguishable in appearance and function from the patient's original teeth.

Types of Dental Implants

There are two main types of dental implants: endosteal implants and subperiosteal implants. Endosteal implants are artificial roots or anchors that are surgically placed into the jawbone. Once they fuse with the bone and the surrounding gum tissue heals, metal posts are connected to the implants to hold tooth restorations. Subperiosteal implants consist of a metal frame that is surgically fitted on the jawbone beneath the gum tissue. Once the frame fuses with the jawbone, metal posts are attached to it to hold tooth restorations.

Dental implants can be used to replace a single tooth, multiple teeth, or an entire upper or lower set of teeth. In single-tooth replacement, a single implant serves as the anchor for a custom-made, artificial tooth form called a "crown." In multiple-tooth replacement, multiple implants serve as the anchors for a permanent, custom-made bridge that contains several artificial teeth. For patients who are missing all of their upper or lower teeth, four to six implants may be used to support a removable denture that snaps or clips into place.

Since dental implants are made of metal, they are not subject to dental decay in the same way as the roots of natural teeth. In addition, crowns, bridges, and other prosthetic tooth restorations can be replaced by a dentist if they suffer excessive wear or damage without affecting the implants supporting them. However, people with dental implants must commit to practicing good oral hygiene to control bacterial biofilm on the tissues surrounding the implants. Otherwise, the patient may develop an inflammatory response called "peri-implantitis," which can cause disintegration of the bone surrounding the implant. Finally, people with dental implants must visit a dentist regularly to ensure the continued stability and function of the implants.

References

1. "Understanding Dental Implants," ICOI, 2016.

2. "What Are Dental Implants?" Colgate Oral Care Center, 2016.

3. "What Types of Dental Implants Are Available?" Gordon West, DDS, 2013.

Chapter 32

Facial Trauma

Facial trauma describes any type of injury to the face, ranging from cuts and bruises to fractures of facial bones, such as the jaw, nose, eye socket, cheek, or forehead. Some of the most common causes of facial trauma include sports injuries, automobile and motorcycle accidents, falls, and violence. Children sustain facial injuries more frequently than adults, but they are less likely to break facial bones.

Symptoms of Facial Trauma

Although many facial injuries are minor, they should always be taken seriously. After all, the face plays a critical role in breathing, eating, speaking, and seeing, as well as personal identity and self-esteem. Prompt treatment of a facial laceration by a cosmetic surgeon, for instance, may prevent the formation of an embarrassing or disfiguring scar. In addition, facial trauma often coincides with injuries to the head, spine, eye, mouth, or teeth, so people who show symptoms of facial trauma should also be evaluated for signs of concussion or other potentially serious injuries.

Some of the common symptoms of facial trauma include bleeding, swelling, bruising, numbness, and facial bones that appear uneven or out of place. If these symptoms are severe, or are accompanied by any of the following symptoms, the patient should seek immediate medical attention:

• Loss of consciousness

"Facial Trauma," © 2017 Omnigraphics. Reviewed July 2019.

- Seizure

- Weakness, numbness, or tingling on one side of the body

- Severe headache

- Dizziness, lightheadedness, or trouble standing or walking

- Confusion, irritability, or abnormal behavior

- Eye pain or vision problems, such as blurring or double vision

- Ear pain or hearing problems

- Missing teeth, tooth pain, or trouble chewing

- Pain or other symptoms that get worse rather than steadily improving

Treatment of Facial Injuries

Minor facial injuries can often be treated at home using basic first aid techniques. To stop bleeding, put firm but gentle pressure on the wound with a sterile gauze pad or clean cloth. Avoid taking aspirin, which may prolong bleeding. Apply an ice or cold pack to relieve pain and minimize swelling. Avoid things that might increase swelling— such as heating pads, hot showers, or drinking hot fluids—for the first 48 hours. Keep the head of the bed elevated while sleeping. Avoid smoking, which can prolong the healing process.

More serious facial injuries should be examined by a physician or treated in an emergency room. An x-ray or computerized tomography (CT) scan of the head and neck may be used to check for fractures in the facial bones. Treatment of facial trauma depends on the location, type, and severity of the injury, as well as the overall health condition of the patient. Surgery may be needed if the injury affects the normal functioning of the eyes, nose, or mouth or if the injury poses a risk of scarring or deformity.

Fractures of the jaw, palate, or cheekbones may require treatment by an oral and maxillofacial surgeon to restore the patient's ability to speak, chew, and swallow. Wiring or plating techniques may be used to hold the facial bones in the correct position until they heal. The jaws may be wired shut for up to six weeks, during which time the patient will need to eat a nutritional liquid or pureed diet.

Prevention of Facial Trauma

Many facial injuries are preventable with proper attention to safety. Some tips for reducing the risk of facial trauma include the following:

- Wear seatbelts and place children in age-appropriate car safety seats.

- Wear a helmet while participating in activities such as bicycling, skateboarding, skiing, snowboarding, horseback riding, or rock climbing.

- Wear a mouthguard while participating in contact sports.

- Wear appropriate protective clothing, such as safety goggles, face shields, or hard hats, while working with power tools.

- Remove loose rugs, fix loose boards, and remove other hazards that could cause a fall in the home.

- Never keep loaded guns in the home.

- Never dive into shallow water.

- Use child safety gates to prevent children from falling down stairs.

- Never allow children to walk around while using a bottle or sippy cup.

- Never leave babies or toddlers unattended on a couch, bed, table, porch, or deck.

References

1. "Facial Injuries," WebMD, November 14, 2014.

2. Jothi, Sumana. "Facial Trauma," MedlinePlus, National Institutes of Health (NIH), August 5, 2015.

3. "Treatment of Facial Injuries," American Association of Oral and Maxillofacial Surgeons (AAOMS), 2016.

Chapter 33

Corrective Jaw Surgery

Corrective jaw surgery—formally known as "orthognathic surgery"—is performed to address skeletal and dental irregularities that cannot be remedied through orthodontic treatment alone. In most cases, corrective jaw surgery is used to adjust the supporting bones of the jaw so that fixed orthodontic braces can effectively align the teeth and bite. Orthognathic surgery can correct a variety of functional problems affecting the teeth and jaws, leading to improvements in chewing, speaking, and breathing as well as appearance. It is performed by an oral and maxillofacial surgeon, a specialist whose training includes four years of surgical residency in addition to four years of dental school.

Some of the problems that are commonly treated with corrective jaw surgery include the following:

- Severe underbites or overbites

- Congenital abnormalities or birth defects affecting jaw development, such as cleft palate

- Facial asymmetries or unbalanced facial appearance

- Protruding jaw or receding chin

- Chronic jaw or temporomandibular joint (TMJ) pain

- Difficulty in biting, chewing, or swallowing food

"Corrective Jaw Surgery," © 2017 Omnigraphics. Reviewed July 2019.

- Facial injury or trauma

- Chronic mouth breathing or dry mouth

- Obstructive sleep apnea

Undergoing Corrective Jaw Surgery

Patients are likely to be referred to an oral and maxillofacial surgeon for corrective jaw surgery by a dentist or orthodontist who has determined that an irregularity in the structure of the jaws makes it impossible for orthodontic treatment alone to provide effective results. The process of orthognathic surgery begins with consultation and planning among members of the dental team, including the oral and maxillofacial surgeon, the orthodontist, and the general or restorative dentist. These professionals will use diagnostic imaging to create three-dimensional models of the patient's mouth and jaws to develop a step-by-step treatment plan.

In preparation for orthognathic surgery, most patients will have fixed orthodontic braces installed to align their teeth and move them into the best possible position for the necessary surgical adjustment to the jaws. The braces are typically applied around 18 months prior to the surgery and remain in place both during and after the procedure. In some cases, patients may also need to have their wisdom teeth extracted prior to surgery if they obstruct the area of the jaw on which the surgeon will be operating. Two weeks before the surgery date, the orthodontist will attach hooks to the braces to facilitate the procedure.

Corrective jaw surgery generally involves making a planned fracture of the jaw in order to reset the bone in a new position. Small plates and screws are inserted into the bone to hold it in the desired position. Wires or strong elastic bands may also be used to help maintain the new jaw position and guide the teeth into alignment. Since the work is completed inside the mouth, there are usually no visible scars on the patient's face. The procedure generally takes three to six hours. It is usually performed in a hospital with the patient under general anesthesia, although in some cases it may be performed in the oral and maxillofacial surgeon's office. Depending on the complexity of the procedure, the patient may remain in the hospital for two to three days.

Recovering from Corrective Jaw Surgery

Immediately after undergoing corrective jaw surgery, patients are likely to experience jaw soreness and stiffness and facial swelling. Pain medications are usually prescribed for the first few weeks to reduce the discomfort. Since it takes four to six weeks for bones in the jaw to heal, patients who undergo orthognathic surgery cannot chew solid food and must follow a nutritional liquid or pureed diet. They should also practice good oral hygiene to reduce the risk of infection and avoid smoking or drinking alcohol, which can prolong the healing process.

Many patients who have surgery on their lower jaw experience numbness in the lower lip or chin, while patients who have surgery on their upper jaw may experience numbness in the upper lip or cheek. The numbness is usually temporary, but it is important to avoid biting or burning the lips during this time. Patients may experience a tingling sensation as the feeling gradually returns to the area over the course of several weeks.

Many patients need at least four weeks of recovery time before they can return to work or school. In addition, people who have orthognathic surgery may need to avoid air travel for at least six weeks due to potential complications from changes in air pressure. Finally, patients should avoid playing contact sports or doing other activities that put strain on the jaw for at least 10 to 12 weeks following surgery.

Beginning about one week after undergoing corrective jaw surgery, patients must make regular visits to the orthodontist to check and adjust the fixed braces. The braces will remain in place for six to nine months after the surgery to further align the teeth and prevent the jaw from moving back to its original position. Even after the braces are removed, the patient will likely need to wear retainers to maintain the alignment of the teeth and jaw. In most cases the plates and screws that were inserted by the oral surgeon will remain in place for life.

References

1. "Corrective Jaw Surgery," Christopher M. Brieden, DDS, 2016.

2. "What Is Corrective Jaw Surgery?" NHS Foundation Trust, 2016.

Part Five

Oral Diseases and Disorders

Chapter 34

Amelogenesis Imperfecta

Amelogenesis imperfecta (AI) (amelogenesis—enamel formation; imperfecta—imperfect) is a disorder that affects the structure and appearance of the enamel of the teeth. This condition causes teeth to be unusually small, discolored, pitted or grooved, and prone to rapid wear and breakage with early tooth decay and loss. These dental problems, which vary among affected individuals, can affect both primary (baby) teeth and permanent teeth. People with this disease may also have problems involving the tissues surrounding teeth (periodontal tissues), such as gums, cementum, ligaments, and alveolar bones in which the tooth root rests. Teeth are also sensitive to either hot or cold exposures, and sometimes both. Severe and continuous pain due to exposed dentin resulting from the enamel defect is present in some cases.

There are 4 main types of AI that are classified based on the symptoms, x-rays appearance and type of enamel defect. The main types are: hypoplastic (type I); hypomaturation (type II); hypocalcified (type III); and hypomaturation/hypoplasia/taurodontism (type IV). These 4 types are divided further into 17 or 18 subtypes, which are distinguished by their specific genetic cause and by their pattern of inheritance. AI can be inherited in an autosomal dominant, autosomal recessive or X-linked recessive pattern. Treatment may include dentures that cap the teeth (full-crown restorations), orthodontic treatment, special toothpaste for the tooth sensitivity, and good oral hygiene.

This chapter includes text excerpted from "Amelogenesis Imperfecta," Genetic and Rare Diseases Information Center (GARD), National Center for Advancing Translational Sciences (NCATS), June 11, 2018.

Symptoms of Amelogenesis Imperfecta

In general, both the primary and permanent teeth are affected. The enamel tends to be soft and weak, and the teeth appear yellow and damage easily.

The defects associated with amelogenesis imperfecta are highly variable and include abnormalities classified as hypoplastic (defects in the amount of enamel), hypomaturation (defect in the final growth and development of the tooth enamel), and hypocalcification (defect in the initial stage of enamel formation followed by defective tooth growth). The enamel in the hypomaturation and hypocalcification types is not mineralized and is thus described as hypomineralized.

Traditionally, the diagnosis and classification of amelogenesis imperfecta is based on the clinical presentation and the mode of inheritance. There are four principal types based on the defects in the tooth enamel. These types are subdivided into 14 different subtypes based on the clinical presentation and the mode of inheritance.

Causes of Amelogenesis Imperfecta

Amelogenesis imperfecta is caused by mutations in the *AMELX*, *ENAM*, and *MMP20* genes. These genes provide instructions for making proteins that are essential for normal tooth development. These proteins are involved in the formation of enamel, which is the hard, calcium-rich material that forms the protective outer layer of each tooth. Mutations in any of these genes alter the structure of these proteins or prevent the genes from making any protein at all. As a result, tooth enamel is abnormally thin or soft and may have a yellow or brown color. Teeth with defective enamel are weak and easily damaged.

In some cases, the genetic cause of amelogenesis imperfecta cannot be identified. Researchers are working to find mutations in other genes that are responsible for this disorder.

Inheritance of Amelogenesis Imperfecta

The different types of amelogenesis imperfecta can have different types of inheritance according to the gene that is altered:

The following types have an autosomal dominant inheritance:

- IA

- IB

- IIIA

- IIIB
- IV

The types that are inherited in an autosomal recessive manner are:

- IC
- IF
- IG or enamel-renal syndrome type
- IH
- IJ
- IIA1
- IIA2
- IIA3
- IIA4
- IIA5
- IIA6

Type 1E is inherited in a dominant pattern linked to the X chromosome.

In autosomal dominant cases, one copy of the altered gene in each cell is sufficient to cause the disorder. Autosomal recessive inheritance means two copies of the gene in each cell have to be altered for the person to have the disease. A condition is considered X-linked if the mutated gene that causes the disorder is located on the X chromosome, one of the two sex chromosomes. In most cases, males with X-linked amelogenesis imperfecta experience more severe dental abnormalities than females with this form of this condition.

Diagnosis of Amelogenesis Imperfecta

A dentist can identify and diagnose amelogenesis imperfecta based on the patient's family history and the signs and symptoms present in the affected individual.

Extraoral x-rays (x-rays taken outside the mouth) can reveal the presence of teeth that never erupted or that were absorbed. Intraoral x-rays (x-rays taken inside the mouth) shows a contrast between the enamel and dentin in cases in which mineralization is affected.

Genetic testing is available for the genes *AMELX, ENAM,* and *MMP20.*

Treatment for Amelogenesis Imperfecta

Treatment depends on the type of amelogenesis imperfecta, the age of the affected person, and the type and severity of enamel abnormality. Treatments include preventative measures, various types of crowns, as well as tooth implants or dentures, orthodontic, periodontal and restorative treatment. The social and emotional impact of this condition should also be addressed.

Chapter 35

Bad Breath (Halitosis)

When you open your mouth to talk, you probably want your friends to think about what you are saying—and not about what you ate for lunch. But, certain strong-smelling foods such as onions and garlic can cause bad breath. So can smoking. And so can bacteria that grow on bits of food that get stuck between your teeth.

Lots of people have bad breath at some point. Do not worry! There are steps you can take to keep your mouth fresh and healthy.

Tips for Preventing Bad Breath

- **Brush your teeth** (and tongue!) for at least two minutes twice a day with a fluoride toothpaste, especially after meals and at bedtime.

- **Ask your dentist how to floss correctly.** Flossing can remove tiny bits of food that can rot and smell bad.

- **Replace your toothbrush** every three to four months.

- **Visit your dentist twice a year.** She or he will help keep your teeth and your mouth healthy.

- **Eat smart.** Avoid foods and drinks that can leave behind strong smells, such as cabbage, garlic, raw onions, and coffee. If you are trying to lose weight, remember that not eating enough or

This chapter includes text excerpted from "Bad Breath," girlshealth.gov, Office on Women's Health (OWH), April 15, 2014. Reviewed July 2019.

cutting out certain foods (such as carbohydrates) can cause bad breath.

- **Do not smoke!** You will smell sweeter—and be lots healthier.

- **Drink enough fluids.** Drinking helps wash away tiny bits of food and bacteria, which can smell bad.

If your bad breath does not go away, be sure to talk to your dentist, doctor, or nurse. It could be a sign of a medical problem, such as a sinus infection or gum disease. You may feel a little funny talking about bad breath, but it is very common and you can get help.

Tips for Keeping Your Mouth Healthy

A lot of the tips for keeping your mouth healthy are the same as the tips for stopping bad breath, such as brushing and flossing. Below are some more tips for good oral hygiene, which is just a fancy way to say taking care of your teeth and mouth. Do you feel like they are a pain? Well, they are a lot less of a pain than the dentist's drill!

Eat smart. Avoid sugary foods and drinks. This helps prevent damage to your teeth and is great for your overall health.

Brush after sweets. If you eat or drink sugary stuff, try to brush right after. If you cannot brush, at least rinse your mouth with water.

Definitely do not smoke. Smoking does not just smell bad and stain your teeth. It also can increase your risk of gum disease and tooth decay.

Chapter 36

Burning Mouth Syndrome

Burning mouth syndrome (BMS) is a painful, complex condition often described as a burning, scalding, or tingling feeling in the mouth that may occur every day for months or longer. Dry mouth or an altered taste in the mouth may accompany the pain.

Burning mouth syndrome is most commonly found in adults over the age of 60. It is estimated to be about five times more frequent in women than in men.

Doctors and dentists do not have a specific test for BMS, which makes it hard to diagnose. No specific treatment works for everyone. However, a doctor can prescribe medications to help you manage the pain, dry mouth, or other symptoms.

Causes of Burning Mouth Syndrome

Primary BMS. If BMS is not caused by an underlying medical problem, it is called "primary BMS." Experts believe that primary BMS is caused by damage to the nerves that control pain and taste.

Secondary BMS. If BMS is caused by an underlying medical problem, it is called "secondary BMS." Treating the medical problem should relieve the symptoms.

This chapter includes text excerpted from "Burning Mouth Syndrome," National Institute of Dental and Craniofacial Research (NIDCR), April 2019.

Common causes of secondary BMS may include:

- Hormonal changes (such as those associated with menopause or thyroid disease)

- Metabolic disorders such as diabetes

- Allergies to dental products, dental materials (usually metals), or foods

- Dry mouth, which can be caused by disorders (such as Sjögren syndrome) and treatments (such as certain drugs and radiation therapy)

- Medications such as those that reduce blood pressure

- Nutritional deficiencies such as a low level of vitamin B_{12} or iron

- Oral infections such as a yeast infection

- Acid reflux

Symptoms of Burning Mouth Syndrome

The main symptom of BMS is a burning, scalding, or tingling pain in the mouth. It can also feel like numbness. Other symptoms include dry mouth or altered taste in the mouth.

Burning mouth syndrome usually affects the tongue, but the pain may also be in the lips, the roof of the mouth, or throughout the mouth.

The pain of BMS can last for a long time. Some people feel constant pain every day. For others, pain increases throughout the day. For many people, pain is reduced when eating or drinking.

Diagnosis of Burning Mouth Syndrome

Burning mouth syndrome is hard to diagnose. It is not something that a doctor or dentist can see during an exam. Your dentist or doctor may refer you to a specialist. Specialists who diagnose BMS include dentists who specialize in oral medicine or oral surgery. Otolaryngologists (ear, nose, and throat specialists), gastroenterologists, dermatologists, or neurologists may also be able to diagnose the disorder.

To diagnose BMS, a dentist or doctor will review your medical history and examine your mouth. Additional tests may be needed such as:

- Blood tests to check for underlying medical problems

- Oral swab tests

- Allergy tests

- Salivary flow test

- Tissue biopsy

- Imaging tests

Treatment of Burning Mouth Syndrome

Burning mouth syndrome is a complex pain disorder. The treatment that works for one person may not work for another. Your dentist or doctor may prescribe medications to help manage the pain, dry mouth, or other symptoms.

Symptoms of secondary BMS may go away when the underlying medical condition, such as diabetes or oral infection, is treated. If a drug is causing the problem, a doctor may switch you to a different medicine.

Helpful Tips

To help ease the pain, sip a cold beverage, suck on ice chips, or chew sugarless gum.

Avoid things that can irritate your mouth, such as:

- Tobacco

- Hot, spicy foods

- Alcoholic beverages

- Mouthwash that contains alcohol

- Products high in acid, such as citrus fruits and juices

Ask your dentist and doctor for other helpful tips.

Chapter 37

Cleft Lip and Cleft Palate

Chapter Contents

Section 37.1

What Are Craniofacial Defects?

This section contains text excerpted from the following sources:
Text in this section begins with excerpts from "Craniofacial
Abnormalities," MedlinePlus, National Institutes of Health (NIH),
July 27, 2016; Text under the heading "Craniofacial Birth Defects"
is excerpted from "Craniofacial Birth Defects," National Institute of
Dental and Craniofacial Research (NIDCR), July 2018.

"Craniofacial" is a medical term that relates to the bones of the skull and face. Craniofacial abnormalities are birth defects of the face or head. Some, like cleft lip and palate, are among the most common of all birth defects. Others are very rare. Most of them affect how a person's face or head looks. These conditions may also affect other parts of the body.

Treatment depends on the type of problem. Plastic and reconstructive surgery may help the person's appearance.

Craniofacial Birth Defects

Craniofacial defects, such as cleft lip and cleft palate are among the most common of all birth defects. They can be isolated or one component of an inherited disease or syndrome. Both genetic and environmental factors contribute to oral clefts. Although clefts can be repaired to varying degrees with surgery, researchers are working toward understanding the developmental processes that lead to clefting and how to prevent the condition or more effectively treat it.

There are no national data for cleft lip or palate. The National Birth Defects Prevention Network (NBDPN) collects cleft lip and palate data annually from 11 states (Alabama, Arkansas, California, Georgia, Hawaii, Iowa, Massachusetts, North Carolina, Oklahoma, Texas, and Utah), which provides a means for estimating national data.

Section 37.2

Facts about Cleft Lip and Cleft Palate

This section includes text excerpted from "Facts about
Cleft Lip and Cleft Palate," Centers for Disease
Control and Prevention (CDC), November 21, 2017.

Cleft lip and cleft palate are birth defects that occur when a baby's lip or mouth does not form properly during pregnancy. Together, these birth defects commonly are called "orofacial clefts."

What Is Cleft Lip?

Cleft lip forms between the fourth and seventh weeks of pregnancy. As a fetus develops during pregnancy, body tissue and special cells from each side of the head grow toward the center of the face and join together to make up the face. This joining of tissue forms the facial features, such as the lips and mouth. A cleft lip happens if the tissue that makes up the lip does not join completely before birth. This results in an opening in the upper lip. The opening in the lip can be a small slit or it can be a large opening that goes through the lip into the nose. A cleft lip can be on one or both sides of the lip or in the middle of the lip, which occurs very rarely. Children with a cleft lip can have a cleft palate.

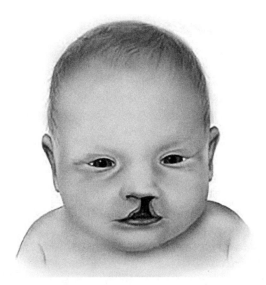

Figure 37.1. *Baby with Cleft Lip*

What Is Cleft Palate?

The roof of the mouth (palate) is formed between the sixth and ninth weeks of pregnancy. A cleft palate happens if the tissue that makes up the roof of the mouth does not join together completely during pregnancy. For some babies, both the front and back parts of the palate are open. For other babies, only part of the palate is open.

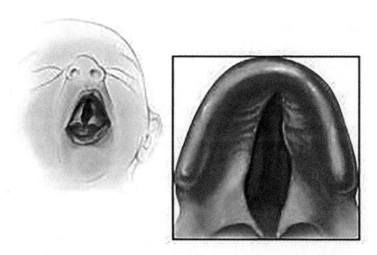

Figure 37.2. *Baby with Cleft Palate and Inner View of Cleft Palate*

Other Problems

Children with cleft lip or those with cleft lip and palate or those with cleft palate alone often have problems with feeding and speaking clearly and can have ear infections. They also might have hearing problems and problems with their teeth.

Occurrence

The Centers for Disease Control and Prevention (CDC) recently estimated that, each year in the United States, about 2,650 babies are born with cleft palate and 4,440 babies are born with cleft lip with or without cleft palate. Isolated orofacial clefts, or clefts that occur with no other major birth defects, are one of the most common types of birth defects in the United States. Depending on the cleft type, the rate of isolated orofacial clefts can vary from 50 to 80 percent of all clefts.

Causes and Risk Factors

The causes of orofacial clefts among most infants are unknown. Some children have a cleft lip or cleft palate because of changes in their genes. Cleft lip and cleft palate are thought to be caused by a combination of genes and other factors, such as things the mother comes in contact within her environment, or what the mother eats or drinks, or certain medications she uses during pregnancy.

Like the many families of children with birth defects, the CDC wants to find out what causes them. Understanding the factors that are more common among babies with a birth defect will help us learn more about the causes. The CDC funds the Centers for Birth Defects Research and Prevention, which collaborate on large studies such as the National Birth Defects Prevention Study (NBDPS; births 1997–2011) and the Birth Defects Study To Evaluate Pregnancy exposureS (BD-STEPS; began with births in 2014) to understand the causes of and risks for birth defects, including orofacial clefts.

The CDC reported on important findings from research studies about some factors that increase the chance of having a baby with an orofacial cleft:

- **Smoking**—Women who smoke during pregnancy are more likely to have a baby with an orofacial cleft than women who do not smoke.

- **Diabetes**—Women with diabetes diagnosed before pregnancy have an increased risk of having a child with a cleft lip with or without cleft palate, compared to women who did not have diabetes.

- **Use of certain medicines**—Women who used certain medicines to treat epilepsy, such as topiramate or valproic acid during the first trimester (the first 3 months) of pregnancy, have an increased risk of having a baby with cleft lip with or without cleft palate, compared to women who did not take these medicines.

The CDC continues to study birth defects, such as cleft lip and cleft palate, and how to prevent them. If you are pregnant or thinking about becoming pregnant, talk with your doctor about ways to increase your chances of having a healthy baby.

Diagnosis

Orofacial clefts, especially cleft lip with or without cleft palate, can be diagnosed during pregnancy by a routine ultrasound. They can also be diagnosed after the baby is born, especially cleft palate. However, sometimes certain types of cleft palate (e.g., submucous cleft palate and bifid uvula) might not be diagnosed until later in life.

Management and Treatment

Services and treatment for children with orofacial clefts can vary depending on the severity of the cleft; the child's age and needs; and the presence of associated syndromes or other birth defects, or both.

Surgery to repair a cleft lip usually occurs in the first few months of life and is recommended within the first 12 months of life. Surgery to repair a cleft palate is recommended within the first 18 months of life or earlier if possible. Many children will need additional surgical procedures as they get older. Surgical repair can improve the look and appearance of a child's face and might also improve breathing, hearing, and speech and language development. Children born with orofacial clefts might need other types of treatments and services, such as special dental or orthodontic care or speech therapy.

Because children with orofacial clefts often require a variety of services that need to be provided in a coordinated manner throughout childhood and into adolescence and sometimes adulthood, the American Cleft Palate–Craniofacial Association recommends services and treatment by cleft and craniofacial teams. Cleft and craniofacial teams provide a coordinated approach to care for children with orofacial clefts. These teams usually consist of experienced and qualified physicians and healthcare providers from different specialties. Cleft and craniofacial teams and centers are located throughout the United States and other countries.

With treatment, most children with orofacial clefts do well and lead a healthy life. Some children with orofacial clefts may have issues with self-esteem if they are concerned with visible differences between themselves and other children. Parent-to-parent support groups can prove to be useful for families of babies with birth defects of the head and face, such as orofacial clefts.

Section 37.3

Breastfeeding Children with Cleft Palate

Cleft palate and cleft lip—known collectively as "orofacial clefts"—rank among the most common types of birth defects in the United States. According to the U.S. Centers for Disease Control and Prevention (CDC), around 2,650 babies are born with a cleft palate in the United States each year, while around 4,440 babies are born with a cleft lip. Orofacial clefts occur early in the gestation process, when the tissues that grow around the sides of the head to form the face fail to meet in the middle. Left untreated, they can have a significant impact on a child's breathing, hearing, eating, and speech. As a result, most babies born with orofacial clefts undergo surgery within the first year of life to repair the cleft and improve the function of the mouth.

Prior to the surgical repair, orofacial clefts can greatly complicate breastfeeding efforts. Experts have compared breastfeeding with a cleft palate to drinking through a straw with a hole in it. The cleft allows air to enter the mouth and prevents the baby from getting adequate suction. The feeding process becomes physically taxing, and the baby may swallow a great deal of air. As a result of these complications, the breastfeeding advocacy group La Leche League International warns that most babies with uncorrected cleft palate are not able to get the nutrition they need through breastfeeding exclusively. Since research has shown that breastfeeding offers a number of important benefits to a baby's health and well-being, this news is upsetting to many mothers of babies with a cleft palate.

Feeding Options for Babies with Cleft Palate

Babies born with a cleft lip only (not a cleft palate) are often able to breastfeed successfully before surgery. The mother usually needs to experiment with different nursing positions to help the baby's lips form a seal over the nipple. Lactation consultants often recommend holding the baby in an upright position, perhaps with the support of a nursing pillow.

Babies born with a cleft palate, on the other hand, are rarely able to breastfeed successfully before surgery. Although this situation can be deeply disappointing for mothers, there are still many options available to help them share the benefits of breastfeeding with their babies. Some of the main options include the following:

- Use a hospital-grade breast pump to express breast milk and feed it to the baby using a cleft palate feeding system, which includes specialized bottles and nipples. Feeding breast milk from a bottle ensures that the baby gets all the nutritional benefits of nursing.

- To experience the physical intimacy and emotional bonding aspects of breastfeeding, make as much eye contact and skin contact with the baby as possible while bottle feeding.

- Once bottle feeding has been established successfully, put the baby on the mother's breast for nonnutritive sucking. This action not only helps develop muscles in the baby's mouth and tongue but can also stimulate milk production in mothers who pump.

- After the baby undergoes surgery to repair the cleft palate, it may be possible to reintroduce breastfeeding.

Using a pump to express milk can be challenging and time consuming for new mothers, as can learning to feed a baby with a cleft palate. It is important that mothers have the support of friends and family members as they figure out the best feeding methods for themselves and their babies. Even though breast milk is widely viewed as the best food for newborns, formula has nourished millions of healthy children. Overwhelmed mothers of babies with orofacial clefts may simply decide that pumping is too difficult given the demands of work and family, and they should not feel guilty about lovingly feeding their babies with formula.

References

1. Condon, Susan. "How Do I Breastfeed a Baby with Cleft Lip or Palate?" Baby Center, April 2015.

2. "What about Breastfeeding?" Cleft Palate Foundation, July 15, 2009.

Section 37.4

Use of Topiramate in Pregnancy and Risk of Oral Clefts

This section includes text excerpted from "FDA Drug Safety Communication: Risk of Oral Clefts in Children Born to Mothers Taking Topamax (Topiramate)," U.S. Food and Drug Administration (FDA), February 7, 2018.

Safety Announcement

In early 2018, the U.S. Food and Drug Administration (FDA) informed the public of new data that show that there is an increased risk for the development of cleft lip and/or cleft palate (oral clefts) in infants born to women treated with topiramate (Topamax and generic products) during pregnancy.

The benefits and the risks of topiramate should be carefully weighed when prescribing this drug to women of childbearing age, particularly for conditions not usually associated with permanent injury or death. Alternative medications that have a lower risk of oral clefts and other adverse birth outcomes should be considered for these patients. If the decision is made to use topiramate in women of childbearing age, effective birth control should be used. Oral clefts occur in the first trimester of pregnancy before many women know they are pregnant.

Topiramate was previously classified as a Pregnancy Category C drug, which means that data from animal studies suggested potential fetal risks, but no adequate data from human clinical trials or studies were available at the time of approval. However, because of new human data that show an increased risk for oral clefts, topiramate is being placed in Pregnancy Category D. Pregnancy Category D means there is positive evidence of human fetal risk based on human data but the potential benefits from the use of the drug in pregnant women may be acceptable in certain situations despite its risks.

Facts about Topiramate

- An anticonvulsant medication FDA-approved for use alone or with other medications to treat patients with epilepsy who have certain types of seizures.

- FDA-approved for use to prevent migraine headaches, but not to relieve the pain of migraine headaches when they occur.

- Has been used off-label (for unapproved uses) for other conditions, some of which may not be considered serious.

- From January 2007 through December 2010, approximately 32.3 million topiramate prescriptions were dispensed and approximately 4.3 million patients filled topiramate prescriptions from the outpatient retail pharmacies in the United States.

Additional Information for Patients

- If you take topiramate during pregnancy, there is a higher risk that your baby will develop a cleft lip and/or cleft palate. Oral clefts happen early in pregnancy, before many women even know they are pregnant. For this reason, women of childbearing age should talk to their healthcare professionals about other treatment options.

- Women of childbearing age who do decide to take topiramate and are not planning a pregnancy should use effective birth control (contraception) while taking topiramate. Women should talk to their healthcare professionals about the best kind of birth control to use while taking topiramate.

- Before you start topiramate, you should tell your healthcare professional if you are pregnant or are planning to become pregnant. Healthcare professionals may discuss other treatment options with you.

- You should tell your healthcare professional right away if you become pregnant while taking topiramate. You and your healthcare provider should decide if you will continue to take topiramate while you are pregnant.

- Topiramate should not be stopped without talking to a healthcare professional, even in pregnant women. Stopping topiramate suddenly can cause serious problems. Not treating epilepsy during pregnancy can be harmful to women and their developing babies.

- If you become pregnant while taking topiramate, you should talk to your healthcare professional about registering with the North American Antiepileptic Drug (AED) Pregnancy Registry. You can enroll in this registry by calling 888-233-2334. The purpose of this registry is to collect additional information about the safety of antiepileptic drugs during pregnancy.

• Topiramate passes into breast milk, but its effects on developing babies remain unknown. You should talk to your healthcare professional about the best way to feed your baby if you take topiramate.

• You should report any side effects you experience to the FDA MedWatch program using the MedWatch Voluntary Reporting Form.

• You should read the Medication Guide when picking up a prescription for topiramate. It will help you understand the potential risks and benefits of this medication.

Chapter 38

Dentinogenesis Imperfecta

What Is Dentinogenesis Imperfecta?

Dentinogenesis imperfecta (DI) is a condition characterized by teeth that are translucent and discolored (most often blue-grey or yellow-brown in color). Individuals with this disorder tend to have teeth that are weaker than normal, which leads to wear, breakage, and loss of teeth. This damage can include teeth fractures or small holes (pitting) in the enamel. Dentinogenesis imperfecta can affect both primary (baby) teeth and permanent teeth. People with this condition may also have speech problems or teeth that are not placed correctly in the mouth. Dentinogenesis imperfecta is caused by mutations in the *DSPP* gene and is inherited in an autosomal dominant manner.

Types of Dentinogenesis Imperfecta

According to the original classification, there are three types of dentinogenesis imperfecta:

Type I: Occurs in people who have osteogenesis imperfecta (OI), a genetic condition in which bones are brittle, causing them to break easily. People with this type of dentinogenesis imperfecta have mutations in *COL1A1* or *COL1A2*.

This chapter includes text excerpted from "Dentinogenesis Imperfecta," Genetic and Rare Diseases Information Center (GARD), National Center for Advancing Translational Sciences (NCATS), March 17, 2017.

Type II: Usually, occurs in people without another inherited disorder. Some families with type II have progressive hearing loss in older age. Type II is the most common type of dentinogenesis imperfecta.

Type III: Usually, occurs in people without another inherited disorder. Type III was first identified in a group of families in southern Maryland and has also been seen in individuals of Ashkenazi Jewish descent.

Some researchers believe that dentinogenesis imperfecta type II and type III, along with a similar condition called "dentin dysplasia type II," are actually just different forms of a single disorder.

Causes of Dentinogenesis Imperfecta

Mutations in the *DSPP* gene cause dentinogenesis imperfecta. The *DSPP* gene provides instructions for making three proteins that are essential for normal tooth development. These proteins are involved in the formation of dentin, which is a bone-like substance that makes up the protective middle layer of each tooth. Mutations in *DSPP* change the proteins made from the gene, leading to the production of abnormally soft dentin. Teeth with defective dentin are discolored, weak, and more likely to decay and break. It is unclear how *DSPP* mutations are related to hearing loss in some families with dentinogenesis imperfecta type II.

Inheritance of Dentinogenesis Imperfecta

Dentinogenesis imperfecta is inherited in an autosomal dominant manner, which means only one changed copy of *DSPP* in each cell is sufficient to cause the disorder. We inherit one copy of each gene from our mother and another copy from our father. In most cases, a person who is affected with dentinogenesis imperfecta has one parent with the condition, although it is possible for the condition to occur for the first time in an individual who does not have an affected parent. In these cases, the change in the gene is known as "de novo" because it was not inherited from either parent.

Diagnosis of Dentinogenesis Imperfecta

Dentinogenesis imperfecta is diagnosed by a clinical exam that is consistent with signs of the condition. A dental x-ray is specifically helpful in diagnosing dentinogenesis imperfecta. The specific signs found in a clinical exam may differ depending on the type of dentino-genesis imperfecta:

Type I: People who have type I dentinogenesis imperfecta also have osteogenesis imperfecta. This will cause them to have other health concerns, so they will typically not be diagnosed by dental x-ray.

Type II: People who have type II dentinogenesis imperfecta will be expected to show signs, such as amber or multicolored (opalescent) dentin, short roots, and missing pulp chambers of the teeth. The pulp chamber is the innermost layer of the tooth.

Type III: People who have type III dentinogenesis imperfecta will be expected to show signs, such as multicolored (opalescent) primary and permanent teeth and large pulp chambers.

Treatment of Dentinogenesis Imperfecta

The aims of treatment for dentinogenesis imperfecta are to remove sources of infection or pain, restore aesthetics, and protect teeth from wear. Treatment varies according to the age of the patient, severity of the problem, and presenting complaint. Treatment options include amalgams as dental fillings, veneers to fix the discoloration of teeth, crowns, caps, and bridges. Dentures or dental implants may be necessary if the majority of teeth are lost. Some dentists may also recommend resin restorations and teeth bleaching.

Chapter 39

Dry Mouth Disorders

Chapter Contents

Section 39.1

Dry Mouth: An Overview

This section includes text excerpted from "Dry Mouth," National Institute of Dental and Craniofacial Research (NIDCR), August 2017.

What Is Dry Mouth?

Dry mouth is a condition when there is not enough saliva in the mouth. Everyone has a dry mouth once in a while—if one is nervous, upset, or under stress. But if one has a dry mouth all or most of the time, it can be uncomfortable and can lead to serious health problems. Dry mouth can also be a sign of certain diseases and conditions. When one has a dry mouth, the following problems are faced:

- Difficulties in tasting, chewing, swallowing, and speaking

- Chances of developing dental decay and other infections in the mouth increase

- Side effects occur due to certain medications or medical treatments

Dry mouth is not a normal part of aging. So if you think you have dry mouth, see your dentist or physician—there are things you can do to get relief.

Symptoms of dry mouth include:

- A sticky, dry feeling in the mouth

- Trouble chewing, swallowing, tasting, or speaking

- A burning feeling in the mouth

- A dry feeling in the throat

- Cracked lips

- A dry, rough tongue

- Mouth sores

- An infection in the mouth

Why Is Saliva So Important?

Saliva does more than keeping the mouth wet.

- It helps digest food.

- It protects teeth from decay.

- It prevents infection by controlling bacteria and fungi in the mouth.

- It makes it possible for you to chew and swallow.

Without enough saliva, you can develop tooth decay or other infections in the mouth. You also might not get the nutrients you need if you cannot chew and swallow certain foods.

What Causes Dry Mouth

People get dry mouth when the glands in the mouth that make saliva are not working properly. Because of this, there might not be enough saliva to keep your mouth wet. There are several reasons why these glands (called "salivary glands") might not work right.

- **Side effects of some medicines.** More than 400 medicines can cause the salivary glands to make less saliva. For example, medicines for high blood pressure and depression often cause dry mouth.

- **Disease.** Some diseases affect the salivary glands. For example, Sjögren syndrome, human deficiency virus (HIV)/acquired immunodeficiency syndrome (AIDS), and diabetes can all cause dry mouth.

- **Radiation therapy.** The salivary glands can be damaged if they are exposed to radiation during cancer treatment.

- **Chemotherapy.** Drugs used to treat cancer can make saliva thicker, causing the mouth to feel dry.

- **Nerve damage.** Injury to the head or neck can damage the nerves that tell salivary glands to make saliva.

What Can Be Done about Dry Mouth?

Dry mouth treatment will depend on what is causing the problem. If you think you have dry mouth, see your dentist or physician. She or he can try to determine what is causing your dry mouth.

- If your dry mouth is caused by medicine, your physician might change your medicine or adjust the dosage.

271

- If your salivary glands are not working right but can still produce some saliva, your physician or dentist might give you a medicine that helps the glands work better.

- Your physician or dentist might suggest that you use artificial saliva to keep your mouth wet.

What Can You Do about Dry Mouth?

- Sip water or sugarless drinks often.

- Avoid drinks with caffeine, such as coffee, tea, and some sodas. Caffeine can dry out the mouth.

- Sip water or a sugarless drink during meals. This will make chewing and swallowing easier. It may also improve the taste of food.

- Chew sugarless gum or suck on sugarless hard candy to stimulate saliva flow; citrus, cinnamon, or mint-flavored candies are good choices. Some sugarless chewing gums and candies contain xylitol and may help prevent cavities.

- Do not use tobacco or alcohol. They dry out the mouth.

- Be aware that spicy or salty foods may cause pain in a dry mouth.

- Use a humidifier at night.

Dry Mouth and Tips for Keeping Your Teeth Healthy

Remember, if you have dry mouth, you need to be extra careful to keep your teeth healthy. Make sure you:

- Gently brush your teeth at least twice a day.

- Floss your teeth regularly.

- Use toothpaste with fluoride in it. Most toothpastes sold at grocery and drug stores have fluoride in them.

- Avoid sticky, sugary foods. If you do eat them, brush immediately afterward.

- Visit your dentist for a checkup at least twice a year. Your dentist might also suggest you use a prescription-strength fluoride gel (which is like a toothpaste) to help prevent dental decay.

Section 39.2

Sialadenitis

This section includes text excerpted from "Sialadenitis," Genetic and Rare Diseases Information Center (GARD), National Center for Advancing Translational Sciences (NCATS), November 8, 2016.

What Is Sialadenitis?

Sialadenitis is an infection of the salivary glands. It is usually caused by a virus or bacteria. The parotid (in front of the ear) and submandibular (under the chin) glands are most commonly affected. Sialadenitis may be associated with pain, tenderness, redness, and gradual, localized swelling of the affected area. Sialadenitis most commonly affects the elderly and chronically ill, especially those with dry mouth or who are dehydrated, but can also affect people of any age including newborn babies. Diagnosis is usually made by clinical exam, but a computed tomography (CT) scan, magnetic resonance imaging (MRI) scan, or ultrasound may be done if the doctor suspects an abscess or wants to look for stones. Treatment may include an antibiotic (if bacterial), warm compresses, increasing fluid intake, and good oral hygiene. Most salivary gland infections go away on their own or are cured with treatment. Complications are not common.

Symptoms of Sialadenitis

Signs and symptoms of sialadenitis may include fever, chills, and unilateral pain and swelling in the affected area. The affected gland may be firm and tender, with redness of the overlying skin. Pus may drain through the gland into the mouth.

Causes of Sialadenitis

Sialadenitis usually occurs after decreased flow of saliva (hyposecretion) or duct obstruction, but may develop without an obvious cause. Saliva flow can be reduced in people who are sick or recovering from surgery, or people who are dehydrated, malnourished, or immunosuppressed. A stone or a kink in the salivary duct can also diminish saliva flow, as can certain medications (such as antihistamines, diuretics, psychiatric medications, beta-blockers, or barbiturates). It often occurs in chronically ill people with dry mouth (xerostomia), people

273

with Sjögren syndrome, and in those who have had radiation therapy (RT) to the oral cavity.

Sialadenitis is most commonly due to bacterial infections caused by *Staphylococcus aureus*. Other bacteria which can cause infections include streptococci, coliforms, and various anaerobic bacteria. Although less common than bacteria, several viruses have also been implicated in sialadenitis. These include the mumps virus, human immunodeficiency virus (HIV), coxsackievirus, parainfluenza types I and II, influenza A, and herpes.

Treatment of Sialadenitis

The treatment of sialadenitis depends on what type of microbe is causing the infection. If the infection is bacterial, an antibiotic effective against whichever bacteria is present will be the treatment of choice. If the infection is due to a virus, such as herpes, treatment is usually symptomatic but may include antiviral medications.

In addition, since sialadenitis usually occurs after decreased flow of saliva (hyposecretion), patients are usually advised to drink plenty of fluids and eat or drink things that trigger saliva flow (such as lemon juice or hard candy). Warm compresses and gland massage may also be helpful if the flow is obstructed in some way. Good oral hygiene is also important. Occasionally an abscess may form which needs to be drained especially if it proves resistant to antibiotics (or antiviral medication). In rare cases of chronic or relapsing sialadenitis, surgery may be needed to remove part or all of the gland. This is more common when there is an underlying condition which is causing the hyposecretion.

Prognosis of Sialadenitis

The prognosis of acute sialadenitis is very good. Most salivary gland infections go away on their own or are easily cured with treatment with conservative medical management (medication, increasing fluid intake and warm compresses or gland massage). Acute symptoms usually resolve within one week; however, edema in the area may last several weeks. Complications are not common, but may occur and can include abscess of the salivary gland or localized spreading of bacterial infection (such as cellulitis or Ludwig angina). In chronic or relapsing sialadenitis, the prognosis depends on the underlying cause of the infection.

Section 39.3

Sjögren Syndrome

This section includes text excerpted from "Sjögren's
Syndrome Information Page," National Institute of
Neurological Disorders and Stroke (NINDS), March 27, 2019.

What Is Sjögren Syndrome?

Sjögren syndrome is an autoimmune disorder in which immune
cells attack and destroy the glands that produce tears and saliva.
Sjögren syndrome is also associated with rheumatic disorders, such
as rheumatoid arthritis (RA).

Symptoms of Sjögren Syndrome

The hallmark symptoms of the disorder are dry mouth and dry
eyes. In addition, Sjogren syndrome may cause skin, nose, and vaginal
dryness and may affect other organs of the body, including the kidneys,
blood vessels, lungs, liver, pancreas, and brain.

Sjögren syndrome affects 1 to 4 million people in the United States.
Most people are more than 40 years old at the time of diagnosis. Women
are 9 times more likely to have Sjögren syndrome than men.

Treatment of Sjögren Syndrome

There is no known cure for Sjögren syndrome, nor is there a specific
treatment to restore gland secretion. Treatment is generally symptomatic and supportive. Moisture replacement therapies may ease the
symptoms of dryness. Nonsteroidal anti-inflammatory drugs (NSAIDs)
may be used to treat musculoskeletal symptoms. For individuals with
severe complications, corticosteroids or immunosuppressive drugs may
be prescribed.

Prognosis of Sjögren Syndrome

Sjögren syndrome can damage vital organs of the body with symptoms that may remain stable, worsen, or go into remission. Some people may experience only mild symptoms of dry eyes and mouth, while
others go through cycles of good health followed by severe disease.
Many patients are able to treat problems symptomatically. Others are

forced to cope with blurred vision, constant eye discomfort, recurrent mouth infections, swollen parotid glands, hoarseness, and difficulty in swallowing and eating. Debilitating fatigue and joint pain can seriously impair quality of life.

Chapter 40

Jaw Problems

Chapter Contents

277

Section 40.1

Temporomandibular Joint and Muscle Disorders

This section includes text excerpted from "TMJ (Temporomandibular Joint and Muscle Disorders)," National Institute of Dental and Craniofacial Research (NIDCR), July 2018.

What Are Temporomandibular Joint and Muscle Disorders?

Temporomandibular joint and muscle disorders, commonly called "TMJ," are a group of conditions that cause pain and dysfunction in the jaw joint and muscles that control jaw movement.

Researchers generally agree that the conditions fall into three main categories:

1. Myofascial pain involves discomfort or pain in the muscles that control jaw function.

2. Internal derangement of the joint involves a displaced disc, dislocated jaw, or injury to the condyle.

3. Arthritis refers to a group of degenerative/inflammatory joint disorders that can affect the temporomandibular joint.

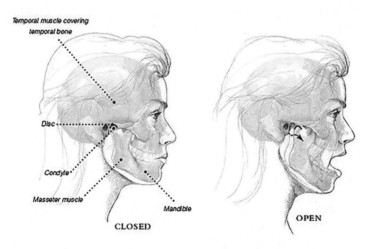

Figure 40.1. *Temporomandibular Joint and Muscle Disorders*

278

A person may have one or more of these conditions at the same time. Some estimates suggest that TMJ disorders affect over 10 million Americans. These conditions appear to be more common in women than in men.

Causes of Temporomandibular Joint and Muscle Disorders

Trauma to the jaw or temporomandibular joint plays a role in some TMJ disorders, but in most cases, the exact cause of the condition is not clear. For many people, symptoms seem to start without an obvious reason. Because TMJ is more common in women than in men, scientists are exploring a possible link between female hormones and TMJ disorders.

Symptoms of Temporomandibular Joint and Muscle Disorders

A variety of symptoms may be linked to TMJ disorders. The most common symptom is pain in the chewing muscles and/or jaw joint. Other symptoms include:

- Radiating pain in the face, jaw, or neck
- Jaw muscle stiffness
- Limited movement or locking of the jaw
- Painful clicking, popping, or grating in the jaw joint when opening or closing the mouth
- A change in the way the upper and lower teeth fit together

Diagnosis of Temporomandibular Joint and Muscle Disorders

There is no widely accepted, standard test now available to correctly diagnose TMJ disorders. Because the exact causes and symptoms are not clear, identifying these disorders can be difficult and confusing.

Your doctor will note your symptoms, take a detailed medical history, and examine problem areas, including the head, neck, face, and jaw for tenderness, clicking, popping, or difficulty with movement. The doctor might also suggest imaging studies such as an x-ray.

You may want to ask your doctor about other causes of pain. Facial pain can be a symptom of many conditions, such as sinus or ear infections, various types of headaches, and facial neuralgias (nerve-related facial pain). Ruling out these problems first helps in identifying TMJ disorders.

Treatment of Temporomandibular Joint and Muscle Disorders

Because more studies are needed on the safety and effectiveness of most treatments for jaw joint and muscle disorders, experts strongly recommend using the most conservative, reversible treatments possible. Conservative treatments do not invade the tissues of the face, jaw, or joint, or involve surgery. Reversible treatments do not cause permanent changes in the structure or position of the jaw or teeth. Even when TMJ disorders have become persistent, most patients still do not need aggressive types of treatment.

Conservative Treatments

Because the most common jaw joint and muscle problems are temporary and do not get worse, simple treatment may be all that is necessary to relieve discomfort. Short-term use of over-the-counter (OTC) pain medicines or nonsteroidal anti-inflammatory drugs (NSAIDs), such as ibuprofen; the use of a stabilization splint, or bite guard, that fits over upper or lower teeth may provide relief. If a stabilization splint is recommended, it should be used only for a short time and should not cause permanent changes in bite. Studies of their effectiveness in providing pain relief have been inconclusive.

Irreversible Treatments

Surgical treatments are controversial, often irreversible, and should be avoided where possible. There have been no long-term clinical trials to study the safety and effectiveness of surgical treatments for TMJ disorders. Additionally, surgical replacement of jaw joints with artificial implants may cause severe pain and permanent jaw damage. Some of these devices may fail to function properly or may break apart in the jaw over time.

Helpful Tips

Self-care practices that may help ease symptoms of TMJ:

- Eating soft foods

- Applying an ice pack

- Avoiding extreme jaw movements, such as wide yawning, loud singing, and gum chewing

- Learning techniques to relax and reduce stress

- Practicing gentle jaw stretching and relaxing exercises that may help increase jaw movement

Section 40.2

Osteonecrosis and Jaw Pain

Osteonecrosis
What Is Osteonecrosis?

Osteonecrosis is a disease of the bones. When there is no blood supply to the bones, the tissues in the bones die and the bones collapse. This will render the surrounding joints unable to function. When such difficulty occurs, a person experiences pain due to stressful joints. The person will find it hard to move due to mild or even severe pain.

What Is Osteonecrosis of the Jaw?

Osteonecrosis of the jaw (ONJ) is a lesion in the mouth that involves the exposure of the maxillary bone or the mandible. This exposure is painful and accompanied by pus discharge. The condition can occur after tooth extraction. When osteonecrosis of the jaw is linked with excessive or prolonged antiresorptive drug use (drugs such as bisphosphonates or denosumab), it is called "medication-related ONJ."

Risk Factors Leading to Medication-Related Osteonecrosis of the Jaw

- Extraction of the tooth

- Denture wearing

- Poor oral hygiene

- Periodontitis (serious infection of the gum that leads to soft tissue damage of the tooth)

- Smoking

How Do Oral Lesions Occur?

Oral lesions are mouth ulcers that occur due to a break in the skin or mucous membrane in the oral cavity. Ulcers form due to a loss of surface tissue or disintegration of epithelial tissue. Ulcers usually occur when the tooth gets weak and begins to break. Sometimes it could even be a broken filling. The sharp edges of a broken tooth begin to hurt the skin inside the oral cavity, which results in sores. These sores get inflamed and ulcerous. When such conditions persist and treatment is delayed, the ulcers can turn into oral cancer.

How Are Oral Lesions and Mouth Ulcers Treated?

Minor ulcers of the mouth require no treatment. If ulcers persist or are recurring, then following these measures may help:

- Rinse the mouth with saltwater and baking soda.

- Rinse the mouth with steroids to reduce swelling.

- Try anesthetic products, such as Orajel™ or Anbesol (over-the-counter (OTC) benzocaine).

- Try supplements, such as vitamin B_6 and vitamin B_{12}, folic acid, and zinc.

- Keep moist tea bags on the ulcers.

Here Are Some Tips for Preventing Mouth Ulcers and Oral Lesions

- Avoid acidic fruits, such as lemons, oranges, grapefruit, and pineapple.

- Avoid spicy food such as chips.

- Eat a balanced diet rich in multivitamins.

- Avoid talking while eating because biting the flesh inside the mouth accidentally can cause sores.

- Get plenty of rest to prevent mouth ulcers.

Jaw Pain
What Is Jaw Pain?

Jaw pain is common among millions of people. Accurate diagnosis of the pain is crucial for successful treatment. Some causes of jaw and facial pain include:

- Arthritis (inflammation of the bone and joints of the mandibular bone), nerve injuries, and physical and blood vessel problems

- Teeth grinding and clenching that occur due to increased emotional stress

- Infection of the tooth tissues, which causes osteomyelitis

- Osteoarthritis and osteoarthrosis that occur due to the wearing away of the jawbones

- Synovitis or capsulitis that occurs when ligaments get inflamed

- Cavities, gum diseases, abscesses, and damaged teeth

- Inflamed sinuses and headaches

- Nerve damage that triggers pain signals

- Lifestyle-related factors, such as emotional problems, disturbances during sleep, lack of nutrients, and extreme fatigue or tiredness

- Rheumatoid arthritis, mental-health conditions, and hypothyroidism

Symptoms of Jaw Pain

Some of the symptoms of jaw pain include:

- Jaw alignment problems

- Restricted movement of the jaw

- Muscle tenderness

- Locking of the upper and lower jaws
- Headaches and earaches and pressure behind the eyes
- Toothache and dizziness
- Burning sensation in the nerves
- Fever accompanied by facial swelling

Complications and Diagnosis

Complications that accompany jaw pain may be dental and surgical, and stem from chronic pain, eating habit changes, emotional distress, and infection. Jaw pain can be diagnosed by physical examination comprising evaluation of the nerves and neck bones, jaw, mouth, and muscles. A complete medical history is taken, including lab tests, such as an erythrocyte sedimentation rate (ESR) blood test, x-rays, and psychological and psychiatric screenings in certain scenarios.

Treatments for Jaw Pain

Treatment methods for jaw pain vary and can include:

- Antidepressants to help alleviate pain
- Antibiotics to combat pain caused by infections
- Muscle tranquilizers prescribed to relax the affected muscles
- Surgery to get rid of the damaged bone
- Root canal treatment to remove infections within teeth

The ones with jaw pain can reduce excessive jaw movement by replacing crunchy food with a softer diet in order to avoid excessive pain.

Preventive Measures for Jaw Pain

Common preventive measures include:

- Avoid chewing hard or crunchy food items (such as ice).
- Add calcium and magnesium supplements, as may be relevant.
- Avoid grinding teeth.
- Take care of teeth with proper dental care.

References

1. "Osteonecrosis," National Institute of Arthritis and Musculoskeletal and Skin Diseases (NIAMS), October 30, 2015.

2. "Oral Health Topics—Osteoporosis Medications and Medication-Related Osteonecrosis of the Jaw," Center for Scientific Information, American Dental Association (ADA) Science Institute, July 3, 2019.

3. Johnson, Shannon. "What Causes Mouth Ulcers and How to Treat Them," Healthline Media, December 20, 2017.

4. "Oral Science Protocols—Oral Lesions," Oral Science, March 5, 2017.

5. "Periodontitis," Mayo Clinic—Mayo Foundation for Medical Education and Research (MFMER), March 6, 2018.

6. Smith, Lori. "Everything You Need to Know about Jaw Pain," MedicalNewsToday, Healthline Media UK Ltd, Brighton, UK, April 27, 2017.

Chapter 41

Leukoplakia

Leukoplakia is a condition in which thickened, white patches form on the tongue, gums, inside of the cheek, or sometimes on the outer female genitals. Although the sores can vary in appearance, they are usually white or gray; thick, and slightly raised with a hard surface. The condition is thought to be caused by irritation, but the cause is not always known. Tobacco is considered to be the main cause of its development in the mouth. Most patches are benign, but a small percentage show early signs of cancer. Removing the source of irritation may cause the condition to go away, but surgery to remove the sore(s) may be necessary in some cases.

Symptoms of Leukoplakia

Early signs of cancer may not be apparent. The clinical appearance of leukoplakia does not generally correlate with its appearance when examined under a microscope. For example, the lesion may appear unchanged for a period of time but may actually show changes when looked at under a microscope. Therefore, a biopsy is typically recommended in all cases to determine which lesions are precancerous. Small lesions may be biopsied and just followed periodically if it is shown to remain benign. However, those that show precancerous or cancerous features should be removed.

This chapter includes text excerpted from "Leukoplakia," Genetic and Rare Diseases Information Center (GARD), National Center for Advancing Translational Sciences (NCATS), May 21, 2012. Reviewed July 2019.

Treatment of Leukoplakia

For most people, removing the source of irritation is important and often causes the lesion to disappear. For example, if tobacco use is thought to be the cause, stopping tobacco use usually clears the condition. Dental causes, such as rough teeth or fillings should be treated as soon as possible. When this is not effective or if the lesions show early signs of cancer, treatment may include removing the patches. The lesion is usually removed in the healthcare provider's office using local anesthesia. Leukoplakia on the vulva is treated in the same way as oral lesions. Recurrences are common, so follow-up visits with a physician are recommended.

Prognosis of Leukoplakia

Leukoplakia usually does not cause complications or permanent damage. Sores often clear up a few weeks or months after the source of irritation is removed. Although most leukoplakia patches are benign (noncancerous), a small percentage show early signs of cancer, and many cancers of the mouth occur next to areas of leukoplakia. Even after leukoplakia patches are removed, the risk of oral cancer remains higher than in the general population. Prognosis is better when leukoplakia is found and treated early.

Chapter 42

Mouth Sores

What Are Mouth Sores?

Mouth sores are common ailments that appear on the soft tissues of your mouth, including the cheeks, lips, tongue, gums, and roof and floor of the mouth. There is also a possibility of developing mouth sores in your esophagus—a muscular tube that carries food and liquids from your mouth to the stomach.

There are many types of mouth sores; however, the most common types are cold sores and canker sores. Cold sores, sometimes called "fever blisters," form around your lips.

Canker sores, also called "aphthous ulcers," are shallow, small lesions that develop on the soft tissues in the mouth or at the base of your gums.

Causes of Mouth Sores

Mostly, mouth sores occur as a result of irritation from:

- Biting your cheek, tongue, or lip
- Burning your mouth from hot drinks or foods
- Chewing tobacco
- A sharp or broken tooth

"Mouth Sores: Causes and Care," © 2019 Omnigraphics. Reviewed July 2019.

- Braces

In other cases, mouth sores can develop due to the following reasons:

- High acidic foods
- Stress
- Hormonal changes during pregnancy
- Vitamin and folate deficiencies

The sores can spread from person to person by close contact (such as kissing).

Cold sores are caused by the herpes simplex virus (HSV) and are contagious. Unlike cold sores, canker sores do not occur on the surface of the lips and are not contagious. The cause of the canker sores remains unclear, but it may be related to:

- Virus
- Irritation
- Minor injury during dental operations
- Overzealous brushing
- Mouth rinses and toothpastes containing lauryl sulfate
- Diet lacking in vitamin B_{12}, zinc, folate, or iron
- Hormonal changes during menstruation

Rarely, mouth sores can be a sign of a tumor or illness. In such cases, they may form in response to:

- Mouth cancer
- Infection (such as hand-foot-mouth syndrome)
- Bleeding disorders
- Weakened immune system
- Autoimmune disorders

Certain drugs and medications, such as aspirin, penicillin, phenytoin, streptomycin, chemotherapeutic agents, and sulfa drugs. tend to cause mouth sores.

Signs and Symptoms of Mouth Sores
Cold Sores

Cold sores are tiny, fluid-filled blisters that occur around your lips. These blisters are often grouped together in patches. The symptoms of cold sores are:

- Blisters, lesions, or ulcers in the mouth
- Pain in the mouth or tongue
- Lip swelling
- Sore throat
- Difficulty swallowing
- Swollen glands
- Fever
- Headache

The signs and symptoms may vary depending on whether this is a recurrence or the first outbreak.

Canker Sores

Canker sores appear either as a single pale or yellow ulcer with a red outer ring or as a cluster of sores. The major symptoms of canker sores are:

- Severe pain
- Fever
- Extreme difficulty eating and drinking

How to Take Care of Your Mouth Sores

Mouth sores can last from 10 to 14 days. Usually, mouth sores do not need any treatment, but persistent, large, and painful sores often do need medical attention. Follow these steps to make yourself feel better:

- Gargle with salt or cold water.
- Apply cool compression.
- Avoid hot beverages.

- Avoid eating spicy and salty foods.

- Avoid citrus fruits.

- Avoid alcohol.

- Take pain relievers, such as acetaminophen.

  For canker sores:

- Apply a thin paste of water and baking soda to the sore.

- For severe cases, anti-inflammatory amlexanox paste (Aphthasol®) or fluocinonide gel (Lidex®) is recommended.

Over-the-counter (OTC) medicines (such as creams, pastes, gels, or liquids) can help relieve the pain caused by mouth sores and to speed up the healing process.

When to See the Doctor

You must consult the doctor, if:

- You have large patches on the tongue or roof of the mouth

- The sore begins after starting a new medication

- The sore lasts more than two weeks

- You have other symptoms, such as a skin rash, drooling, fever, or difficulty swallowing

What to Expect during a Doctor's Visit

The doctor will perform a physical examination of your tongue and mouth and review your medical history and symptoms.
The treatment will consist of the following:

- Antiviral medication to treat the sores that are caused by the HSV virus

- Medicine to numb the area that is causing extreme pain; this medicine may be prescribed as an ointment, such as lidocaine (which must not be used for children)

- Steroid gel to apply to the mouth sore

- A paste that stops swelling and inflammation (Aphthasol®)

The doctor will prescribe a mouthwash, such as chlorhexidine gluconate (Peridex®), or a solution to use to rinse the mouth. This will help you to heal and prevent further infections. The doctor may recommend a nutritional supplement, such as folate, zinc, or vitamin B_{12}, if you are low on nutrients.

Prevention of Mouth Sores

Mouth sores are common and can be prevented from spreading.

The following steps can be followed to prevent mouth sores from spreading:

- Avoid close contact with people who have sores. The virus spreads more quickly when the sores secrete moisture from blisters.

- Avoid sharing items. Towels, utensils, and lip balms can spread the virus when blisters are present.

- Keep your hands clean.

References

1. "Cold Sore," Mayo Clinic, December 20, 2018.

2. "Canker Sore," Mayo Clinic, April 3, 2018.

3. Fletcher, Jenna. "Mouth Sores: Everything You Need to Know," Medical News Today, March 12, 2019.

4. Nordqvist, Christian. "Everything You Need to Know about Cold Sores," Medical News Today, May 19, 2017.

Chapter 43

Oral Allergy Syndrome

Allergies are a common chronic disease that occurs when the body's immune system fights off foreign substances that it identifies as harmful. The immune system, a defense mechanism of the body, generates antibodies that help get rid of these foreign substances. When the body sounds an alarm about a substance being harmful, this is called an "allergic reaction." The substances can be found in food, as well as in the environment. Skin irritation, watery eyes, or sneezing are common allergic reactions. Sometimes a more severe condition called "anaphylaxis," which is discussed later in this chapter, can also occur, and it is life-threatening.

What Is Oral Allergy Syndrome?

Oral allergy syndrome (OAS) occurs in adults and children. This allergy is related to food. A person can develop this allergy after consuming certain herbs, nuts or seeds, vegetables, and fresh fruits. Research shows that if the food contains particular proteins that have a structure similar to that of pollen grains, then allergic reactions can get triggered. That is, when the body mistakes a fruit protein for pollen, the immunoglobulin E antibody present in the immune system reacts and the allergic reaction occurs. Therefore, OAS is sometimes referred to as "pollen–fruit allergy syndrome."

"Oral Allergy Syndrome," © 2019 Omnigraphics. Reviewed July 2019.

Common Symptoms of Oral Allergy Syndrome

Oral allergy syndrome symptoms are usually oral (observed in the mouth), but they can affect the rest of the body too in rare cases. The following symptoms are associated with OAS:

- Itchy tongue
- Itchy roof of the mouth (palate)
- Tingling feelings on the tongue
- Swollen lips
- Numb lips
- Scratchy throat
- Sneezing and nasal congestion

What Foods Trigger Oral Allergy Syndrome

People react differently to different food. These common foods can trigger OAS:

- Fresh fruits, such as cherries, apples, oranges, peaches, and bananas
- Fresh vegetables, such as carrots, cucumbers, bell peppers, and tomatoes
- Herbs, such as parsley and cilantro
- Sunflower seeds
- Hazelnuts and almonds (although the allergy caused by these nuts is not as severe or fatal as other nut allergies)
- Generally, OAS is not so serious. However, there is a slight chance of the allergy getting worse and anaphylaxis occurring. Studies have shown that less than two percent of the population experiences anaphylaxis.

Reducing Risks of Oral Allergy Syndrome

Avoiding foods that cause OAS is the best and most straightforward method to not develop OAS. However, practice the below ways to reduce the risks of OAS.

- Peel vegetables or fruit to get rid of allergy-causing proteins that are present in the skin.

- Cook vegetables and heat food to eliminate allergens. Deploying heat while preparing food causes chemical changes in the food, which in turn makes the food allergen-free.

- Buy canned or preserved fruits and vegetables.

Treatment of Oral Allergy Syndrome

Some common ways to reduce OAS symptoms follow:

- Use ice packs to reduce swelling and itching.

- Use over-the-counter (OTC) histamine blockers, such as diphenhydramine (Benadryl®) and fexofenadine (Allegra®) and decongestants to help relieve itchiness in the mouth. These drugs sometimes suppress other reactions caused by OAS as well.

  - Antihistamines and decongestants can help prevent symptoms, such as hives by ensuring that your body does not react to allergens.

  - Decongestants can help clear the nose.

  - Antihistamines and decongestants are available in the form of tablets, nasal sprays, and eye drops.

  - The side effects of OTC drugs cause drowsiness. Therefore, avoid driving and rest.

  - Do not take antihistamines and decongestants for more than three consecutive days.

Who Is Vulnerable to Oral Allergy Syndrome?

Oral allergy syndrome is common in people who are allergic to ragweed pollen, birch pollen, and grass pollen, as reported by the American College of Allergy, Asthma, and Immunology (ACAAI). The season of pollination (April through June) is the peak time for allergies, such as OAS. Also, the autumn months (September and October), when trees lose their leaves and seeds, can cause OAS symptoms.

What Is Anaphylaxis?

About two percent of Americans are at risk for anaphylaxis, and children are particularly prone to medicine allergies. They are also allergic to certain foods, insects, and latex. Anaphylaxis can result in shock, a sudden blood pressure fluctuation, and choking. It could even lead to cardiac arrest. Symptoms of anaphylaxis are concentrated on the skin, and in the mouth and eyes; severe cases also involve the lungs, heart, gut, and brain.

Symptoms of Anaphylaxis

- Itchiness and hives
- Skin rashes
- Swollen lips, tongue, and throat
- Mild-to-severe breathing difficulties
- Fainting
- Severe stomach pain
- Vomiting or diarrhea

Treatment of Anaphylaxis

- Call 911 immediately.
- Keep the person calm.
- Slowly ease the person into lying on her or his back.
- Raise the feet 10 to 12 inches.
- Cover the person with a blanket, and make sure that clothing is loose and comfortable.
- Do not give any oral medicine if the person is having trouble breathing.
- If you know how to administer epinephrine to the patient, then look for the patient's auto-injector, which is a safe and easy way to reduce symptoms.

You can help a person who is choking, coughing, and finding it difficult to breathe because of with anaphylaxis by using cardiopulmonary resuscitation (CPR). You do not have to be formally trained to assist with CPR. The affected person should be given chest presses at a rate of approximately 100 per minute until emergency services arrives.

References

1. "Living with Food Allergies," Kids with Food Allergies—A Division of the Asthma and Allergy Foundation of America (AAFA), June 15, 2014.

2. "What Is Oral Allergy Syndrome?" Healthline Media, May 8, 2019.

Chapter 44

Oral Cancer

Chapter Contents

Section 44.1

What You Need to Know about Oral Cancer

This section includes text excerpted from "Lip and Oral
Cavity Cancer Treatment (Adult) (PDQ®)—Patient Version,"
National Cancer Institute (NCI), March 7, 2019.

Lip and oral cavity cancer is a disease in which malignant (cancer)
cells form in the lips or mouth.

The oral cavity includes the following:

- The front two-thirds of the tongue

- The gingiva (gums)

- The buccal mucosa (the lining of the inside of the cheeks)

- The floor (bottom) of the mouth under the tongue

- The hard palate (the roof of the mouth)

- The retromolar trigone (the small area behind the wisdom teeth)

Most lip and oral cavity cancers start in squamous cells, the thin,
flat cells lining the inside of the lips and oral cavity. These are called
"squamous cell carcinomas (SCC)." Cancer cells may spread into deeper
tissue as the cancer grows. Squamous cell carcinoma usually develops
in areas of leukoplakia (white patches of cells that do not rub off).

Lip and oral cavity cancer is a type of head and neck cancer.

Risks of Lip and Oral Cavity Cancer due to Tobacco and Alcohol Use

Anything that increases your risk of getting a disease is called a
"risk factor." Having a risk factor does not mean that you will get cancer; not having risk factors does not mean that you will not get cancer.
Talk with your doctor if you think you may be at risk. Risk factors for
lip and oral cavity cancer include the following:

- Using tobacco products

- Heavy alcohol use

- Being exposed to natural sunlight or artificial sunlight (such as
  from tanning beds) over long periods of time

- Being male

Signs of Lip and Oral Cavity Cancer

Signs of lip and oral cavity cancer include a sore or lump on the lips or in the mouth.

These and other signs and symptoms may be caused by lip and oral cavity cancer or by other conditions. Check with your doctor if you have any of the following:

- A sore on the lip or in the mouth that does not heal

- A lump or thickening on the lips or gums or in the mouth

- A white or red patch on the gums, tongue, or lining of the mouth

- Bleeding, pain, or numbness in the lip or mouth

- Change in voice

- Loose teeth or dentures that no longer fit well

- Trouble chewing or swallowing or moving the tongue or jaw

- Swelling of the jaw

- Sore throat or feeling that something is caught in the throat

Lip and oral cavity cancer may not have any symptoms and is sometimes found during a regular dental exam.

Diagnosis of Lip and Oral and Cavity Cancer

Tests that examine the mouth and throat are used to detect (find), diagnose, and stage lip and oral cavity cancer. The following tests and procedures may be used:

- **Physical exam of the lips and oral cavity:** An exam to check the lips and oral cavity for abnormal areas. The medical doctor or dentist will feel the entire inside of the mouth with a gloved finger and examine the oral cavity with a small long-handled mirror and lights. This will include checking the insides of the cheeks and lips; the gums; the roof and floor of the mouth; and the top, bottom, and sides of the tongue. The neck will be felt for swollen lymph nodes. A history of the patient's health habits and past illnesses and medical and dental treatments will also be taken.

- **Endoscopy:** A procedure to look at organs and tissues inside the body to check for abnormal areas. An endoscope is inserted through an incision (cut) in the skin or opening in the body, such as the mouth. An endoscope is a thin, tube-like instrument with a light and a lens for viewing. It may also have a tool to remove tissue or lymph node samples, which are checked under a microscope for signs of disease.

- **Biopsy:** The removal of cells or tissues so they can be viewed under a microscope by a pathologist. If leukoplakia is found, cells taken from the patches are also checked under the microscope for signs of cancer.

- **Exfoliative cytology:** A procedure to collect cells from the lip or oral cavity. A piece of cotton, a brush, or a small wooden stick is used to gently scrape cells from the lips, tongue, mouth, or throat. The cells are viewed under a microscope to find out if they are abnormal.

- **Magnetic resonance imaging (MRI):** A procedure that uses a magnet, radio waves, and a computer to make a series of detailed pictures of areas inside the body. This procedure is also called "nuclear magnetic resonance imaging" (NMRI).

- **Computed tomography (CT) scan (computed axial tomography (CAT) scan):** A procedure that makes a series of detailed pictures of areas inside the body, taken from different angles. The pictures are made by a computer linked to an x-ray machine. A dye may be injected into a vein or swallowed to help the organs or tissues show up more clearly. This procedure is also called "computed tomography," "computerized tomography," or "computerized axial tomography."

- **Barium swallow:** A series of x-rays of the esophagus and stomach. The patient drinks a liquid that contains barium (a silver-white metallic compound). The liquid coats the esophagus and x-rays are taken. This procedure is also called an "upper gastrointestinal (GI) series."

- **Positron emission tomography (PET) scan:** A procedure to find malignant tumor cells in the body. A small amount of radioactive glucose (sugar) is injected into a vein. The PET scanner rotates around the body and makes a picture of where glucose is being used in the body. Malignant tumor cells show up brighter in the picture because they are more active and take up more glucose than normal cells do.

- **Bone scan:** A procedure to check if there are rapidly dividing cells, such as cancer cells, in the bone. A very small amount of radioactive material is injected into a vein and travels through the bloodstream. The radioactive material collects in the bones with cancer and is detected by a scanner.

Factors Affecting Prognosis and Treatment Options

Certain factors affect prognosis (chance of recovery) and treatment options.

The prognosis (chance of recovery) depends on the following:

- The stage of cancer

- Where the tumor is in the lip or oral cavity

- Whether the cancer has spread to blood vessels

For patients who smoke, the chance of recovery is better if they stop smoking before beginning radiation therapy (RT).

Treatment options depend on the following:

- The stage of the cancer

- The size of the tumor and where it is in the lip or oral cavity

- Whether the patient's appearance and ability to talk and eat can stay the same

- The patient's age and general health

Patients who have had lip and oral cavity cancer have an increased risk of developing a second cancer in the head or neck. Frequent and careful follow-up is important.

Two types of standard treatment are used:

Surgery

Surgery (removing the cancer in an operation) is a common treatment for all stages of lip and oral cavity cancer. Surgery may include the following:

- **Wide local excision:** Removal of the cancer and some of the healthy tissue around it. If the cancer has spread into bone, surgery may include removal of the involved bone tissue.

305

- **Neck dissection:** Removal of lymph nodes and other tissues in the neck. This is done when cancer may have spread from the lip and oral cavity.

- **Plastic surgery:** An operation that restores or improves the appearance of parts of the body. Dental implants, a skin graft, or other plastic surgery may be needed to repair parts of the mouth, throat, or neck after removal of large tumors.

After the doctor removes all the cancer that can be seen at the time of the surgery, some patients may be given chemotherapy or radiation therapy after surgery to kill any cancer cells that are left. Treatment given after the surgery, to lower the risk that the cancer will come back, is called "adjuvant therapy."

Radiation Therapy

Radiation therapy (RT) is a cancer treatment that uses high-energy x-rays or other types of radiation to kill cancer cells or keep them from growing. There are two types of radiation therapy:

- External radiation therapy uses a machine outside the body to send radiation toward the cancer.

- Internal radiation therapy uses a radioactive substance sealed in needles, seeds, wires, or catheters that are placed directly into or near the cancer.

The way the radiation therapy is given depends on the type and stage of the cancer being treated. External and internal radiation therapy are used to treat lip and oral cavity cancer.

Radiation therapy may work better in patients who have stopped smoking before beginning treatment. It is also important for patients to have a dental exam before radiation therapy begins, so that existing problems can be treated.

Section 44.2

Smokeless Tobacco's Connection to Cancer

This section includes text excerpted from "Smokeless Tobacco: Health Effects," Centers for Disease Control and Prevention (CDC), January 17, 2018.

Smokeless tobacco is associated with many health problems. Using smokeless tobacco:

- Can lead to nicotine addiction

- Causes cancer of the mouth, esophagus (the passage that connects the throat to the stomach), and pancreas (a gland that helps with digestion and maintaining proper blood sugar levels)

- Is associated with diseases of the mouth

- Can increase risks for early delivery and stillbirth when used during pregnancy

- Can cause nicotine poisoning in children

- May increase the risk for death from heart disease and stroke

Using smokeless products can cause serious health problems. Protect your health; do not start. If you do use them, quit.

Addiction to Smokeless Tobacco

- Smokeless tobacco contains nicotine, which is highly addictive.

- Because young people who use smokeless tobacco can become addicted to nicotine, they may be more likely to also become cigarette smokers.

Smokeless Tobacco and Cancer

- Many smokeless tobacco products contain cancer-causing chemicals.

  - The most harmful chemicals are tobacco-specific nitrosamines, which form during the growing, curing, fermenting, and aging of tobacco. The amount of these chemicals varies by product.

- The higher the levels of these chemicals, the greater the risk for cancer.

- Other chemicals found in tobacco can also cause cancer. These include:

  - A radioactive element (polonium-210) found in tobacco fertilizer

  - Chemicals formed when tobacco is cured with heat (polynuclear aromatic hydrocarbons—also known as "polycyclic aromatic hydrocarbons")

  - Harmful metals (arsenic, beryllium, cadmium, chromium, cobalt, lead, nickel, mercury)

  - Smokeless tobacco causes cancer of the mouth, esophagus, and pancreas.

Smokeless Tobacco and Oral Disease

- Smokeless tobacco can cause white or gray patches inside the mouth (leukoplakia) that can lead to cancer.

- Smokeless tobacco can cause gum disease, tooth decay, and tooth loss.

Reproductive and Developmental Risks

- Using smokeless tobacco during pregnancy can increase the risk for early delivery and stillbirth.

- Nicotine in smokeless tobacco products that are used during pregnancy can affect how a baby's brain develops before birth.

Other Risks

- Using smokeless tobacco increases the risk for death from heart disease and stroke.

- Smokeless tobacco can cause nicotine poisoning in children.

- Additional research is needed to examine long-term effects of newer smokeless tobacco products, such as dissolvables and the U.S. snus.

Chapter 45

Taste Disorders

Your Sense of Taste[1]

There are tiny taste buds inside your mouth—on your tongue, in your throat, even on the roof of your mouth. What we call "flavor" is based on five basic tastes: sweet, salty, bitter, sour, and savory. Along with how it tastes, how food smells is also part of what makes up its flavor.

When food tastes bland, many people try to improve the flavor by adding more salt or sugar. This may not be healthy for older people, especially if you have medical problems, such as high blood pressure or diabetes (high blood sugar).

People who have lost some of their sense of taste may not eat the foods they need to stay healthy. This can lead to other issues such as:

- Weight loss

- Malnutrition (not getting the calories, protein, carbohydrates, vitamins, and minerals you need from the food)

- Social isolation

- Depression

This chapter includes text excerpted from documents published by two public domain sources. Text under the headings marked 1 are excerpted from "How Smell and Taste Change as You Age," National Institute on Aging (NIA), National Institutes of Health (NIH), April 1, 2015. Reviewed July 2019; Text under the headings marked 2 are excerpted from "Taste Disorders," National Institute on Deafness and Other Communication Disorders (NIDCD), May 12, 2017.

309

Eating food that is good for you is important to your health. If you have a problem with how food tastes, be sure to talk with your doctor.

What Are Taste Disorders?[2]

The most common taste disorder is phantom taste perception: a lingering, often unpleasant taste even though there is nothing in your mouth. People can also experience a reduced ability to taste sweet, sour, bitter, salty, and umami—a condition called "hypogeusia." Some people cannot detect any tastes, which is called "ageusia." True taste loss, however, is rare. Most often, people are experiencing a loss of smell instead of a loss of taste.

In other disorders of the chemical senses, an odor, taste, or a flavor may be distorted. Dysgeusia is a condition in which a foul, salty, rancid, or metallic taste sensation persists in the mouth. Dysgeusia is sometimes accompanied by burning mouth syndrome, a condition in which a person experiences a painful burning sensation in the mouth. Although it can affect anyone, burning mouth syndrome is most common in middle-aged and older women.

How Common Are Taste Disorders?[2]

Many of us take our sense of taste for granted, but a taste disorder can have a negative effect on your health and quality of life (QOL). If you are having a problem with your sense of taste, you are not alone. More than 200,000 people visit a doctor each year for problems with their ability to taste or smell. Scientists believe that up to 15 percent of adults might have a taste or smell problem, but many do not seek a doctor's help.

The senses of taste and smell are very closely related. Most people who go to the doctor because they think they have lost their sense of taste are surprised to learn that they have a smell disorder instead.

How Does Your Sense of Taste Work?[2]

Your ability to taste comes from tiny molecules released when you chew, drink, or digest food; these molecules stimulate special sensory cells in the mouth and throat. These taste cells, or gustatory cells, are clustered within the taste buds of the tongue and roof of the mouth, and along the lining of the throat. Many of the small bumps on the tip of your tongue contain taste buds. At birth, you have about 10,000 taste buds, but after age 50, you may start to lose them.

When the taste cells are stimulated, they send messages through three specialized taste nerves to the brain, where specific tastes are identified. Taste cells have receptors that respond to one of at least five basic taste qualities: sweet, sour, bitter, salty, and umami. Umami, or savory, is the taste you get from glutamate, which is found in chicken broth, meat extracts, and some cheeses. A common misconception is that taste cells that respond to different tastes are found in separate regions of the tongue. In humans, the different types of taste cells are scattered throughout the tongue.

Taste quality is just one way that you experience a certain food. Another chemosensory mechanism, called the "common chemical sense," involves thousands of nerve endings, especially on the moist surfaces of the eyes, nose, mouth, and throat. These nerve endings give rise to sensations, such as the coolness of mint and the burning or irritation of chili peppers. Other specialized nerves create the sensations of heat, cold, and texture. When you eat, the sensations from the five taste qualities, together with the sensations from the common chemical sense and the sensations of heat, cold, and texture, combine with a food's aroma to produce a perception of flavor. It is the flavor that lets you know whether you are eating a pear or an apple.

Most people who think they have a taste disorder actually have a problem with smell. When you chew food, aromas are released that activate your sense of smell by way of a special channel that connects the roof of the throat to the nose. If this channel is blocked, such as when your nose is stuffed up by a cold or flu, odors cannot reach sensory cells in the nose that are stimulated by smells. As a result, you lose much of our enjoyment of flavor. Without smell, foods tend to taste bland and have little or no flavor.

Colors and Spices Can Help[1]

If you are having trouble smelling and tasting your food, try adding color and texture to make your food more interesting. For example, try eating brightly colored vegetables, such as carrots, sweet potatoes, broccoli, and tomatoes. Also, if your diet allows, flavor your food with a little butter, olive oil, cheese, nuts, or fresh herbs, such as sage, thyme, or rosemary. To put some zing in your food, add mustard, hot pepper, onions, garlic, ginger, different spices, or lemon or lime juice. Choose foods that look good to you.

A Special Doctor for Taste[1]

If the foods you enjoy do not smell or taste the way you think they should talk to your doctor. She or he might suggest you see a specialist who treats people with smell and taste problems. This kind of doctor is called an "otolaryngologist," also known as an "ENT" (which stands for ear, nose, and throat). An otolaryngologist works on problems related to the ear, nose, and throat, as well as the larynx (voice box), mouth, and parts of the neck and face. The doctor may ask:

- Can you smell anything at all?

- Can you taste any food?

- When did you first notice the problem?

- Is the problem getting worse?

- Have you been told that you have allergies or chronic sinus problems?

- What medicines do you take?

There are likely ways to help fix the problem. If not, the doctor can help you cope with the changes in smell and taste.

How Are Taste Disorders Diagnosed?[2]

Both taste and smell disorders are diagnosed by an otolaryngologist (sometimes called an "ENT"), a doctor of the ear, nose, throat, head, and neck. An otolaryngologist can determine the extent of your taste disorder by measuring the lowest concentration of a taste quality that you can detect or recognize. You may be asked to compare the tastes of different substances or to note how the intensity of a taste grows when a substance's concentration is increased.

Scientists have developed taste tests in which the patient responds to different chemical concentrations. This may involve a simple "sip, spit, and rinse" test, or chemicals may be applied directly to specific areas of the tongue.

An accurate assessment of your taste loss will include, among other things, a physical examination of your ears, nose, and throat; a dental examination and assessment of oral hygiene; a review of your health history; and a taste test supervised by a healthcare professional.

What Causes Taste Disorders[2]

Some people are born with taste disorders, but most develop them after an injury or illness. Among the causes of taste problems are:

- Gum disease

- Poor oral hygiene and dental problems

- Smoking

- Alcohol consumption

- Exposure to certain chemicals, such as insecticides and some medications, including some common antibiotics and antihistamines

- Head injury

- Upper respiratory and middle ear infections

- Radiation therapy for cancers of the head and neck

- Some surgeries to the ear, nose, and throat (such as middle ear surgery) or extraction of the third molar (wisdom tooth)

Can Taste Disorders Be Treated?[2]

Diagnosis by an otolaryngologist is important to identify and treat the underlying cause of your disorder. If a certain medication is the cause, stopping or changing your medicine may help eliminate the problem. (Do not stop taking your medications unless directed by your doctor, however.) Often, the correction of a general medical problem can correct the loss of taste. For example, people who lose their sense of taste because of respiratory infections or allergies may regain it when these conditions resolve. Occasionally, a person may recover her or his sense of taste spontaneously. Proper oral hygiene is important to regaining and maintaining a well-functioning sense of taste. If your taste disorder cannot be successfully treated, counseling may help you adjust to your problem.

If you lose some or all of your sense of taste, there are things you can try to make your food taste better:

- Prepare foods with a variety of colors and textures.

- Use aromatic herbs and hot spices to add more flavor; however, avoid adding more sugar or salt to foods.

- If your diet permits, add small amounts of cheese, bacon bits, butter, olive oil, or toasted nuts on vegetables.

- Avoid combination dishes, such as casseroles, that can hide individual flavors and dilute the taste.

Chapter 46

Thrush (Oropharyngeal Candidiasis)

Candidiasis is an infection caused by a yeast (a type of fungus) called *"Candida." Candida* normally lives inside the body (in places such as the mouth, throat, gut, and vagina) and on the skin without causing any problems. Sometimes, *Candida* can multiply and cause an infection if the environment inside the mouth, throat, or esophagus changes in a way that encourages fungal growth.

Candidiasis in the mouth and throat is also called "thrush" or "oropharyngeal candidiasis." Candidiasis in the esophagus (the tube that connects the throat to the stomach) is called "esophageal candidiasis" or *"Candida* esophagitis." Esophageal candidiasis is one of the most common infections in people living with human immunodeficiency virus (HIV)/acquired immunodeficiency syndrome (AIDS).

Symptoms

Candidiasis in the mouth and throat can have many different symptoms, including:

- White patches on the inner cheeks, tongue, the roof of the mouth, and throat (photo showing candidiasis in the mouth)

- Redness or soreness

This chapter includes text excerpted from "Fungal Diseases—*Candida* Infections of the Mouth, Throat, and Esophagus," Centers for Disease Control and Prevention (CDC), April 12, 2019.

315

- Cotton-like feeling in the mouth
- Loss of taste
- Pain while eating or swallowing
- Cracking and redness at the corners of the mouth

Symptoms of candidiasis in the esophagus usually include pain when swallowing and difficulty swallowing.

Risk and Prevention
Who Gets Candidiasis in the Mouth, Throat, or Esophagus

Candidiasis in the mouth, throat, or esophagus is uncommon in healthy adults. People who are at higher risk of getting candidiasis in the mouth and throat include babies, especially those younger than one month old, and people who:

- Wear dentures
- Have diabetes
- Have cancer
- Have HIV/AIDS
- Take antibiotics or corticosteroids, including inhaled corticosteroids for conditions, such as asthma
- Take medications that cause dry mouth or have medical conditions that cause dry mouth
- Smoke

Most people who get candidiasis in the esophagus have weakened immune systems, meaning that their bodies do not fight infections well. This includes people living with HIV/AIDS and people who have blood cancers, such as leukemia and lymphoma. People who get candidiasis in the esophagus often also have candidiasis in the mouth and throat.

How Can I Prevent Candidiasis in the Mouth, Throat, or Esophagus?

Ways to help prevent candidiasis in the mouth and throat include:

- Maintain good oral health
- Rinse your mouth or brush your teeth after using inhaled corticosteroids

Sources

Candida normally lives in the mouth, throat, and the rest of the digestive tract without causing any problems. Sometimes, *Candida* can multiply and cause an infection if the environment inside the mouth, throat, or esophagus changes in a way that encourages its growth. This can happen when a person's immune system becomes weakened if antibiotics affect the natural balance of microbes in the body, or for a variety of other reasons in other groups of people.

Diagnosis and Testing

Healthcare providers can usually diagnose candidiasis in the mouth or throat simply by looking inside. Sometimes a healthcare provider will take a small sample from the mouth or throat. The sample is sent to a laboratory for testing, usually to be examined under a microscope.

Healthcare providers usually diagnose candidiasis in the esophagus by doing an endoscopy. An endoscopy is a procedure to examine the digestive tract using a tube with a light and a camera. A healthcare provider might prescribe antifungal medication without doing an endoscopy to see if the patient's symptoms get better.

Treatment

Candidiasis in the mouth, throat, or esophagus is usually treated with antifungal medicine. The treatment for mild to moderate infections in the mouth or throat is usually an antifungal medicine applied to the inside of the mouth for 7 to 14 days. These medications include clotrimazole, miconazole, or nystatin. For severe infections, the treatment is usually fluconazole or another type of antifungal medicine given by mouth or through a vein for people who do not get better after taking fluconazole. The treatment for candidiasis in the esophagus is usually fluconazole. Other types of prescription antifungal medicines can also be used for people who cannot take fluconazole or who do not get better after taking fluconazole.

Statistics

The exact number of cases of candidiasis in the mouth, throat, and esophagus in the United States is difficult to determine because there is no national surveillance for these infections. The risk of these infections varies based on the presence of certain underlying medical conditions. For example, candidiasis in the mouth, throat, or esophagus is uncommon in healthy adults. However, they are some of the most common infections in people living with HIV/AIDS. In one study, approximately one-third of patients with advanced HIV infection had candidiasis in the mouth and throat.

Chapter 47

Tongue Disorders

Chapter Contents

Section 47.1

Giant Tongue (Macroglossia)

This section includes text excerpted from "Macroglossia,"
Genetic and Rare Diseases Information Center (GARD), National
Center for Advancing Translational Sciences (NCATS),
September 16, 2015. Reviewed July 2019.

Macroglossia is the abnormal enlargement of the tongue in proportion to other structures in the mouth. It usually occurs secondary to an underlying disorder that may be present from birth (congenital) or acquired. In rare cases, it is an isolated, congenital feature. Symptoms associated with macroglossia may include drooling; speech impairment; difficulty eating; stridor; snoring; airway obstruction; abnormal growth of the jaw and teeth; ulceration; and/or dying tissue on the tip of the tongue. The tongue may protrude from the mouth. Inherited or congenital disorders associated with macroglossia include Down syndrome, Beckwith-Wiedemann syndrome (BWS), primary amyloidosis, and congenital hypothyroidism. Acquired causes may include trauma, cancer, endocrine disorders, and inflammatory or infectious diseases. Isolated, congenital macroglossia can be genetic, inherited in an autosomal dominant manner. Treatment depends upon the underlying cause and severity and may range from speech therapy in mild cases, to surgical reduction in more severe cases.

Causes of Macroglossia

Macroglossia can be associated with a wide range of congenital (present from birth) and acquired conditions, or it can occur as an isolated feature (with no other abnormalities). In most cases, it is due to vascular malformations (blood vessel abnormalities) and muscular hypertrophy (an increase in muscle mass).

Congenital or inherited causes of macroglossia may include various syndromes (e.g., Beckwith-Wiedemann syndrome or Down syndrome); hemangioma; congenital hypothyroidism; mucopolysaccharidosis; and neurofibromatosis.

Acquired causes may include metabolic or endocrine conditions, such as hypothyroidism, amyloidosis, and acromegaly; inflammatory/ infectious diseases, such as pemphigus vulgaris, diphtheria, tuberculosis (TB), and sarcoidosis; and trauma.

Neoplastic conditions (involving abnormal or uncontrolled cell growth) may also cause macroglossia, such as lymphangioma or various malignancies (cancers).

In some cases, macroglossia occurs as an isolated hereditary trait that is inherited in an autosomal dominant manner.

Treatment of Macroglossia

Medical therapy for macroglossia is useful when the underlying cause is identified, and the cause is medically treatable—such as hypothyroidism, infection, or amyloidosis. No medical treatments have been proven useful when the cause is unclear. Surgery to reduce the size of the tongue may be an option for people with macroglossia. Most studies have shown that surgical procedures for macroglossia lead to improved physical appearance, speech, chewing and feeding.

Section 47.2

Tongue Tie (Ankyloglossia)

This section includes text excerpted from "Treatments for Ankyloglossia and Ankyloglossia with Concomitant Lip-Tie," Effective Health Care Program, Agency for Healthcare Research and Quality (AHRQ), May 2015. Reviewed July 2019.

Ankyloglossia is a congenital condition characterized by an abnormally short, thickened, or tight lingual frenulum, or an anterior attachment of the lingual frenulum, that restricts the mobility of the tongue. It variably causes reduced anterior tongue mobility and has been associated with functional limitations in breastfeeding; swallowing; articulation; orthodontic problems, including malocclusion, open bite, and separation of lower incisors; mechanical problems related to oral clearance; and psychological stress. One review including studies of infants, children, and adults reported rates of ankyloglossia ranging from 0.1 to 10.7 percent, but definitive incidence and prevalence statistics are elusive due to an absence of a criterion standard or clinically practical diagnostic criteria.

Recognition of potential benefits of breastfeeding in recent years has resulted in a renewed interest in the functional sequelae of ankyloglossia. In infants with anterior or posterior ankyloglossia, there is a reported 25 to 80 percent incidence of breastfeeding difficulties, including failure to thrive, maternal nipple damage, maternal breast pain, poor milk supply, maternal breast engorgement, and refusing the breast. An ineffective latch is hypothesized to underlie these problems.

Mechanistically, infants with restrictive ankyloglossia cannot extend their tongues over the lower gumline to form a proper seal and, therefore, use their jaws to keep the breast in the mouth for breastfeeding.

Adequate tongue mobility is required for breastfeeding, and infants with ankyloglossia often cannot overcome their deficiency with conservative measures, such as positioning and latching techniques, thereby requiring surgical correction.

Nonetheless, the consensus on ankyloglossia's role in breastfeeding difficulties is lacking. A minority of surveyed pediatricians (10%) and otolaryngologists (30%) believe it commonly affects feeding, while 69 percent of lactation consultants feel that it frequently causes breastfeeding problems. Therefore, depending on the audience, enthusiasm for its treatment varies. Currently, the U.K. National Health Service (NHS) and the Canadian Paediatric Society (CPS) recommend treatment only if it interferes with breastfeeding. A standard definition of "interference" with breastfeeding is not provided, leaving room for interpretation and variation in treatment thresholds. The absence of data on the natural history of untreated ankyloglossia further promulgates uncertainty. Some propose that a short frenulum elongates spontaneously due to progressive stretching and thinning of the frenulum with age and use. However, there are no prospective longitudinal data on the congenitally short lingual frenulum. Without this information it is difficult to inform parents fully about the long-term implications of ankyloglossia, thereby complicating the decision-making process.

Although most ankyloglossia research is focused on the infant and breastfeeding issues, concerns beyond infancy include speech-related issues, such as difficulty with articulation, and social concerns related to limited tongue mobility. Individuals with untreated ankyloglossia may experience difficulty with oral mechanism, particularly in relation to licking ice cream, kissing, drooling, playing wind instruments, and licking the lips. Self-esteem or psychological issues may also be a concern for affected older patients.

Treatment Strategies

Ankyloglossia may be treated with surgical or nonsurgical approaches. Surgical modalities include frenotomy, frenulectomy, and frenuloplasty. These interventions involve clipping or cutting of the lingual frenulum, generally without sedation. Laser frenotomy or frenulotomy has also been described, and proponents argue that its use is more exact and provides better hemostasis than standard frenotomy or frenulotomy. Frenuloplasty, more technically involved than frenotomy or frenulotomy, generally refers to rearranging tissue or adding grafts after making incisions and closing the resultant wound in a specific pattern to lengthen the anterior tongue. Frenuloplasty is most commonly performed under a general anesthetic and used in older infants and children or in more complex frenulum repairs. Nonsurgical approaches include speech therapy, lactation interventions, and observation to determine if intervention is warranted.

Part Six

Health Conditions That Affect Oral Health

Chapter 48

Cancer Treatment and Oral Complications

Chapter Contents

Section 48.1

Three Good Reasons to See a Dentist before Cancer Treatment

This section includes text excerpted from "Three Good Reasons to See a Dentist before Cancer Treatment," National Institute of Dental and Craniofacial Research (NIDCR), September 2015. Reviewed July 2019.

Three good reasons to see a dentist before cancer treatment:

1. **Feel better:** Cancer treatment can cause side effects in your mouth. A dental checkup before treatment starts can help prevent painful mouth problems.

2. **Save teeth and bones:** A dentist will help protect your mouth, teeth, and jawbones from damage caused by head and neck radiation and chemotherapy. Children also need special protection for their growing teeth and facial bones.

3. **Fight cancer:** Serious side effects in the mouth can delay, or even stop, cancer treatment. To fight cancer best, your cancer care team should include a dentist.

Protect Your Mouth during Cancer Treatment
Brush Gently, Brush Often

- Brush your teeth—and your tongue—gently with an extra-soft toothbrush.
- Soften the bristles in warm water if your mouth is very sore.
- Brush after every meal and at bedtime.

Floss Gently—Do It Daily

- Floss once a day to remove plaque.
- Avoid areas of your gums that are bleeding or sore, but keep flossing your other teeth.

Keep Your Mouth Moist

- Rinse often with water.
- Do not use mouthwashes that contain alcohol.

328

- Use a saliva substitute to help moisten your mouth

Eat and Drink with Care

- Choose soft, easy-to-chew foods.

- Protect your mouth from spicy, sour, or crunchy foods.

- Choose lukewarm foods and drinks instead of hot or icy-cold ones.

- Avoid alcoholic drinks.

Stop Using Tobacco

- Ask your cancer care team to help you stop smoking or chewing tobacco. People who quit smoking or chewing tobacco have fewer mouth problems.

Tips to Help You Care for Mouth Problems

- **Sore mouth, sore throat:** To help keep your mouth clean, rinse often with ¼ teaspoon of salt and ¼ teaspoon of baking soda in 1 quart (4 cups) of warm water. Follow with a plain water rinse. Ask your cancer care team about medicines that can help with the pain.

- **Dry mouth:** Rinse your mouth often with water, use sugar-free gum or candy, and talk to your dentist about saliva substitutes.

- **Infections:** Call your cancer care team right away if you see a sore, swelling, bleeding, or a sticky, white film in your mouth.

- **Eating problems:** Your cancer care team can help by giving you medicines to numb the pain from mouth sores and showing you how to choose foods that are easy to swallow.

- **Bleeding:** If your gums bleed or hurt, avoid flossing the areas that are bleeding or sore, but keep flossing other teeth. Soften the bristles of your toothbrush in warm water.

- **Stiffness in chewing muscles:** Three times a day, open and close your mouth as far as you can without pain. Repeat 20 times.

- **Vomiting:** Rinse your mouth after vomiting with ¼ teaspoon of baking soda in 1 cup of warm water.

- **Cavities:** Brush your teeth after meals and before bedtime. Your dentist might have you put fluoride gel on your teeth to help prevent cavities.

When Should You Call Your Cancer Care Team about Mouth Problems?

Take a moment each day to check how your mouth looks and feels. Call your cancer care team when:

- You first notice a mouth problem.

- An old problem gets worse.

- You notice any changes you are not sure about.

Section 48.2

Chemotherapy and Your Mouth

This section includes text excerpted from "Chemotherapy and Your Mouth," National Institute of Dental and Craniofacial Research (NIDCR), August 2013. Reviewed July 2019.

Are You Being Treated with Chemotherapy for Cancer?

While chemotherapy helps treat cancer, it can also cause other things to happen in your body called "side effects." Some of these problems affect the mouth and could cause you to delay or stop treatment.

To help prevent serious problems, see a dentist ideally one month before starting chemotherapy.

How Does Chemotherapy Affect the Mouth?

Chemotherapy is the use of drugs to treat cancer. These drugs kill cancer cells, but they may also harm normal cells, including cells in the mouth. Side effects include problems with your teeth and gums; the soft, moist lining of your mouth; and the glands that make saliva (spit).

It is important to know that side effects in the mouth can be serious.

- The side effects can hurt and make it hard to eat, talk, and swallow.

- You are more likely to get an infection, which can be dangerous when you are receiving cancer treatment.

- If the side effects are bad, you may not be able to keep up with your cancer treatment. Your doctor may need to cut back on your cancer treatment or may even stop it.

What Mouth Problems Does Chemotherapy Cause?

You may have certain side effects in your mouth from chemotherapy. Another person may have different problems. The problems depend on the chemotherapy drugs and how your body reacts to them. You may have these problems only during treatment or for a short time after treatment ends.

- Painful mouth and gums

- Dry mouth

- Burning, peeling, or swelling tongue

- Infection

- Change in taste

Why Should I See a Dentist?

You may be surprised that your dentist is important in your cancer treatment. If you go to the dentist before chemotherapy begins, you can help prevent serious mouth problems. Side effects often happen because a person's mouth is not healthy before chemotherapy starts. Not all mouth problems can be avoided but the fewer side effects you have, the more likely you will stay on your cancer treatment schedule.

It is important for your dentist and cancer doctor to talk to each other about your cancer treatment. Be sure to give your dentist your cancer doctor's phone number.

You need to see the dentist one month, if possible, before chemotherapy begins. If you have already started chemotherapy and did not go to a dentist, see one as soon as possible.

What Will the Dentist and Dental Hygienist Do?

- Check and clean your teeth
- Take x-rays
- Take care of mouth problems
- Show you how to take care of your mouth to prevent side effects

What Can I Do to Keep My Mouth Healthy?

You can do a lot to keep your mouth healthy during chemotherapy. The first step is to see a dentist before you start cancer treatment. Once your treatment starts, it is important to look in your mouth every day for sores or other changes. These tips can help prevent and treat a sore mouth:

Keep Your Mouth Moist

- Drink a lot of water.
- Suck ice chips.
- Use sugarless gum or sugar-free hard candy.
- Use a saliva substitute to help moisten your mouth.

Clean Your Mouth, Tongue, and Gums

- Brush your teeth, gums, and tongue with an extra-soft toothbrush after every meal and at bedtime. If brushing hurts, soften the bristles in warm water.
- Use a fluoride toothpaste.
- Do not use mouthwashes with alcohol in them.
- Floss your teeth gently every day. If your gums bleed and hurt, avoid the areas that are bleeding or sore, but keep flossing your other teeth.
- Rinse your mouth several times a day with a solution of ¼ teaspoon of salt or 1 teaspoon of baking soda in 1 cup (8 ounces) of warm water. Follow with a plain water rinse.
- Dentures that do not fit well can cause problems. Talk to your cancer doctor or dentist about your dentures.

If Your Mouth Is Sore, Watch What You Eat and Drink

- Choose foods that are good for you and easy to chew and swallow.
- Take small bites of food, chew slowly, and sip liquids with your meals.
- Eat soft, moist foods, such as cooked cereals, mashed potatoes, and scrambled eggs.
- If you have trouble swallowing, soften your food with gravy, sauces, broth, yogurt, or other liquids.

Call Your Doctor or Nurse When Your Mouth Hurts

- Work with them to find medicines to help control the pain.
- If the pain continues, talk to your cancer doctor about stronger medicines.

Remember to Stay Away From

- Sharp, crunchy foods, like taco chips, that could scrape or cut your mouth
- Foods that are hot, spicy, or high in acid, like citrus fruits and juices, which can irritate your mouth
- Sugary foods, like candy or soda, that could cause cavities
- Toothpicks, because they can cut your mouth
- All tobacco products
- Alcoholic drinks

Do Children Get Mouth Problems, Too?

Chemotherapy causes other side effects in children, depending on the child's age.

Problems with teeth are the most common. Permanent teeth may be slow to come in and may look different from normal teeth. Teeth may fall out. The dentist will check your child's jaws for any growth problems.

Before chemotherapy begins, take your child to a dentist. The dentist will check your child's mouth carefully and pull loose teeth or those that may become loose during treatment. Ask the dentist or hygienist what you can do to help your child with mouth care.

Section 48.3

Head and Neck Radiation Treatment and Your Mouth

This section includes text excerpted from "Head and Neck Radiation Treatment and Your Mouth," National Institute of Dental and Craniofacial Research (NIDCR), April 2013. Reviewed July 2019.

Doctors use head and neck radiation to treat cancer because it kills cancer cells. But radiation to the head and neck can harm normal cells, including cells in the mouth. Side effects include problems with your teeth and gums; the soft, moist lining of your mouth; glands that make saliva (spit); and jawbones.

It Is Important to Know That Side Effects in the Mouth Can Be Serious

- The side effects can hurt and make it hard to eat, talk, and swallow.
- You are more likely to get an infection, which can be dangerous when you are receiving cancer treatment.
- If the side effects are bad, you may not be able to keep up with your cancer treatment. Your doctor may need to cut back on your cancer treatment or may even stop it.

What Mouth Problems Does Head and Neck Radiation Cause?

You may have certain side effects in your mouth from head and neck radiation. Another person may have different problems. Some problems go away after treatment. Others last a long time, while some may never go away.

- Dry mouth
- A lot of cavities
- Loss of taste
- Sore mouth and gums
- Infections

- Jaw stiffness

- Jawbone changes

Why Should I See a Dentist?

You may be surprised that your dentist is important in your cancer treatment. If you go to the dentist before head and neck radiation begins, you can help prevent serious mouth problems. Side effects often happen because a person's mouth is not healthy before radiation starts. Not all mouth problems can be avoided but the fewer side effects you have, the more likely you will stay on your cancer treatment schedule.

It is important for your dentist and cancer doctor to talk to each other before your radiation treatment begins. Be sure to give your dentist your cancer doctor's phone number.

You need to see the dentist one month, if possible, before your first radiation treatment. If you have already started radiation and did not go to a dentist, see one as soon as possible.

What Will the Dentist and Dental Hygienist Do?

- Check and clean your teeth

- Take x-rays

- Take care of mouth problems

- Show you how to take care of your mouth to prevent side effects

- Show you how to prevent and treat jaw stiffness by exercising the jaw muscles three times a day. Open and close the mouth as far as possible (without causing pain) 20 times.

What Can I Do to Keep My Mouth Healthy?

You can do a lot to keep your mouth healthy during head and neck radiation. The first step is to see a dentist before you start cancer treatment. Once your treatment starts, it is important to look in your mouth every day for sores or other changes. These tips can help prevent and treat a sore mouth:

Keep Your Mouth Moist

- Drink a lot of water.

- Suck ice chips.

- Use sugarless gum or sugar-free hard candy.

- Use a saliva substitute to help moisten your mouth.

Clean Your Mouth, Tongue, and Gums

Brush your teeth, gums, and tongue with an extra-soft toothbrush after every meal and at bedtime. If it hurts, soften the bristles in warm water.

- Use a fluoride toothpaste.

- Use the special fluoride gel that your dentist prescribes.

- Do not use mouthwashes with alcohol in them.

- Floss your teeth gently every day. If your gums bleed and hurt, avoid the areas that are bleeding or sore, but keep flossing your other teeth.

- Rinse your mouth several times a day with a solution of ¼ teaspoon each of baking soda and salt in one quart of warm water. Follow with a plain water rinse.

- Dentures that do not fit well can cause problems. Talk to your cancer doctor or dentist about your dentures.

If Your Mouth Is Sore, Watch What You Eat and Drink

- Choose foods that are good for you and easy to chew and swallow.

- Take small bites of food, chew slowly, and sip liquids with your meals.

- Eat moist, soft foods, such as cooked cereals, mashed potatoes, and scrambled eggs.

- If you have trouble swallowing, soften your food with gravy, sauces, broth, yogurt, or other liquids.

Call Your Doctor or Nurse When Your Mouth Hurts

- Work with them to find medicines to help control the pain.

- If the pain continues, talk to your cancer doctor about stronger medicines.

Remember to Stay Away From

- Sharp, crunchy foods, like taco chips, that could scrape or cut your mouth

- Foods that are hot, spicy, or high in acid, like citrus fruits and juices, which can irritate your mouth

- Sugary foods, like candy or soda, that could cause cavities

- Toothpicks, because they can cut your mouth

- All tobacco products

- Alcoholic drinks

Do Children Get Mouth Problems, Too?

Head and neck radiation causes other side effects in children, depending on the child's age. Problems with teeth are the most common. Permanent teeth may be slow to come in and may look different from normal teeth. Teeth may fall out. The dentist will check your child's jaws for any growth problems. Before radiation begins, take your child to a dentist. The dentist will check your child's mouth carefully and pull loose teeth or those that may become loose during treatment. Ask the dentist or hygienist what you can do to help your child with mouth care.

Section 48.4

What the Dental Team Can Do

This section includes text excerpted from "Dental Team—Oral Complications of Cancer Treatment," National Institute of Dental and Craniofacial Research (NIDCR), September 2009. Reviewed July 2019.

Oral complications from radiation to the head and neck or chemotherapy for any malignancy can compromise patients' health and quality of life, and affect their ability to complete planned cancer treatment. For some patients, the complications can be so debilitating that they may tolerate only lower doses of therapy, postpone scheduled treatments, or discontinue treatment entirely. Oral complications can also lead to serious systemic infections. Medically necessary oral care before, during, and after cancer treatment can prevent or reduce the incidence and severity of oral complications, enhancing both patient survival and quality of life (QOL).

Special Considerations for Hematopoietic Stem Cell Transplant Patients

The intensive conditioning regimens of transplantation can result in pronounced immunosuppression, greatly increasing a patient's risk of mucositis, ulceration, hemorrhage, infection, and xerostomia. The complications begin to resolve when hematologic status improves. Although the complete blood count and differential may be normal, immunosuppression may last for up to a year after the transplant, along with the risk of infections. Also, the oral cavity and salivary glands are commonly involved in graft-versus-host disease in allograft recipients. This can result in mucosal inflammation, ulceration, and xerostomia, so continued monitoring is necessary. Careful attention to oral care in the immediate and long-term posttransplant period is important to patients' overall health.

Chapter 49

Celiac Disease and Dental Enamel Defects

What Is Celiac Disease?

Celiac disease is a digestive disorder that damages the small intestine. The disease is triggered by eating foods containing gluten. Gluten is a protein found naturally in wheat, barley, and rye, and is common in foods, such as bread, pasta, cookies, and cakes. Many prepackaged foods, lip balms and lipsticks, hair and skin products, toothpastes, vitamin and nutrient supplements, and, rarely, medicines, contain gluten.

Celiac disease can be very serious. The disease can cause long-lasting digestive problems and keep your body from getting all the nutrients it needs. Celiac disease can also affect the body outside the intestine.

Celiac disease is different from gluten sensitivity or wheat intolerance. If you have gluten sensitivity, you may have symptoms similar to those of celiac disease, such as abdominal pain and tiredness. Unlike celiac disease, gluten sensitivity does not damage the small intestine.

This chapter contains text excerpted from the following sources: Text beginning with the heading "What Is Celiac Disease?" is excerpted from "Definition and Facts for Celiac Disease," National Institute of Diabetes and Digestive and Kidney Diseases (NIDDK), June 2016; Text beginning with the heading "Dental Enamel Defects and Celiac Disease" is excerpted from "Dental Enamel Defects and Celiac Disease," National Institute of Diabetes and Digestive and Kidney Diseases (NIDDK), September 2014. Reviewed July 2019.

Celiac disease is also different from a wheat allergy. In both cases, your body's immune system reacts to wheat. However, some symptoms in wheat allergies, such as having itchy eyes or a hard time breathing, are different from celiac disease. Wheat allergies also do not cause long-term damage to the small intestine.

How Common Is Celiac Disease?

As many as one in 141 Americans has celiac disease, although most do not know it.

Who Is More Likely to Develop Celiac Disease?

Although celiac disease affects children and adults in all parts of the world, the disease is more common in Caucasians and more often diagnosed in females. You are more likely to develop celiac disease if someone in your family has the disease. Celiac disease also is more common among people with certain other diseases, such as Down syndrome, Turner syndrome, and type 1 diabetes.

Dental Enamel Defects and Celiac Disease

Celiac disease manifestations can extend beyond the classic gastrointestinal problems, affecting any organ or body system. One manifestation—dental enamel defects—can help dentists and other healthcare providers identify people who may have celiac disease and refer them to a gastroenterologist. For some people with celiac disease, a dental visit, rather than a trip to the gastroenterologist, was the first step toward discovering their condition.

Not all dental enamel defects are caused by celiac disease, although the problem is fairly common among people with the condition, particularly children, according to Alessio Fasano, M.D., medical director at the Massachusetts General Hospital for Celiac Research and Treatment. And dental enamel defects might be the only presenting manifestations of celiac disease.

Dental enamel problems stemming from celiac disease involve permanent dentition and include tooth discoloration—white, yellow, or brown spots on the teeth—poor enamel formation, pitting or banding of teeth, and mottled or translucent-looking teeth. The imperfections are symmetrical and often appear on the incisors and molars.

Tooth defects resulting from celiac disease are permanent and do not improve after adopting a gluten-free diet—the primary treatment for celiac disease. However, dentists may use bonding, veneers, and other cosmetic solutions to cover dental enamel defects in older children and adults.

Similar Symptoms, Different Problem

Tooth defects that result from celiac disease may resemble those caused by too much fluoride or a maternal or early childhood illness.

"Dentists mostly say it is from fluoride, that the mother took tetracycline, or that there was an illness early on," said Peter H.R. Green, M.D., Director of the Celiac Disease Center at Columbia University. "Celiac disease is not on the radar screen of dentists in this country. Dentists should be made aware of these manifestations to help them identify people and get them to see their doctors so they can exclude celiac disease."

Green just completed a U.S. study with his dental colleague Ted Malahias, D.D.S., that demonstrates celiac disease is highly associated with dental enamel defects in childhood—most likely due to the onset of celiac disease during enamel formation. The study, which did not identify a similar association in adults, concluded that all physician education about celiac disease should include information about the significance of dental enamel defects.

Other Oral Symptoms

Checking a patient's mouth is something primary care physicians also can do to help identify people who might have celiac disease. While dental enamel defects are the most prominent, a number of other oral problems are related to celiac disease, according to Green. These include:

- Recurrent aphthous stomatitis, or canker sores or ulcers that recur inside the mouth

- Atrophic glossitis, a condition characterized by a red, smooth, shiny tongue

- Dry mouth syndrome

- Squamous cell carcinoma—a type of cancer—of the pharynx and mouth

Chapter 50

Diabetes and Oral Health

What Is Diabetes?

Diabetes is a disease that occurs when your blood glucose, also called "blood sugar," is too high. Blood glucose is your main source of energy and comes from the food you eat. Insulin, a hormone made by the pancreas, helps glucose from food get into your cells to be used for energy. Sometimes your body doesn't make enough—or any—insulin or does not use insulin well. Glucose then stays in your blood and does not reach your cells.

Over time, having too much glucose in your blood can cause health problems. Although diabetes has no cure, you can take steps to manage your diabetes and stay healthy.

Sometimes people call diabetes "a touch of sugar" or "borderline diabetes." These terms suggest that someone does not really have diabetes or has a less serious case, but every case of diabetes is serious.

This chapter contains text excerpted from the following sources: Text under the heading "What Is Diabetes?" is excerpted from "Diabetes Overview," National Institute of Diabetes and Digestive and Kidney Diseases (NIDDK), November 2016; Text beginning with the heading "How Can Diabetes Affect My Mouth?" is excerpted from "Diabetes, Gum Disease, and Other Dental Problems," National Institute of Diabetes and Digestive and Kidney Diseases (NIDDK), September 2014. Reviewed July 2019.

How Can Diabetes Affect My Mouth?

Too much glucose, also called "sugar," in your blood from diabetes can cause pain, infection, and other problems in your mouth. Your mouth includes:

- Your teeth

- Your gums

- Your jaw

- Tissues, such as your tongue, the roof and bottom of your mouth, and the inside of your cheeks

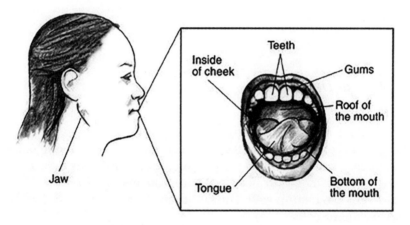

Figure 50.1. *Anatomy of the Mouth*

Glucose is present in your saliva—the fluid in your mouth that makes it wet. When diabetes is not controlled, high glucose levels in your saliva help harmful bacteria grow. These bacteria combine with food to form a soft, sticky film called "plaque." Plaque also comes from eating foods that contain sugars or starches. Some types of plaque cause tooth decay or cavities. Other types of plaque cause gum disease and bad breath.

Gum disease can be more severe and take longer to heal if you have diabetes. In turn, having gum disease can make your blood glucose hard to control.

What Happens If You Have a Plaque

Plaque that is not removed hardens over time into tartar and collects above your gum line. Tartar makes it more difficult to brush and clean between your teeth. Your gums become red and swollen, and bleed easily—signs of unhealthy or inflamed gums, called "gingivitis."

When gingivitis is not treated, it can advance to gum disease called "periodontitis." In periodontitis, the gums pull away from the teeth and form spaces, called "pockets," which slowly become infected. This infection can last a long time. Your body fights the bacteria as the plaque spreads and grows below the gum line. Both the bacteria and your body's response to this infection start to break down the bone and the tissue that hold the teeth in place. If periodontitis is not treated, the gums, bones, and tissue that support the teeth are destroyed. Teeth may become loose and might need to be removed. If you have periodontitis, your dentist may send you to a periodontist, an expert in treating gum disease.

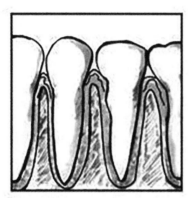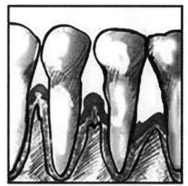

Figure 50.2. *Differences between Healthy Gums and Gums Affected by Peridontitis*

What Are the Most Common Mouth Problems from Diabetes?

The following table shows the most common mouth problems from diabetes.

Table 50.1. Common Mouth Problems from Diabetes

Problem	What It Is	Symptoms	Treatment
Gingivitis	• Unhealthy or inflamed gums	• Red, swollen, and bleeding gums	• Daily brushing and flossing • Regular cleanings at the dentist
Periodontitis	• Gum disease, which can change from mild to severe	• Red, swollen, and bleeding gums • Gums that have pulled away from the teeth • Long-lasting infection between the teeth and gums • Bad breath that would not go away • Permanent teeth that are loose or moving away from one another • Changes in the way your teeth fit together when you bite • Sometimes pus between the teeth and gums • Changes in the fit of dentures, which are teeth you can remove	• Deep cleaning at your dentist • Medicine that your dentist prescribes • Gum surgery in severe cases
Thrush, called "candidiasis"	• The growth of a naturally occurring fungus that the body is unable to control	• Sore, white—or sometimes red—patches on your gums, tongue, cheeks, or the roof of your mouth • Patches that have turned into open sores	• Medicine that your doctor or dentist prescribes to kill the fungus • Cleaning dentures • Removing dentures for part of the day or night, and soaking them in medicine that your doctor or dentist prescribes

Table 50.1. Continued

Problem	What It Is	Symptoms	Treatment
Dry mouth, called "xerostomia"	• A lack of saliva in your mouth, which raises your risk for tooth decay and gum disease	• Dry feeling in your mouth, often or all of the time • Dry, rough tongue • Pain in the mouth • Cracked lips • Mouth sores or infection problems • Chewing, eating, swallowing, or talking	• Taking medicine to keep your mouth wet that your doctor or dentist prescribes • Rinsing with a fluoride mouth rinse to prevent cavities • Using sugarless gum or mints to increase saliva flow • Taking frequent sips of water • Avoiding tobacco, caffeine, and alcoholic beverages • Using a humidifier, a device that raises the level of moisture in your home, at night • Avoiding spicy or salty foods that may cause pain in a dry mouth
Oral burning	• A burning sensation inside the mouth caused by uncontrolled blood glucose levels	• Burning feeling in the mouth • Dry mouth • Bitter taste • Symptoms may worsen throughout the day	• Seeing your doctor, who may change your diabetes medicine • Once your blood glucose is under control, the oral burning will go away

More symptoms of a problem in your mouth are:

- A sore, or an ulcer, that does not heal
- Dark spots or holes in your teeth
- Pain in your mouth, face, or jaw that does not go away
- Loose teeth
- Pain when chewing
- A changed sense of taste or a bad taste in your mouth
- Bad breath that does not go away when you brush your teeth

How Will I Know If I Have Mouth Problems from Diabetes?

Check your mouth for signs of problems from diabetes. If you notice any problems, see your dentist right away. Some of the first signs of gum disease are swollen, tender, or bleeding gums. Sometimes you would not have any signs of gum disease. You may not know you have it until you have serious damage. Your best defense is to see your dentist twice a year for a cleaning and checkup.

How Can I Prepare for a Visit to My Dentist?

Plan ahead. Talk with your doctor and dentist before the visit about the best way to take care of your blood glucose during dental work.

You may be taking a diabetes medicine that can cause low blood glucose, also called "hypoglycemia." If you take insulin or other diabetes medicines, take them and eat as usual before visiting the dentist. You may need to bring your diabetes medicines and your snacks or meal with you to the dentist's office.

You may need to postpone any nonemergency dental work if your blood glucose is not under control.

If you feel nervous about visiting the dentist, tell your dentist and the staff about your feelings. Your dentist can adapt the treatment to your needs. Do not let your nerves stop you from having regular checkups. Waiting too long to take care of your mouth may make things worse.

What If My Mouth Is Sore after My Dental Work?

A sore mouth is common after dental work. If this happens, you might not be able to eat or chew the foods you normally eat for several hours or days. For guidance on how to adjust your usual routine while your mouth is healing, ask your doctor:

- What foods and drinks you should have

- If you should change the time when you take your diabetes medicines

- If you should change the dose of your diabetes medicines

- How often you should check your blood glucose

How Does Smoking Affect My Mouth?

Smoking makes problems with your mouth worse. Smoking raises your chances of getting gum disease, oral and throat cancers, and oral fungal infections. Smoking also discolors your teeth and makes your breath smell bad.

Smoking and diabetes are a dangerous mix. Smoking raises your risk for many diabetes problems. If you quit smoking:

- You will lower your risk for heart attack, stroke, nerve disease, kidney disease, and amputation

- Your cholesterol and blood pressure levels might improve

- Your blood circulation will improve

If you smoke, stop smoking. Ask for help so that you do not have to do it alone. You can start by calling 800-QUIT-NOW or 800-784-8669.

How Can I Keep My Mouth Healthy?

You can keep your mouth healthy by taking these steps:

- Keep your blood glucose numbers as close to your target as possible. Your doctor will help you set your target blood glucose numbers and teach you what to do if your numbers are too high or too low.

- Eat healthy meals and follow the meal plan that you and your doctor or dietitian have worked out.

- Brush your teeth at least twice a day with fluoride toothpaste. Fluoride protects against tooth decay.

  - Aim for brushing first thing in the morning, before going to bed, and after each meal and sugary or starchy snack.

349

- Use a soft toothbrush.
- Gently brush your teeth with the toothbrush angled towards the gum line.
- Use small, circular motions.
- Brush the front, back, and top of each tooth. Brush your tongue, too.
- Change your toothbrush every three months or sooner if the toothbrush looks worn or the bristles spread out. A new toothbrush removes more plaque.

- Drink water that contains added fluoride or ask your dentist about using a fluoride mouth rinse to prevent tooth decay.
- Ask your dentist about using an antiplaque or antigingivitis mouth rinse to control plaque or prevent gum disease.
- Use dental floss to clean between your teeth at least once a day. Flossing helps prevent plaque from building up on your teeth. When flossing,
  - Slide the floss up and down and then curve it around the base of each tooth under the gums
  - Use clean sections of floss as you move from tooth to tooth
- Another way of removing plaque between teeth is to use a dental pick or brush—thin tools designed to clean between the teeth. You can buy these picks at drug stores or grocery stores.
- If you wear dentures, keep them clean and take them out at night. Have them adjusted if they become loose or uncomfortable.
- Call your dentist right away if you have any symptoms of mouth problems.
- See your dentist twice a year for a cleaning and checkup. Your dentist may suggest more visits if you need them.
- See your dentist twice a year for a cleaning and checkup.
- Follow your dentist's advice.
  - If your dentist tells you about a problem, take care of it right away.
  - Follow any steps or treatments from your dentist to keep your mouth healthy.

- Tell your dentist that you have diabetes.

    - Tell your dentist about any changes in your health or medicines.

    - Share the results of some of your diabetes blood tests, such as the A1C test or the fasting blood glucose test.

    - Ask if you need antibiotics before and after dental treatment if your diabetes is uncontrolled.

- If you smoke, stop smoking.

Chapter 51

Disabilities and Oral Care

Chapter Contents

Section 51.1

Special Care in Oral Health

This section includes text excerpted from
"Developmental Disabilities," National Institute of
Dental and Craniofacial Research (NIDCR), July 2018.

A disability is any condition of the body or mind (impairment) that makes it more difficult for the person with the condition to do certain activities (activity limitation) and interact with the world around them (participation restrictions).

Disabilities, such as autism, cerebral palsy, Down syndrome, and other cognitive disabilities create challenges in accomplishing daily activities, especially self-care activities. People with these disabilities may need extra help to achieve and maintain good health, which includes oral health. To achieve and maintain good oral health, people with mild or moderate disabilities often require a special approach to dental care.

Health Challenges

- **Mental capabilities** will vary from person to person and may have an impact upon how well someone can follow the directions in a dental office and at home.

- **Behavior problems** can complicate oral healthcare. For example, anxiety caused by a disability may make someone uncooperative.

- **Mobility problems** may require a person to use a wheelchair or a walker to move around. Access to the dental operatory and chair may require special arrangements and assistance with patient transfer. Longer appointment times may be needed.

- **Neuromuscular problems** can affect the mouth. Some people with disabilities have persistently rigid or loose chewing muscles, or have drooling, gagging, and swallowing problems that complicate oral care.

- **Uncontrolled body movements** can jeopardize safety and the ability to deliver oral care.

- **Cardiac disorders,** particularly mitral valve prolapse and heart valve damage, are common in people with disabilities such as Down syndrome. Consult a cardiologist to determine the need for pretreatment antibiotics.

- **Gastroesophageal reflux** sometimes affects people with central nervous system disorders, such as cerebral palsy. Teeth may be sensitive or display signs of erosion.

- **Seizures** accompany many disabilities. Patients may chip teeth or bite the tongue or cheeks during a seizure.

- **Visual impairments and hearing loss and deafness** may also be present in people with disabilities.

- **Latex allergies** may be more likely in people with disabilities.

Oral Health Problems

- **Tooth decay** is common in people with disabilities.

- **Periodontal (gum) disease** occurs more often and at a younger age in people with disabilities. Difficulty performing effective brushing and flossing may be an obstacle to successful treatment and outcomes.

- **Malocclusion** occurs in many people with disabilities, which can make chewing and speaking difficult and increase the risk of periodontal (gum) disease, dental caries, and oral trauma.

- **Damaging oral habits,** such as teeth grinding and clenching, food pouching, mouth breathing, and tongue thrusting can be a problem for people with disabilities.

- **Oral malformations** may cause enamel defects, high lip lines with dry gums, and variations in the number, size, and shape of teeth.

- **Delayed tooth eruption** may occur in children with disabilities, such as Down syndrome. Children may not get their first baby tooth until they are 2 years old.

- **Trauma and injury** to the mouth from falls or accidents may occur in people with seizure disorders or cerebral palsy.

Tips for Caregivers

Taking care of someone with a disability requires patience and skill. As a caregiver, you know this as well as anyone does. You also know how challenging it is to help that person with oral healthcare. It takes planning, time, and the ability to manage physical, mental, and behavioral problems. Oral care is not always easy, but you can make it work for you and the person you help.

- **Brush every day.** Depending on whether the person you care for is able to brush her or his teeth, you may need to take on the job of brushing their teeth yourself, or modify the toothbrush to accommodate physical limitations to allow the person to continue brushing her or his own teeth.

- **Floss regularly.** Some people with disabilities may find flossing a real challenge. You may need to do the flossing yourself, or obtain aids such as floss holders or floss picks.

- **Visit a dentist regularly.** Professional cleanings are an important part of maintaining good oral health. It may take time for the person you care for to become comfortable at the dental office. A "get-acquainted" visit with no treatment provided might help to familiarize them with the office and the exam routine before a real visit.

Tips for Dental Professionals

Providing oral care to patients with disabilities requires adaptation of the skills you use every day. Most people with mild or moderate disabilities can be treated successfully in the general practice setting. As a dental professional, you also need to be aware of the special challenges—behavioral, physical, and cognitive—that someone who arrives at the dental office with disabilities may have. Learning appropriate skills and techniques to meet the unique oral health needs of people with disabilities will help you be successful in delivering care to these patients.

- **Determine your patient's mental capabilities and communication skills.** Talk with the patient and their caregivers about how the patient's abilities might affect oral healthcare. Be receptive to their thoughts and ideas on how to make the experience a success.

- **Set the stage for a successful visit.** Involve the entire dental team—from the receptionist to the dental assistant.

- **Observe if physical manifestations of the disability(ies) are present.** How does the patient move? Look for challenges, such as uncontrolled body movements or problems with sitting in the dentist's chair.

- **Ask if the patient has an allergy to latex before you begin treatment.** Latex allergies can be life-threatening.

Section 51.2

Practical Oral Care for People with Autism

This section includes text excerpted from "Practical Oral Care for People with Autism," National Institute of Dental and Craniofacial Research (NIDCR), July 2009. Reviewed July 2019.

Autism is a complex disability that impairs communication and social, behavioral, and intellectual functioning. Some people with the disorder appear distant, aloof, or detached from other people or from their surroundings. Others do not react appropriately to common verbal and social cues, such as a parent's tone of voice or smile. Obsessive routines, repetitive behaviors, unpredictable body movements, and self-injurious behavior may all be symptoms that complicate dental care. Autism varies widely in symptoms and severity, and some people have coexisting conditions, such as intellectual disability or epilepsy. Autism varies widely in symptoms and severity, and some people have coexisting conditions, such as intellectual disability or epilepsy.

Providing oral care to people with autism requires adaptation of the skills you use every day. In fact, most people with mild or moderate forms of autism can be treated successfully in the general practice setting.

Health Challenges in Autism and Strategies for Care

Before the appointment, obtain and review the patient's medical history. Consultation with physicians, family, and caregivers is essential to assembling an accurate medical history. Also, determine who can legally provide informed consent for treatment.

Communication problems and mental capabilities are central concerns when treating people with autism.

- Talk with the parent or caregiver to determine your patient's intellectual and functional abilities, and then communicate with the patient at a level she or he can understand.

- Use a "tell-show-do" approach to providing care. Start by explaining each procedure before it occurs. Take the time to show what you have explained, such as the instruments you will use and how they work. Demonstrations can encourage some patients to be more cooperative.

Behavior problems—which may include hyperactivity and quick frustration—can complicate oral healthcare for patients with autism. The invasive nature of oral care may trigger violent and self-injurious behavior, such as temper tantrums or head banging.

- Plan a desensitization appointment to help the patient become familiar with the office, staff, and equipment through a step-by-step process. These steps may take several visits to accomplish.

  - Have the patient sit alone in the dental chair to become familiar with the treatment setting. Some patients may refuse to sit in the chair and choose instead to sit on the operator's stool.

  - Once your patient is seated, begin a cursory examination using your fingers.

  - Next, use a toothbrush to brush the teeth and gain additional access to the patient's mouth. The familiarity of a toothbrush will help your patient feel comfortable and provide you with an opportunity to further examine the mouth.

- When the patient is prepared for treatment, make the appointment short and positive.

- Pay special attention to the treatment setting. Keep dental instruments out of sight and light out of your patient's eyes.

- Praise and reinforce good behavior after each step of a procedure. Ignore inappropriate behavior as much as you can.

- Try to gain cooperation in the least restrictive manner. Some patients' behavior may improve if they bring comfort items, such as a stuffed animal or a blanket. Asking the caregiver to sit nearby or hold the patient's hand may be helpful as well.

- Use immobilization techniques only when absolutely necessary to protect the patient and staff during dental treatment—not as a convenience. There are no universal guidelines on immobilization that apply to all treatment settings. Before employing any kind of immobilization, it may help to consult available guidelines on federally funded care, your state department of mental health/ disabilities, and your State Dental Practice Act. Guidelines on behavior management published by the American Academy of Pediatric Dentistry (AAPD) may also be useful. Obtain consent from your patient's legal guardian and choose the least restrictive technique that will allow you to provide care safely. Immobilization should not cause physical injury or undue discomfort.

- If all other strategies fail, pharmacological options are useful in managing some patients. Others need to be treated under general anesthesia. However, caution is necessary because some patients with developmental disabilities can have unpredictable reactions to medications.

People with autism often engage in perseveration, a continuous, meaningless repetition of words, phrases, or movements. Your patient may mimic the sound of the suction, for example, or repeat an instruction over and again. Avoid demonstrating dental equipment if it triggers perseveration, and note this in the patient's record.

Unusual responses to stimuli can create distractions and interrupt treatment. People with autism need consistency and can be especially sensitive to changes in their environment. They may exhibit unusual sensitivity to sensory stimuli, such as sound, bright colors, and touch. Reactions vary: Some people with autism may overreact to noise and touch, while exposure to pain and heat may not provoke much reaction at all.

- Use the same staff, dental operatory, and appointment time to sustain familiarity. These details can help make dental treatment seem less threatening.

- Minimize the number of distractions. Try to reduce unnecessary sights, sounds, odors, or other stimuli that might be disruptive. Use an operatory that is somewhat secluded instead of one in the middle of a busy office. Also, consider lowering ambient light and asking the patient's caregiver whether soft music would help.

- Allow time for your patient to adjust and become desensitized to the noise of a dental setting. Some patients may be hypersensitive to the sound of dental instruments.

- Talk to the caregiver to get a sense of the patient's level of tolerance. People with autism differ in how they accept physical contact. Some are defensive and refuse any contact in or around the mouth, or cradling of the head or face. Others find such cradling comforting.

- Note your findings and experiences in the patient's chart.

Unusual and unpredictable body movements are sometimes observed in people with autism. These movements can jeopardize safety as well as your ability to deliver oral healthcare.

- Make sure the path from the reception area to the dental chair is clear.

- Observe the patient's movements and look for patterns. Try to anticipate the movements, either blending your movements with those of your patient or working around them.

Seizures may accompany autism but can usually be controlled with anticonvulsant medications. The mouth is always at risk during a seizure: Patients may chip teeth or bite the tongue or cheeks. People with controlled seizure disorders can easily be treated in the general dental office.

- Consult your patient's physician. Record information in the chart about the frequency of seizures and the medications used to control them. Determine before the appointment whether medications have been taken as directed. Know and avoid any factors that trigger your patient's seizures.

- Be prepared to manage a seizure. If one occurs during oral care, remove any instruments from the mouth and clear the area around the dental chair. Attaching dental floss to rubber dam clamps and mouth props when treatment begins can help you remove them quickly. Do not attempt to insert any objects between the teeth during a seizure.

- Stay with your patient, turn her or him to one side, and monitor the airway to reduce the risk of aspiration.

Oral Health Problems in Autism and Strategies for Care

People with autism experience few unusual oral health conditions. Although commonly used medications and damaging oral habits can cause problems, the rates of caries and periodontal disease in people with autism are comparable to those in the general population. Communication and behavioral problems pose the most significant challenges in providing oral care.

Damaging oral habits are common and include bruxism; tongue thrusting; self-injurious behavior, such as picking at the gingiva or biting the lips; and pica—eating objects and substances, such as gravel, cigarette butts, or pens. If a mouthguard can be tolerated, prescribe one for patients who have problems with self-injurious behavior or bruxism.

Dental caries risk increases in patients who have a preference for soft, sticky, or sweet foods; damaging oral habits; and difficulty brushing and flossing.

- Recommend preventive measures, such as fluorides and sealants.

- Caution patients or their caregivers about medicines that reduce saliva or contain sugar. Suggest that patients drink water often, take sugar-free medicines when available, and rinse with water after taking any medicine.

- Advise caregivers to offer alternatives to cariogenic foods and beverages as incentives or rewards.

- Encourage independence in daily oral hygiene. Ask patients to show you how they brush, and follow up with specific recommendations. Perform hands-on demonstrations to show patients the best way to clean their teeth. If appropriate, show patients and caregivers how a modified toothbrush or floss holder might make oral hygiene easier.

- Some patients cannot brush and floss independently. Talk to caregivers about daily oral hygiene and do not assume that they know the basics. Use your experiences with each patient to demonstrate oral hygiene techniques and sitting or standing positions for the caregiver. Emphasize that a consistent approach to oral hygiene is important— caregivers should try to use the same location, timing, and positioning.

Periodontal disease occurs in people with autism in much the same way it does in persons without developmental disabilities.

- Some patients benefit from the daily use of an antimicrobial agent, such as chlorhexidine.

- Stress the importance of conscientious oral hygiene and frequent prophylaxis.

Tooth eruption may be delayed due to phenytoin-induced gingival hyperplasia. Phenytoin is commonly prescribed for people with autism.

Trauma and injury to the mouth from falls or accidents occur often in people with seizure disorders. Suggest a tooth-saving kit for group homes. Emphasize to caregivers that traumas require immediate professional attention and explain the procedures to follow if a permanent tooth is knocked out. Also, instruct caregivers to locate any missing pieces of a fractured tooth, and explain that radiographs of the patient's chest may be necessary to determine whether any fragments have been aspirated.

Physical abuse often presents as oral trauma. Abuse is reported more frequently in people with developmental disabilities than in the general population. If you suspect that a child is being abused or neglected, State laws require that you call your Child Protective Services agency. Assistance is also available from the Childhelp® National Child Abuse Hotline at 800-422-4453 or the Child Welfare Information Gateway (www.childwelfare.gov).

Section 51.3

Practical Oral Care for People with Cerebral Palsy

This section includes text excerpted from "Practical Oral Care for People with Cerebral Palsy," National Institute of Dental and Craniofacial Research (NIDCR), July 2009. Reviewed July 2019.

Cerebral palsy is a complex group of motor abnormalities and functional impairments that affect muscle coordination. This developmental disability may be associated with uncontrolled body movements, seizure disorders, balance-related abnormalities, sensory dysfunction, and intellectual disability. For some, the disorder is mild, causing movements to appear merely clumsy or awkward. These patients may need little or no day-to-day supervision. Others, however, experience such severe forms of cerebral palsy that they require a wheelchair and a lifetime of personal care.

Providing oral care to people with cerebral palsy requires adaptation of the skills you use every day. In fact, most people with mild or moderate forms of cerebral palsy can be treated successfully in the general practice setting.

Health Challenges in Cerebral Palsy and Strategies for Care

People with cerebral palsy may present with physical and mental challenges that have implications for oral care. Before the appointment, obtain and review the patient's medical history. Consultation with physicians, family, and caregivers is essential to assembling an accurate medical history. Also, determine who can legally provide informed consent for treatment.

Cerebral palsy types are classified according to associated motor impairments:

Spastic palsy presents with stiff or rigid muscles on one side of the body or in all four limbs, sometimes including the mouth, tongue, and pharynx. People with this form of cerebral palsy may have legs that turn inward and scissor as they walk, or arms that are flexed and positioned against their bodies. Many also have intellectual disability, seizures, and dysarthria (difficulty speaking).

Dyskinetic or **athetoid palsy** is characterized by hypotonia and slow, uncontrolled writhing movements. People with this type of cerebral palsy experience frequent changes in muscle tone in all areas of their bodies; muscles may be rigid during waking hours and normal during sleep. Dysarthria is also associated with this type.

Ataxic palsy is marked by problems with balance and depth perception, as well as an unsteady, wide-based gait. Hypotonia and tremors sometimes occur in people with this rare type of cerebral palsy.

Combined palsy reflects a combination of these types.

Everyone who has cerebral palsy has problems with movement and posture. Observe each patient, then tailor your care accordingly.

- Maintain clear paths for movement throughout the treatment setting. Keep instruments and equipment out of the patient's way.

- Some patients cannot be moved into the dental chair but instead must be treated in their wheelchairs. Some wheelchairs recline or are specially molded to fit people's bodies. Lock the wheels, then slip a sliding board (also called a "transfer board") behind the patient's back to support the head and neck.

- If you need to transfer your patient from a wheelchair to the dental chair, ask about special preferences, such as padding, pillows, or other things you can provide to ease the transition. The patient or caregiver can often explain how to make a smooth transfer.

Uncontrolled body movements are common in people with cerebral palsy. Their limbs move often, so providing oral care can be difficult. When patients with cerebral palsy attempt to move in order to help, their muscles often tense, increasing uncontrolled movements.

- Make the treatment environment calm and supportive. Try to help your patient relax. Relaxation will not stop uncontrolled body movements, but it may reduce their frequency or intensity.

- Place and maintain your patient in the center of the dental chair. Do not force arms and legs into unnatural positions, but allow the patient to settle into a position that is comfortable and will not interfere with dental treatment.

- Observe your patient's movements and look for patterns to help you anticipate direction and intensity. Trying to stop these movements may only intensify the involuntary response. Try instead to anticipate the movements, blending your movements with those of your patient or working around them.

- Softly cradle your patient's head during treatment. Be gentle and slow if you need to turn the patient's head.

- Exert gentle but firm pressure on your patient's arm or leg if it begins to shake.

- Try to keep appointments short, take frequent breaks, or consider prescribing muscle relaxants when long procedures are needed. People with cerebral palsy may need sedation, general anesthesia, or hospitalization if extensive dental treatment is required.

Primitive reflexes are common in many people with cerebral palsy and may complicate oral care. These reflexes often occur when the head is moved or the patient is startled, and efforts to control them may make them more intense. Three types of reflexes are most commonly observed during oral care.

Asymmetric tonic neck reflex: When a patient's head is turned, the arm and leg on that side stiffen and extend. The arm and leg on the opposite side flex.

Tonic labyrinthine reflex: If the neck is extended while a patient is lying on her or his back, the legs and arms also extend, and the back and neck arch.

Startle reflex: Any surprising stimuli, such as noises, lights, or a sudden movement on your part, can trigger uncontrolled, often forceful movements involving the whole body.

- Be empathic about your patient's concerns and frustrations.

- Minimize the number of distractions in the treatment setting. Movements, lights, sounds, or other stimuli can make it difficult for your patient to cooperate. Tell her or him about any such stimulus before it appears. For example, tell the patient before you move the dental chair.

Mental capabilities vary. Many people with cerebral palsy have mild or moderate intellectual disability, but only 25 percent have a severe form. Some have normal intelligence.

- Talk with the parent or caregiver to determine your patient's intellectual and functional abilities, then explain each procedure at a level the patient can understand. Allow extra time to explain oral health issues, instructions, or procedures.

- Use simple, concrete instructions and repeat them often to compensate for any short-term memory problems. Speak slowly and give only one direction at a time.

- Demonstrations can make patients more cooperative. For example, turn on the saliva ejector so the patient can hear it and feel it at the corner of the mouth. Then slowly introduce it inside the mouth, being careful not to trigger a gag reflex.

- Be consistent in all aspects of oral care. Use the same staff and dental operatory each time to help sustain familiarity. Consistency leads to improved cooperation.

- Listen actively, since communicating clearly is difficult for some — show your patient whether you understand. Be sensitive to the methods she or he uses to communicate, including gestures and verbal or nonverbal requests.

Seizures may accompany cerebral palsy, but can usually be controlled with anticonvulsant medications. The mouth is always at risk during a seizure: Patients may chip teeth or bite the tongue or cheeks. Patients with controlled seizure disorders can easily be treated in the general dental office.

- Consult your patient's physician. Record information in the chart about the frequency of seizures and the medications used to control them. Determine before the appointment whether medications have been taken as directed. Know and avoid any factors that trigger your patient's seizures.

- Be prepared to manage a seizure. If one occurs during oral care, remove any instruments from the mouth and clear the area around the dental chair. Attaching dental floss to rubber dam clamps and mouth props when treatment begins can help you remove them quickly. Do not attempt to insert any objects between the teeth during a seizure.

- Stay with your patient, turn her or him to one side, and monitor the airway to reduce the risk of aspiration.

Visual impairments affect a large number of people with cerebral palsy. The most common of these defects is strabismus, a condition in which the eyes are crossed or misaligned. People with cerebral palsy may develop visual motor skills, such as hand-eye coordination, later than other people.

- Determine the level of assistance your patient requires to move safely through the dental office.

- Use your patients' other senses to connect with them, establish trust, and make treatment a good experience. Tactile feedback, such as a warm handshake, can make your patients feel comfortable.

- Face your patients when you speak and keep them apprised of each upcoming step, especially when water will be used. Rely on clear, descriptive language to explain procedures and demonstrate how equipment might feel and sound. Provide written instructions in large print (16 point or larger).

Hearing loss and deafness can be accommodated with careful planning. Patients with a hearing problem may appear to be stubborn because of their seeming lack of response to a request.

- Patients may want to adjust their hearing aids or turn them off, since the sound of some instruments may cause auditory discomfort.

- If your patient reads lips, speak in a normal cadence and tone. If your patient uses a form of sign language, ask the interpreter to come to the appointment. Speak with this person in advance to discuss dental terms and your patient's needs.

- Visual feedback is helpful. Maintain eye contact with your patient. Before talking, eliminate background noise (turn off the radio and the suction). Sometimes people with a hearing loss simply need you to speak clearly in a slightly louder voice than normal. Remember to remove your face mask first or wear a clear face shield.

Dysarthria is common in people with cerebral palsy, due to problems involving the muscles that control speech and mastication.

- Be patient. Allow time for your patient to express himself or herself. Remember that many people with dysarthria have normal intelligence.

- Consult with the caregiver if you have difficulty understanding your patient's speech.

Gastroesophageal reflux sometimes affects people with cerebral palsy, including those who are tube-fed. Teeth may be sensitive or display signs of erosion. Consult your patient's physician about the management of reflux.

- Place patients in a slightly upright position for treatment.

- Talk with patients and caregivers about rinsing with plain water or a water and baking soda solution. Doing so at least four times a day can help mitigate the effects of gastric acid. Stress that using a fluoride gel, rinse, or toothpaste every day is essential.

Oral Health Problems in Cerebral Palsy and Strategies for Care

Cerebral palsy itself does not cause any unique oral abnormalities. However, several conditions are more common or more severe in people with cerebral palsy than in the general population.

Periodontal disease is common in people with cerebral palsy due to poor oral hygiene and complications of oral habits, physical abilities, and malocclusion. Another factor is the gingival hyperplasia caused by medications.

Encourage independence in daily oral hygiene. Ask patients to show you how they brush, and follow up with specific recommendations on brushing methods or toothbrush adaptations. Involve your patients in hands-on demonstrations of brushing and flossing.

- Some patients cannot brush and floss independently because of impaired physical coordination or cognitive skills. Talk to caregivers about daily oral hygiene. Do not assume that all caregivers know the basics; demonstrate proper brushing and flossing techniques. A power toothbrush or a floss holder can simplify oral care. Also, use your experiences with each patient to demonstrate sitting or standing positions for the caregiver. Emphasize that a consistent approach to oral hygiene is important—caregivers should try to use the same location, timing, and positioning.

- Explain that some patients benefit from the daily use of an antimicrobial agent, such as chlorhexidine. Recommend an appropriate delivery method based on your patient's abilities. Rinsing, for example, may not work for a patient with swallowing difficulties or one who cannot expectorate. Chlorhexidine applied using a spray bottle or toothbrush is equally efficacious.

- If the use of particular medications has led to gingival hyperplasia, monitor for possible delayed tooth eruption and emphasize the importance of daily oral hygiene and frequent professional cleanings.

Dental caries is prevalent among people with cerebral palsy, primarily because of inadequate oral hygiene. Other risk factors include mouth breathing, the effects of medication, enamel hypoplasia, and food pouching.

- Caution patients or their caregivers about medicines that reduce saliva or contain sugar. Suggest that patients drink water often, take sugar-free medicines when available, and rinse with water after taking any medicine.

- Advise caregivers to offer alternatives to cariogenic foods and beverages as incentives or rewards.

- For people who pouch food, talk to caregivers about inspecting the mouth after each meal or dose of medicine. Remove food or medicine from the mouth by rinsing with water, sweeping the mouth with a finger wrapped in gauze, or using a disposable foam applicator swab.

- Recommend preventive measures, such as fluorides and sealants.

Malocclusion in people with cerebral palsy usually involves more than just misaligned teeth—it is also a musculoskeletal problem. An open bite with protruding anterior teeth is common and is typically associated with tongue thrusting. The inability to close the lips because of an open bite also contributes to excessive drooling.

Unfortunately, correcting malocclusion is almost impossible in people with moderate or severe cerebral palsy. Orthodontic treatment may not be an option because of the risk of caries and enamel hypoplasia. However, a developmental disability in and of itself should not be perceived as a barrier to orthodontic treatment.

- The ability of the patient or the caregiver to maintain good daily oral hygiene is critical to the feasibility and success of orthodontic treatment.

- Inform caregivers of emergency procedures for accidents involving oral trauma, since protruding anterior teeth are more likely to be displaced, fractured, or avulsed.

Dysphagia, difficulty with swallowing, is often a problem in people with cerebral palsy. Food may stay in the mouth longer than usual, increasing the risk for caries. Additionally, the semi-soft foods caregivers may prepare for people with this problem tend to adhere to the teeth. Coughing, gagging, choking, and aspiration are other related concerns.

- Keep the breathing passages open by placing your patient in a slightly upright position with the head turned to one side during oral care.

- Use suction frequently or as tolerated by the patient. Use a rubber dam when indicated, but make sure you introduce it slowly, perhaps over a few appointments.

- Advise the caregiver to inspect the patient's mouth after eating and remove any residual food.

Drooling affects daily oral care as well as social interaction. Hypotonia contributes to drooling, as does an open bite and the inability to close the lips.

Bruxism is common in people with cerebral palsy, especially those with severe forms of the disorder. Bruxism can be intense and persistent and cause the teeth to wear prematurely. Before recommending mouth guards or bite splints, consider that gagging or swallowing problems may make them uncomfortable or unwearable.

Hyperactive bite and gag reflexes call for introducing instruments gently into the mouth. Consider using a mouth prop. A patient with a gagging problem benefits from an early morning appointment, before eating or drinking. Help minimize the gag reflex by placing your patient's chin in a neutral or downward position.

Trauma and injury to the mouth from falls or accidents occur in people with cerebral palsy. Suggest a tooth-saving kit for group homes. Emphasize to caregivers that traumas require immediate professional attention and explain the procedures to follow if a permanent tooth is knocked out. Also, instruct caregivers to locate any missing pieces of a fractured tooth, and explain that radiographs of the patient's chest may be necessary to determine whether any fragments have been aspirated.

Physical abuse often presents as oral trauma. Abuse is reported more frequently in people with developmental disabilities than in the general population. If you suspect that a child is being abused or neglected, state laws require that you call your Child Protective Services agency. Assistance is also available from the Childhelp® National Child Abuse Hotline at 800-422-4453 or the Child Welfare Information Gateway (www.childwelfare.gov).

Section 51.4

Practical Oral Care for People with Developmental Disabilities

This section includes text excerpted from "Practical Oral Care for People with Developmental Disabilities," National Institute of Dental and Craniofacial Research (NIDCR), July 2009. Reviewed July 2019.

Developmental disabilities, such as autism, cerebral palsy, Down syndrome, and intellectual disability are present during childhood or adolescence and last a lifetime. They affect the mind, the body, and the skills people use in everyday life: thinking, talking, and self-care. People with disabilities often need extra help to achieve and maintain good health. Oral health is no exception.

Over the past three decades, a trend toward deinstitutionalization has brought people of all ages and levels of disability into the fabric of our communities. Approximately 80 percent of those with developmental disabilities are living in community-based group residences or at home with their families. People with disabilities and their caregivers now look to providers in the community for dental services.

Providing oral care to patients with developmental disabilities requires adaptation of the skills you use every day. In fact, most people with mild or moderate developmental disabilities can be treated successfully in the general practice setting.

Health Challenges and Strategies for Care

Before the appointment, obtain and review the patient's medical history. Consultation with physicians, family, and caregivers is essential to assembling an accurate medical history. Also, determine who can legally provide informed consent for treatment.

Mental capabilities vary in people with developmental disabilities and influence how well they can follow the directions in the operatory and at home.

- Determine each patient's mental capabilities and communication skills. Talk with caregivers about how the patient's abilities might affect oral healthcare. Be receptive to their thoughts and ideas on how to make the experience a success.

371

- Allow time to introduce concepts in language that patients can understand.

- Communicate respectfully with your patients and comfort those who resist dental care. Repeat instructions when necessary and involve your patients in hands-on demonstrations.

Behavior problems can complicate oral healthcare. Anxiety and fear about dental treatment can cause some patients to be uncooperative. Behaviors may range from fidgeting or temper tantrums to violent, self-injurious behavior such as head banging. This is challenging for everyone, but the following strategies can help reduce behavior problems:

Set the stage for a successful visit by involving the entire dental team—from the receptionist's friendly greeting to the caring attitude of the dental assistant in the operatory.

Arrange for a desensitizing appointment to help the patient become familiar with the office, staff, and equipment before treatment begins.

Try to gain cooperation in the least restrictive manner. Some patients' behavior may improve if they bring comfort items, such as a stuffed animal or a blanket. Asking the caregiver to sit nearby or hold the patient's hand may be helpful as well.

Make appointments short whenever possible, providing only the treatment that the patient can tolerate. Praise and reinforce good behavior and try to end each appointment on a good note.

Use immobilization techniques only when absolutely necessary to protect the patient and staff during dental treatment—not as a convenience. There are no universal guidelines on immobilization that apply to all treatment settings. Before employing any kind of immobilization, it may help to consult available guidelines on federally funded care, your state department of mental health/disabilities, and your State Dental Practice Act.

Guidelines on behavior management published by the American Academy of Pediatric Dentistry (AAPD) may also be useful. Obtain consent from your patient's legal guardian and choose the least restrictive technique that will allow you to provide care safely. Immobilization should not cause physical injury or undue discomfort.

Mobility problems are a concern for many people with disabilities; some rely on a wheelchair or a walker to move around.

- Observe the physical impact a disability has and how a particular patient moves. Look for challenges, such as uncontrolled body movements or concerns about posture.

- Maintain a clear path for movement throughout the treatment setting.

- If you need to transfer your patient from a wheelchair to the dental chair, ask the patient or caregiver about special preferences, such as padding, pillows, or other things you can provide. Often the patient or caregiver can explain how to make a smooth transfer.

- Certain patients cannot be moved into the dental chair but instead must be treated in their wheelchairs. Some wheelchairs recline or are specially molded to fit people's bodies. Lock the wheels, then slip a sliding board (also called a "transfer board") behind the patient's back

- To support the head and neck.

Neuromuscular problems can affect the mouth. Some people with disabilities have persistently rigid or loose masticatory muscles. Others have drooling, gagging, and swallowing problems that complicate oral care.

If a patient has a gagging problem, schedule an early morning appointment, before eating or drinking. Help minimize the gag reflex by placing your patient's chin in a neutral or downward position.

If your patient has swallowing problems, tilt the head slightly to one side and place her or his body in a more upright position.

If you use local anesthesia, be sure your patient does not chew the tongue or cheek. A short-lasting form of anesthesia may work well.

Uncontrolled body movements can jeopardize safety and your ability to deliver dental care. Pay special attention to the following:

- **Treatment setting:** Make the treatment setting calm and supportive. Place dental instruments behind the patient and carefully position other objects, such as cords and the light above the dental chair.

- **Patient's position:** Determine in advance whether a patient will need to be treated in her or his wheelchair. If not, keep the patient in the center of the dental chair. Pillows can help maintain a comfortable position.

- **Your position:** Observe the patient's movements and look for patterns to help anticipate direction. Place yourself behind the patient and gently cradle the head to provide support. Rest your hand around the mandible.

Cardiac disorders, particularly mitral valve prolapse and heart valve damage, are common in people with developmental disabilities such as Down syndrome. Consult the patient's physician if you have questions about the medical history and the need for antibiotic prophylaxis.

Gastroesophageal reflux sometimes affects people with central nervous system disorders, such as cerebral palsy. Teeth may be sensitive or display signs of erosion. Consult your patient's physician about the management of reflux.

- Place patients in a slightly upright position for treatment.

- Talk with patients and caregivers about rinsing with plain water or a water and baking soda solution. Doing so at least four times a day can help mitigate the effects of gastric acid. Stress that using a fluoride gel, rinse, or toothpaste every day is essential.

Seizures accompany many developmental disabilities. The mouth is always at risk during a seizure: Patients may chip teeth or bite the tongue or cheeks. Persons with controlled seizure disorders can easily be treated in the general dental office.

- Consult your patient's physician. Record information in the chart about the frequency of seizures and the medications used to control them. Determine before the appointment whether medications have been taken as directed. Know and avoid any factors that trigger your patient's seizures.

- Be prepared to manage a seizure. If one occurs during oral care, remove any instruments from the mouth and clear the area around the dental chair. Attaching dental floss to rubber dam clamps and mouth props when treatment begins can help you remove them quickly. Do not attempt to insert any objects between the teeth during a seizure.

- Stay with your patient, turn her or him to one side, and monitor the airway to reduce the risk of aspiration.

Visual impairments affect many people with developmental disabilities.

- Determine the level of assistance your patient requires to move safely through the office.

- Use your patients' other senses to connect with them, establish trust, and make treatment a good experience. Tactile feedback, such as a warm handshake, can make your patients feel comfortable.

- Face your patients when you speak and keep them apprised of each upcoming step, especially when water will be used. Rely on clear, descriptive language to explain procedures and demonstrate how equipment might feel and sound. Provide written instructions in large print (16-point or larger).

Hearing loss and deafness sometimes occur in people with developmental disabilities.

- Patients may want to adjust their hearing aids or turn them off, since the sound of some instruments may cause auditory discomfort.

- If your patient reads lips, speak in a normal cadence and tone. If your patient uses a form of sign language, ask the interpreter to come to the appointment. Speak with this person in advance to discuss dental terms and your patient's needs.

- Visual feedback is helpful. Maintain eye contact with your patient. Before talking, eliminate background noise (turn off the radio and the suction). Sometimes people with a hearing loss simply need you to speak clearly in a slightly louder voice than normal. Remember to remove your face mask first or wear a clear face shield.

Latex allergies can be a serious problem. People who have spina bifida or who have had frequent surgeries are especially prone to developing an allergic reaction or a sensitivity to latex. An allergic reaction can be life-threatening.

- Ask patients and caregivers about the presence of a latex allergy before you begin treatment.

- Schedule appointments for your latex-allergic or latex-sensitive patients at the beginning of the day when there are fewer airborne allergens circulating through the office.

- Use latex-free gloves and equipment and keep an emergency medical kit handy.

Oral Health Problems and Strategies for Care

People with developmental disabilities typically have more oral health problems than the general population. Focusing on each person's specific needs is the first step toward achieving better oral health.

Dental caries is common in people with developmental disabilities. In addition to discussing the problems associated with diet and oral hygiene, caution patients and caregivers about the cariogenic nature of prolonged bottle feeding and the adverse side effects of certain medications.

- Recommend preventive measures, such as fluorides and sealants.

- Caution patients or their caregivers about medicines that reduce saliva or contain sugar. Suggest that patients drink water frequently, take sugar-free medicines when available, and rinse with water after taking any medicine.

- Advise caregivers to offer alternatives to cariogenic foods and beverages as incentives or rewards.

- Educate caregivers about preventing early childhood caries.

- Encourage independence in daily oral hygiene. Ask patients to show you how they brush, and follow up with specific recommendations. Perform hands-on demonstrations to show patients the best way to clean their teeth.

- If necessary, adapt a toothbrush to make it easier to hold. For example, place a tennis ball or bicycle grip on the handle, wrap the handle in tape, or bend the handle by softening it under hot water. Explain that floss holders and power toothbrushes are also helpful.

- Some patients cannot brush and floss independently. Talk to caregivers about daily oral hygiene and do not assume that they know the basics. Use your experiences with each patient to demonstrate oral care techniques and sitting or standing positions for the caregiver. Emphasize that a consistent approach to oral hygiene is important—caregivers should try to use the same location, timing, and positioning.

Periodontal disease occurs more often and at a younger age in people with developmental disabilities. Contributing factors include poor oral hygiene, damaging oral habits, and physical or mental disabilities. Gingival hyperplasia caused by medications, such as some anticonvulsants, antihypertensives, and immunosuppressants also increases the risk for periodontal disease.

- Some patients benefit from the daily use of an antimicrobial agent, such as chlorhexidine.

- Stress the importance of conscientious oral hygiene and frequent prophylaxis.

Malocclusion occurs in many people with developmental disabilities and may be associated with intraoral and perioral muscular abnormalities, delayed tooth eruption, underdevelopment of the maxilla, and oral habits such as bruxism and tongue thrusting. Malocclusion can make chewing and speaking difficult and increase the risk of periodontal disease, dental caries, and oral trauma. Orthodontic treatment may not be an option for many, but a developmental disability in and of itself should not be perceived as a barrier to orthodontic care. The ability of the patient or the caregiver to maintain good daily oral hygiene is critical to the feasibility and success of orthodontic treatment.

Damaging oral habits can be a problem for people with developmental disabilities. Some of the most common of these habits are bruxism, food pouching, mouth breathing, and tongue thrusting. Other oral habits include self-injurious behavior, such as picking at the gingiva or biting the lips; rumination, where food is chewed, regurgitated, and swallowed again; and pica—eating objects and substances, such as gravel, sand, cigarette butts, or pens.

- For people who pouch food, talk to caregivers about inspecting the mouth after each meal or dose of medicine. Remove food or medicine from the mouth by rinsing with water, sweeping the mouth with a finger wrapped in gauze, or using a disposable foam applicator swab.

- If a mouthguard can be tolerated, prescribe one for patients who have problems with self-injurious behavior or bruxism.

Oral malformations affect many people with developmental disabilities. Patients may present with enamel defects, high lip lines with dry gingiva, and variations in the number, size, and shape of teeth. Craniofacial anomalies, such as facial asymmetry and hypoplasia of the midfacial region are also seen in this population. Identify any malformations and explain to the caregiver the implications for daily oral hygiene and future treatment planning.

Tooth eruption may be delayed in children with developmental disabilities. Eruption times are different for each child, and some children may not get their first primary tooth until they are 2 years old.

Delays are often characteristic of certain disabilities, such as Down syndrome. In other cases, eruption problems are attributable to the gingival hyperplasia that can result from medications, such as phenytoin and cyclosporine. Dental examination by a child's first birthday and regularly thereafter can help identify atypical patterns of eruption.

Trauma and injury to the mouth from falls or accidents occur in people with seizure disorders or cerebral palsy. Suggest a tooth-saving kit for group homes. Emphasize to caregivers that traumas require immediate professional attention and explain the procedures to follow if a permanent tooth is knocked out. Also, instruct caregivers to locate any missing pieces of a fractured tooth, and explain that radiographs of the patient's chest may be necessary to determine whether any fragments have been aspirated.

Physical abuse often presents as oral trauma. Abuse is reported more frequently in people with developmental disabilities than in the general population. If you suspect that a child is being abused or neglected, state laws require that you call your Child Protective Services agency. Assistance is also available from the Childhelp® National Child Abuse Hotline at 800- 422-4453 or the Child Welfare Information Gateway (www.childwelfare.gov).

Section 51.5

Practical Oral Care for People with Down Syndrome

This section includes text excerpted from "Practical Oral Care for People with Down Syndrome," National Institute of Dental and Craniofacial Research (NIDCR), July 2009. Reviewed July 2019.

Down syndrome, a common genetic disorder, ranges in severity and is usually associated with medical and physical problems. For example, people with this developmental disability may have cardiac disorders, infectious diseases, hypotonia, and hearing loss. Additionally, most people with this disorder have mild or moderate intellectual disability, while a small percentage are severely affected. Developmental delays, such as in speech and language, are common.

Providing oral care to people with Down syndrome requires adaptation of the skills you use every day. In fact, most people with mild or moderate Down syndrome can be successfully treated in the general practice setting.

Health Challenges in Down Syndrome and Strategies for Care

People with Down syndrome may present with mental and physical challenges that have implications for oral care. Before the appointment, obtain and review the patient's medical history. Consultation with physicians, family, and caregivers is essential to assembling an accurate medical history. Also, determine who can legally provide informed consent for treatment.

Intellectual disability. Although the mental capability of people with Down syndrome varies widely, many have mild or moderate intellectual disability that limits their ability to learn, communicate, and adapt to their environment. Language development is often delayed or impaired in people with Down syndrome; they understand more than they can verbalize. Also, ordinary activities of daily living and understanding the behavior of others as well as their own can present challenges.

- Listen actively, since speaking may be difficult for people with Down syndrome. Show your patient whether you understand.

- Talk with the parent or caregiver to determine your patient's intellectual and functional abilities, then explain each procedure at a level the patient can understand. Allow extra time to explain oral health issues or instructions and demonstrate the instruments you will use.

- Use simple, concrete instructions, and repeat them often to compensate for any short-term memory problems.

Behavior management is not usually a problem in people with Down syndrome because they tend to be warm and well behaved. Some can be stubborn or uncooperative, but most just need a little extra time and attention to feel comfortable. Gaining the patient's trust is the key to successful treatment.

- Talk to the caregiver or physician about techniques they have found to be effective in managing the patient's behavior. Share your ideas with them, and find out what motivates the patient.

It may be that a new toothbrush at the end of each appointment is all it takes to ensure cooperation. Schedule patients with Down syndrome early in the day if possible. Early appointments can help ensure that everyone is alert and attentive and that waiting time is reduced.

- Set the stage for a successful visit by involving the entire dental team—from the receptionist's friendly greeting to the caring attitude of the dental assistant in the operatory.

- Provide oral care in an environment with few distractions. Try to reduce unnecessary sights, sounds, or other stimuli that might make it difficult for your patient to cooperate. Many people with Down syndrome, however, enjoy music and may be comforted by hearing it in the dental office during treatment.

- Plan a step-by-step evaluation, starting with seating the patient in the dental chair. If this is successful, perform an oral examination using only your fingers. If this, too, goes well, begin using dental instruments. Prophylaxis is the next step, followed by dental radiographs. Several visits may be needed to accomplish these tasks.

- Try to be consistent in all aspects of providing oral healthcare. Use the same staff, dental operatory, appointment times, and other details to help sustain familiarity. The more consistency you provide for your patients, the more likely that they will be cooperative.

- Comfort people who resist oral care and reward cooperative behavior with compliments throughout the appointment.

- Use immobilization techniques only when absolutely necessary to protect the patient and staff during dental treatment— not as a convenience. There are no universal guidelines on immobilization that apply to all treatment settings. Before employing any kind of immobilization, it may help to consult available guidelines on federally funded care, your state department of mental health/disabilities, and your State Dental Practice Act. Guidelines on behavior management published by the American Academy of Pediatric Dentistry (www.aapd. org) may also be useful. Obtain consent from your patient's legal guardian and choose the least restrictive technique that will allow you to provide care safely. Immobilization should not cause physical injury or undue discomfort.

Medical conditions. Though their average life expectancy has risen to the mid-50s, people with Down syndrome are still at risk for problems in nearly every system in the body. Some problems are manifested in the mouth. For example, oral findings such as persistent gingival lesions, prolonged wound healing, or spontaneous gingival hemorrhaging may suggest an underlying medical condition and warrant consultation with the patient's physician.

Cardiac disorders are common in Down syndrome. In fact, mitral valve prolapse occurs in more than half of all adults with this developmental disability. Many others are at risk of developing valve dysfunction that leads to congestive heart failure, even if they have no known cardiac disease. Consult the patient's physician if you have questions about the medical history and the need for antibiotic prophylaxis (www.heart.org).

Compromised immune systems lead to more frequent oral and systemic infections and a high incidence of periodontal disease in people with Down syndrome. Aphthous ulcers, oral *Candida* infections, and acute necrotizing ulcerative gingivitis are common. Chronic respiratory infections contribute to mouth breathing, xerostomia, and fissured lips and tongue.

- Treat acute necrotizing ulcerative gingivitis and other infections aggressively.
- Talk to patients and their caregivers about preventing oral infections with regular dental appointments and daily oral care.
- Stress the importance of using fluoride to prevent dental caries associated with xerostomia.
- Use lip balm during treatment to ease the strain on your patient's lips.

Hypotonia affects the muscles in various areas of the body, including the mouth and large skeletal muscles. When it involves the mouth, it leads to an imbalance of forces on the teeth and contributes to an open bite. If the muscles controlling facial expression and mastication are affected, problems with chewing, swallowing, drooling, and speaking can result. A related problem is atlantoaxial instability, a spinal defect that increases the mobility of the cervical vertebrae and often leads to an unsteady gait and neck pain.

- Maintain a clear path for movement throughout the treatment setting.

- Determine the best position for your patient in the dental chair and the safest way to move her or his body, especially the head and neck. Talk with the physician or caregiver about ways to protect the spinal cord. Use pillows to stabilize your patient and make her or him more comfortable.

Seizures sometimes occur in this population, especially among infants, but can usually be controlled with anticonvulsant medications. The mouth is always at risk during a seizure: Patients may chip teeth or bite the tongue or cheeks. People with controlled seizure disorders can easily be treated in the general dental office.

- Consult your patient's physician. Record information in the chart about the frequency of seizures and the medications used to control them. Determine before the appointment whether medications have been taken as directed. Know and avoid any factors that trigger your patient's seizures.

- Be prepared to manage a seizure. If one occurs during oral care, remove any instruments from the mouth and clear the area around the dental chair. Attaching dental floss to rubber dam clamps and mouth props when treatment begins can help you remove them quickly. Do not attempt to insert any objects between the teeth during a seizure.

- Stay with your patient, turn her or him to one side, and monitor the airway to reduce the risk of aspiration.

Hearing loss and deafness may further complicate poor communication skills, but these, too, can be accommodated with planning. Patients with a hearing problem may appear to be stubborn because of their seeming lack of response to a request.

- Patients may want to adjust their hearing aids or turn them off, since the sound of some instruments may cause auditory discomfort.

- If your patient reads lips, speak in a normal cadence and tone. If your patient uses a form of sign language, ask the interpreter to come to the appointment. Speak with this person in advance to discuss dental terms and your patient's needs.

- Visual feedback is helpful. Maintain eye contact with your patient. Before talking, eliminate background noise (turn off the radio and the suction). Sometimes people with a hearing loss simply need you to speak clearly in a slightly louder voice than normal. Remember to remove your face mask first or wear a clear face shield.

Visual impairments, such as strabismus (crossed or misaligned eyes), glaucoma, and cataracts can affect people with Down syndrome.

- Determine the level of assistance your patient requires to move safely through the dental office. Use your patients' other senses to connect with them, establish trust, and make treatment a better experience. Tactile feedback, such as a warm handshake, can make your patients feel comfortable.

- Face your patients when you speak and keep them apprised of each upcoming step, especially when water will be used. Rely on clear, descriptive language to explain procedures and demonstrate how equipment might feel and sound. Provide written instructions in large print (16-point or larger).

Oral Health Problems in Down Syndrome and Strategies for Care

People with Down syndrome have no unique oral health problems. However, some of the problems they have tend to be frequent and severe. Early professional treatment and daily care at home can mitigate their severity and allow people with Down syndrome to enjoy the benefits of a healthy mouth.

Periodontal disease is the most significant oral health problem in people with Down syndrome. Children experience rapid, destructive periodontal disease. Consequently, large numbers of them lose their permanent anterior teeth in their early teens. Contributing factors include poor oral hygiene, malocclusion, bruxism, conical-shaped tooth roots, and abnormal host response because of a compromised immune system.

- Some patients benefit from the daily use of an antimicrobial agent, such as chlorhexidine. Recommend an appropriate delivery method based on your patient's abilities. Rinsing, for example, may not work for a person who has swallowing difficulties or one who cannot expectorate. Chlorhexidine applied using a spray bottle or toothbrush is equally efficacious.

- If the use of particular medications has led to gingival hyperplasia, emphasize the importance of daily oral hygiene and frequent professional cleanings.

- Encourage independence in daily oral hygiene. Ask patients to show you how they brush, and follow up with specific recommendations on brushing methods or toothbrush adaptations. Involve patients in hands-on demonstrations of brushing and flossing.

- Some people with Down syndrome can brush and floss independently, but many need help. Talk to their caregivers about daily oral hygiene. Do not assume that all caregivers know the basics; demonstrate proper brushing and flossing techniques. A power toothbrush or a floss holder can simplify oral care. Also, use your experiences with each patient to demonstrate sitting or standing positions for the caregiver. Emphasize that a consistent approach to oral hygiene is important—caregivers should try to use the same location, timing, and positioning.

Dental caries. Children and young adults who have Down syndrome have fewer caries than people without this developmental disability. Several associated oral conditions may contribute to this fact: delayed eruption of primary and permanent teeth; missing permanent teeth; and small-sized teeth with wider spaces between them, which make it easier to remove plaque. Additionally, the diets of many children with Down syndrome are closely supervised to prevent obesity; this helps reduce consumption of cariogenic foods and beverages.

By contrast, some adults with Down syndrome are at an increased risk of caries due to xerostomia and cariogenic food choices. Also, hypotonia contributes to chewing problems and inefficient natural cleansing action, which allow food to remain on the teeth after eating.

- Advise patients taking medicines that cause xerostomia to drink water often. Suggest taking sugar-free medicines if available and rinsing with water after dosing.

- Recommend preventive measures, such as topical fluoride and sealants. Suggest fluoride toothpaste, gel, or rinse, depending on your patient's needs and abilities.

- Emphasize noncariogenic foods and beverages as snacks. Advise caregivers to avoid using sweets as incentives or rewards.

Several **orofacial features** are characteristic of people with Down syndrome. The midfacial region may be underdeveloped, affecting the appearance of the lips, tongue, and palate.

- **The maxilla,** the bridge of the nose, and the bones of the midface region are smaller than in the general population, creating a prognathic occlusal relationship. Mouth breathing may occur because of smaller nasal passages, and the tongue may protrude because of a smaller midface region. People with Down syndrome often have a strong gag reflex due to the placement of the tongue, as well as the anxiety associated with any oral stimulation.

- **The palate,** although normal sized, may appear highly vaulted and narrow. This deceiving appearance is due to the unusual thickness of the sides of the hard palate. This thickness restricts the amount of space the tongue can occupy in the mouth and affects the ability to speak and chew.

- **The lips** may grow large and thick. Fissured lips may result from chronic mouth breathing. Additionally, hypotonia may cause the mouth to droop and the lower lip to protrude. Increased drooling, compounded by a chronically open mouth, contributes to angular cheilitis.

- **The tongue** also develops cracks and fissures with age; this condition can contribute to halitosis.

Malocclusion is found in most people with Down syndrome because of the delayed eruption of permanent teeth and the underdevelopment of the maxilla. A smaller maxilla contributes to an open bite, leading to poor positioning of teeth and increasing the likelihood of periodontal disease and dental caries.

- Orthodontia should be carefully considered in people with Down syndrome. Some may benefit, while others may not.

- In and of itself, Down syndrome is not a barrier to orthodontic care. The ability of the patient or caregiver to maintain good daily oral hygiene is critical to the feasibility and success of treatment.

Tooth anomalies are common in Down syndrome.

- **Congenitally missing teeth** occur more often in people with Down syndrome than in the general population. Third molars, laterals, and mandibular second bicuspids are the most common missing teeth.

- **Delayed eruption of teeth,** often following an abnormal sequence, affects some children with Down syndrome. Primary teeth may not appear until age 2, with complete dentition delayed until age 4 or 5. Primary teeth are then retained in some children until they are 14 or 15.

- **Irregularities in tooth formation,** such as microdontia and malformed teeth, are also seen in people with Down syndrome. Crowns tend to be smaller, and roots are often small and conical, which can lead to tooth loss from periodontal disease. Severe illness or prolonged fevers can lead to hypoplasia and hypocalcification.

  - Examine a child by her or his first birthday and regularly thereafter to help identify unusual tooth formation and patterns of eruption.

  - Consider using a panoramic radiograph to determine whether teeth are congenitally missing. Patients often find this technique less threatening than individual films.

  - Maintain primary teeth as long as possible. Consider placing space maintainers where teeth are missing.

Trauma and injury to the mouth from falls or accidents occur in people with Down syndrome. Suggest a tooth-saving kit for group homes. Emphasize to caregivers that traumas require immediate professional attention and explain the procedures to follow if a permanent tooth is knocked out. Also, instruct caregivers to locate any missing pieces of a fractured tooth, and explain that radiographs of the patient's chest may be necessary to determine whether any fragments have been aspirated.

Physical abuse often presents as oral trauma. Abuse is reported more frequently in people with developmental disabilities than in the general population. If you suspect that a child is being abused or neglected, state laws require that you call your Child Protective Services agency. Assistance is also available from the Childhelp® National Child Abuse Hotline at 800- 422-4453 or the Child Welfare Information Gateway (www.childwelfare.gov).

Section 51.6

Practical Oral Care for People with Intellectual Disability

This section includes text excerpted from "Practical Oral Care for People with Intellectual Disability," National Institute of Dental and Craniofacial Research (NIDCR), July 2009. Reviewed July 2019.

Providing oral care to people with intellectual disability requires adaptation of the skills you use every day. In fact, most people with mild or moderate intellectual disability can be treated successfully in the general practice setting. Intellectual disability is a disorder of mental and adaptive functioning, meaning that people who are affected are challenged by the skills they use in everyday life. Intellectual disability is not a disease or a mental illness; it is a developmental disability that varies in severity and is usually associated with physical problems. While one person with intellectual disability may have slight difficulty thinking and communicating, another may face major challenges with basic self-care and physical mobility.

Health Challenges in Intellectual Disability and Strategies for Care

Many people with intellectual disability also have other conditions, such as cerebral palsy, seizure or psychiatric disorders, attention deficit hyperactivity disorder, or problems with vision, communication, and eating. Though language and communication problems are common in anyone with intellectual disability, motor skills are typically more affected when a person has coexisting conditions.

Before the appointment, obtain and review the patient's medical history. Consultation with physicians, family, and caregivers is essential to assembling an accurate medical history. Also, determine who can legally provide informed consent for treatment.

Mental challenges. People with intellectual disability learn slowly and often with difficulty. Ordinary activities of daily living, such as brushing teeth and getting dressed, and understanding the behavior of others as well as their own, can all present challenges to a person with intellectual disability.

- Set the stage for a successful visit by involving the entire dental team—from the receptionist's friendly greeting to the caring

387

attitude of the dental assistant in the operatory. All should be aware of your patient's mental challenges.

- Reduce distractions in the operatory, such as unnecessary sights, sounds, or other stimuli, to compensate for the short attention spans commonly observed in people with intellectual disability.

- Talk with the parent or caregiver to determine your patient's intellectual and functional abilities, then explain each procedure at a level the patient can understand. Allow extra time to explain oral health issues or instructions and demonstrate the instruments you will use.

- Address your patient directly and with respect to establishing a rapport. Even if the caregiver is in the room, direct all questions and comments to your patient.

- Use simple, concrete instructions and repeat them often to compensate for any short-term memory problems. Speak slowly and give only one direction at a time.

- Be consistent in all aspects of oral care, since long-term memory is usually unaffected. Use the same staff and dental operatory each time to help sustain familiarity. The more consistency you provide for your patients, the more likely they will cooperate.

- Listen actively, since communicating clearly is often difficult for people with intellectual disability. Show your patient whether you understand. Be sensitive to the methods she or he uses to communicate, including gestures and verbal or nonverbal requests.

Behavior challenges. While most people with intellectual disability do not pose significant behavior problems that complicate oral care, anxiety about dental treatment occurs frequently. People unfamiliar with a dental office and its equipment and instruments may exhibit fear. Some react to fear with uncooperative behavior, such as crying, wiggling, kicking, aggressive language, or anything that will help them avoid treatment. You can make oral healthcare a better experience by comforting your patients and acknowledging their anxiety.

- Talk to the caregiver or physician about techniques they have found to be effective in managing the patient's behavior.

- Schedule patients with intellectual disability early in the day if possible. Early appointments can help ensure that everyone is alert and attentive and that waiting time is reduced.

- Keep appointments short and postpone difficult procedures until after your patient is familiar with you and your staff.

- Allow extra time for your patients to get comfortable with you, your office, and the entire oral healthcare team. Invite patients and their families to visit your office before beginning treatment. Permit the parents or caregiver to come into the treatment setting to provide familiarity, help with communication, and offer a calming influence by holding your patient's hand during treatment. Some patients' behavior may improve if they bring comfort items, such as a stuffed animal or blanket.

- Reward cooperative behavior with compliments throughout the appointment.

- Consider nitrous oxide/oxygen sedation to reduce anxiety and fear and improve cooperation. Obtain informed consent from the legal guardian before administering any kind of sedation.

- Use immobilization techniques only when absolutely necessary to protect the patient and staff during dental treatment — not as a convenience. There are no universal guidelines on immobilization that apply to all treatment settings. Before employing any kind of immobilization, it may help to consult available guidelines on federally funded care, your state department of mental health/ disabilities, and your State Dental Practice Act. Guidelines on behavior management published by the American Academy of Pediatric Dentistry (www.aapd. org) may also be useful. Obtain consent from your patient's legal guardian and choose the least restrictive technique that will allow you to provide care safely. Immobilization should not cause physical injury or undue discomfort.

People with intellectual disability often engage in perseveration, a continuous, meaningless repetition of words, phrases, or movements. Your patient may mimic the sound of the suction, for example, or repeat an instruction over and again. Avoid demonstrating dental equipment if it triggers perseveration, and note this in the patient's record.

Physical challenges. Intellectual disability does not always include a specific physical trait, although many people have distinguishing

389

features, such as orofacial abnormalities, scoliosis, unsteady gait, or hypotonia due to coexisting conditions. Countering physical challenges requires attention to detail.

Maintain clear paths for movement throughout the treatment setting. Keep instruments and equipment out of the patient's way.

Place and maintain your patient in the center of the dental chair to minimize the risk of injury. Placing pillows on both sides of the patient can provide stability.

If you need to transfer your patient from a wheelchair to the dental chair, ask the patient or caregiver about special preferences, such as padding, pillows, or other things you can provide to ease the transition. The patient or caregiver can often explain how to make a smooth transfer.

Some patients cannot be moved into the dental chair but instead must be treated in their wheelchairs. Some wheelchairs recline or are specially molded to fit people's bodies. Lock the wheels, then slip a sliding board (also called a "transfer board") behind the patient's back to provide support for the head and neck during care.

Cerebral palsy occurs in one-fourth of those who have intellectual disability and tends to affect motor skills more than cognitive skills. Uncontrolled body movements and reflexes associated with cerebral palsy can make it difficult to provide care.

- Place and maintain your patient in the center of the dental chair. Do not force arms and legs into unnatural positions, but allow your patient to settle into a position that is comfortable and will not interfere with dental treatment.

- Observe your patient's movements and look for patterns to help you anticipate direction and intensity. Trying to stop these movements may only intensify the involuntary response. Try instead to anticipate the movements, blending your movements with those of your patient or working around them.

- Softly cradle your patient's head during treatment. Be gentle and slow if you need to turn the patient's head.

- Help minimize the gag reflex by placing your patient's chin in a neutral or downward position. Stay alert and work efficiently in short appointments.

- Exert gentle but firm pressure on your patient's arm or leg if it begins to shake.

- Take frequent breaks or consider prescribing muscle relaxants when long procedures are needed. People with cerebral palsy may need sedation, general anesthesia, or hospitalization if extensive dental treatment is required.

Cardiovascular anomalies such as heart murmurs and damaged heart valves occur frequently in people with intellectual disability, especially those with Down syndrome or multiple disabilities. Consult the patient's physician to determine if antibiotic prophylaxis (www. americanheart.org) is necessary for dental treatment.

Seizures are common in this population but can usually be controlled with anticonvulsant medications. The mouth is always at risk during a seizure: Patients may chip teeth or bite the tongue or cheeks. Persons with controlled seizure disorders can easily be treated in the general dental office.

- Consult your patient's physician. Record information in the chart about the frequency of seizures and the medications used to control them. Determine before the appointment whether medications have been taken as directed. Know and avoid any factors that trigger your patient's seizures.

- Be prepared to manage a seizure. If one occurs during oral care, remove any instruments from the mouth and clear the area around the dental chair. Attaching dental floss to rubber dam clamps and mouth props when treatment begins can help you remove them quickly. Do not attempt to insert any objects between the teeth during a seizure.

- Stay with your patient, turn her or him to one side, and monitor the airway to reduce the risk of aspiration.

Visual impairments, most commonly strabismus (crossed or misaligned eyes) and refractive errors, can be managed with careful planning.

- Determine the level of assistance your patient requires to move safely through the dental office.

- Use your patients' other senses to connect with them, establish trust, and make treatment a good experience. Tactile feedback, such as a warm handshake, can make your patients feel comfortable.

- Face your patients when you speak and keep them apprised of each upcoming step, especially when water will be used.

391

Rely on clear, descriptive language to explain procedures and demonstrate how equipment might feel and sound. Provide written instructions in large print (16-point or larger).

Hearing loss and deafness can also be accommodated with careful planning. Patients with a hearing problem may appear to be stubborn because of their seeming lack of response to a request.

- Patients may want to adjust their hearing aids or turn them off, since the sound of some instruments may cause auditory discomfort.

- If your patient reads lips, speak in a normal cadence and tone. If your patient uses a form of sign language, ask the interpreter to come to the appointment. Speak with this person in advance to discuss dental terms and your patient's needs.

- Visual feedback is helpful. Maintain eye contact with your patient. Before talking, eliminate background noise (turn off the radio and the suction). Sometimes people with a hearing loss simply need you to speak clearly in a slightly louder voice than normal. Remember to remove your face mask first or wear a clear face shield.

Oral Health Problems in Intellectual Disability and Strategies for Care

In general, people with intellectual disability have poorer oral health and oral hygiene than those without this condition. Data indicate that people who have intellectual disability have more untreated caries and a higher prevalence of gingivitis and other periodontal diseases than the general population.

Periodontal disease. Medications, malocclusion, multiple disabilities, and poor oral hygiene combine to increase the risk of periodontal disease in people with intellectual disability.

- Encourage independence in daily oral hygiene. Ask patients to show you how they brush, and follow up with specific recommendations on brushing methods or toothbrush adaptations. Involve your patients in hands-on demonstrations of brushing and flossing.

- Some patients cannot brush and floss independently due to impaired physical coordination or cognitive skills. Talk to their caregivers about daily oral hygiene. Do not assume that all caregivers know the basics; demonstrate proper brushing and flossing techniques. A power toothbrush or a floss holder can simplify oral care. Also, use your experiences with each patient to demonstrate sitting or standing positions for the caregiver. Emphasize that a consistent approach to oral hygiene is important—caregivers should try to use the same location, timing, and positioning.

- Some patients benefit from the daily use of an antimicrobial agent, such as chlorhexidine. Recommend an appropriate delivery method based on your patient's abilities. Rinsing, for example, may not work for a patient who has swallowing difficulties or one who cannot expectorate. Chlorhexidine applied using a spray bottle or toothbrush is equally efficacious.

- If the use of particular medications has led to gingival hyperplasia, emphasize the importance of daily oral hygiene and frequent professional cleanings.

Dental caries. People with intellectual disability develop caries at the same rate as the general population. The prevalence of untreated dental caries, however, is higher among people with intellectual disability, particularly those living in noninstitutional settings.

- Emphasize noncariogenic foods and beverages as snacks. Advise caregivers to avoid using sweets as incentives or rewards.

- Advise patients taking medicines that cause xerostomia to drink water often. Suggest sugar-free medicine if available and stress the importance of rinsing with water after dosing.

- Recommend preventive measures, such as fluorides and sealants.

Malocclusion. The prevalence of malocclusion in people with intellectual disability is similar to that found in the general population, except for those with coexisting conditions, such as cerebral palsy or Down syndrome. A developmental disability in and of itself should not be perceived as a barrier to orthodontic treatment. The ability of the patient or caregiver to maintain good daily oral hygiene is critical to the feasibility and success of treatment.

Missing permanent teeth, delayed eruption, and enamel hypoplasia are more common in people with intellectual disability and coexisting conditions than in people with intellectual disability alone.

- Examine a child by her or his first birthday and regularly thereafter to help identify unusual tooth formation and patterns of eruption.

- Consider using a panoramic radiograph to determine whether teeth are congenitally missing. Patients often find this technique less threatening than individual films.

- Take appropriate steps to reduce sensitivity and risk of caries in your patients with enamel hypoplasia.

Damaging oral habits are a problem for some people with intellectual disability. Common habits include bruxism; mouth breathing; tongue thrusting; self-injurious behavior, such as picking at the gingiva or biting the lips; and pica—eating objects and substances, such as gravel, cigarette butts, or pens. If a mouthguard can be tolerated, prescribe one for patients who have problems with self-injurious behavior or bruxism.

Trauma and injury to the mouth from falls or accidents occur in people with intellectual disability. Suggest a tooth-saving kit for group homes. Emphasize to caregivers that traumas require immediate professional attention and explain the procedures to follow if a permanent tooth is knocked out. Also, instruct caregivers to locate any missing pieces of a fractured tooth, and explain that radiographs of the patient's chest may be necessary to determine whether any fragments have been aspirated.

Physical abuse often presents as oral trauma. Abuse is reported more frequently in people with developmental disabilities than in the general population. If you suspect that a child is being abused or neglected, state laws require that you call your Child Protective Services agency. Assistance is also available from the Childhelp® National Child Abuse Hotline at 800-422-4453 or the Child Welfare Information Gateway (www.childwelfare.gov).

Section 51.7

Dental Care Steps for People with Disability

This section includes text excerpted from "Practical Oral Care for People with Developmental Disabilities. Dental Care Every Day. A Caregiver's Guide," National Institute of Dental and Craniofacial Research (NIDCR), February 2012. Reviewed July 2019.

Taking care of someone with a disability requires patience and skill. As a caregiver, you know this as well as anyone does. You also know how challenging it is to help that person with dental care. It takes planning, time, and the ability to manage physical, mental, and behavioral problems. Dental care is not always easy, but you can make it work for you and the person you help. Everyone needs dental care every day. Brushing and flossing are crucial activities that affect our health. In fact, dental care is just as important to your client's health and daily routine as taking medications and getting physical exercise. A healthy mouth helps people eat well, avoid pain and tooth loss, and feel good about themselves.

Getting Started

Location. The bathroom is not the only place to brush one's teeth. For example, the kitchen or dining room may be more comfortable. Instead of standing next to a bathroom sink, allow the person to sit at a table. Place the toothbrush, toothpaste, floss, and a bowl and a glass of water on the table within easy reach.

No matter what location you choose, make sure you have good light. You cannot help someone brush unless you can see inside that person's mouth. As you read on, you will find ideas on how to sit or stand when you help someone brush and floss.

Behavior. Problem behavior can make dental care difficult. Try these ideas and see what works for you.

- At first, dental care can be frightening to some people. Try the "tell-show-do" approach to deal with this natural reaction. Tell your client about each step before you do it. For example, explain how you will help her or him brush and what it feels like. Show how you are going to do each step before you do it. Also, it might help to let your client hold and feel the toothbrush and floss. Do the steps in the same way that you have explained them.

395

- Give your client time to adjust to dental care. Be patient as that person learns to trust you working in and around her or his mouth.

- Use your voice and body to communicate that you care. Give positive feedback often to reinforce good behavior.

- Have a routine for dental care. Use the same technique at the same time and place every day. Many people with disabilities accept dental care when it is familiar. A routine might soothe fears or help eliminate problem behavior.

- Be creative. Some caregivers allow their client to hold a favorite toy or special item for comfort. Others make dental care a game or play a person's favorite music. If none of these ideas help, ask your client's dentist or dental hygienist for advice.

Three Steps to a Healthy Mouth

Like everyone else, people with disabilities can have a healthy mouth if these three steps are followed:

1. Brush every day.

2. Floss every day.

3. Visit a dentist regularly.

Step 1. Brush Every Day

If the person you care for is unable to brush, these suggestions might be helpful.

- First, wash your hands and put on disposable gloves. Sit or stand where you can see all of the surfaces of the teeth.

- Be sure to use a regular or power toothbrush with soft bristles.

- Use a pea-size amount of toothpaste with fluoride, or none at all. Toothpaste bothers people who have swallowing problems. If this is the case for the person you care for, brush with water instead.

- Brush the front, back, and top of each tooth. Gently brush back and forth in short strokes.

- Gently brush the tongue after you brush the teeth.

- Help the person rinse with plain water. Give people who cannot rinse a drink of water or consider sweeping the mouth with a finger wrapped in gauze.

Get a new toothbrush with soft bristles every 3 months, after a contagious illness, or when the bristles are worn. If the person you care for can brush but needs some help, the ideas listed on the next page might work for you. You may think of other creative ways to solve brushing problems based on your client's special needs.

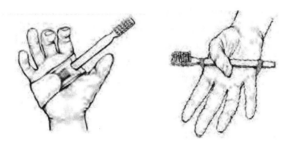

Figure 51.1. *Make Your Toothbrush Easier to Hold*

The same kind of Velcro® strap used to hold food utensils is helpful for some people. Others attach the brush to the hand with a wide elastic or rubber band. Make sure the band is not too tight.

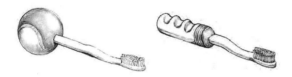

Figure 51.2. *Make Your Toothbrush Handle Bigger*

You can also cut a small slit in the side of a tennis ball and slide it onto the handle of the toothbrush.

You can buy a toothbrush with a large handle, or you can slide a bicycle grip onto the handle. Attaching foam tubing, available from home healthcare catalogs, is also helpful.

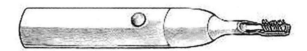

Figure 51.3. *Try Other Toothbrush Options*

A power toothbrush might make brushing easier. Take the time to help your client get used to one.

Guide the Toothbrush. Help brush by placing your hand very gently over your client's hand and guiding the toothbrush. If that does not work, you may need to brush the teeth yourself.

Step 2. Floss Every Day

Flossing cleans between the teeth where a toothbrush cannot reach. Many people with disabilities need a caregiver to help them floss. Flossing is a tough job that takes a lot of practice. Waxed, unwaxed, flavored, or plain floss all do the same thing. The person you care for might like one more than another, or a certain type might be easier to use.

- Use a string of floss 18 inches long. Wrap that piece around the middle finger of each hand.

- Grip the floss between the thumb and index finger of each hand.

- Start with the lower front teeth, then floss the upper front teeth. Next, work your way around to all the other teeth.

- Work the floss gently between the teeth until it reaches the gumline. Curve the floss around each tooth and slip it under the gum. Slide the floss up and down. Do this for both sides of every tooth, one side at a time.

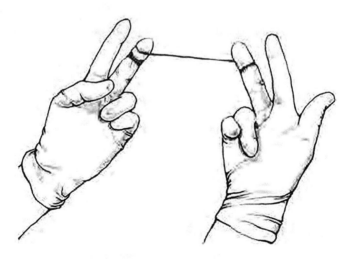

Figure 51.4. *How to Use a String of Floss*

- Adjust the floss a little as you move from tooth to tooth so the floss is clean for each one.

- If you have trouble flossing, try using a floss holder instead of holding the floss with your fingers.

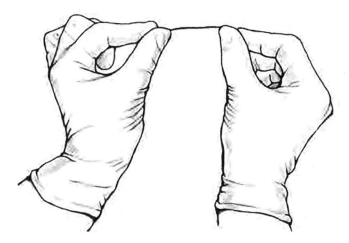

Figure 51.5. *Gripping the String of floss*

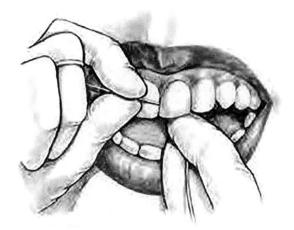

Figure 51.6. *How to Work the Floss*

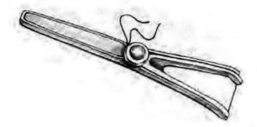

Figure 51.7. *Floss Holder*

The dentist may prescribe a special rinse for your client. Fluoride rinses can help prevent cavities. Chlorhexidine rinses fight germs that cause gum disease. Follow the dentist's instructions and tell your client not to swallow any of the rinse. Ask the dentist for creative ways to use rinses for a client with swallowing problems.

Positioning Your Body: Where to Sit or Stand

Keeping people safe when you clean their mouth is important. Experts in providing dental care for people with disabilities recommend the following positions for caregivers. If you work in a group home or related facility, get permission from your supervisor before trying any of these positions.

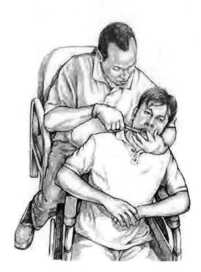

Figure 51.8. *Sitting and Helping a Person in a Wheelchair*

If the person you are helping is in a wheelchair, sit behind it. Lock the wheels, then tilt the chair into your lap.

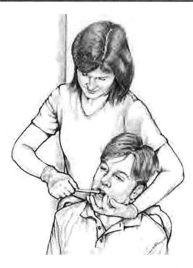

Figure 51.9. *Standing and Helping a Person in a Wheelchair*

Stand behind the person or lean against a wall for additional support. Use your arm to hold the person's head gently against your body.

Step 3. Visit a Dentist Regularly

Your client should have regular dental appointments. Professional cleanings are just as important as brushing and flossing every day. Regular examinations can identify problems before they cause unnecessary pain.

As is the case with dental care at home, it may take time for the person you care for to become comfortable at the dental office. A "get acquainted" visit with no treatment provided might help: The person can meet the dental team, sit in the dental chair if she or he wishes, and receive instructions on how to brush and floss. Such a visit can go a long way toward making dental appointments easier.

Prepare for Every Dental Visit: Your Role

Be prepared for every appointment. You are an important source of information for the dentist. If you have questions about what the dentist will need to know, call the office before the appointment.

- **Know the person's dental history.** Keep a record of what happens at each visit. Talk to the dentist about what occurred at the last appointment. Remind the dental team of what worked and what did not.

- **Bring a complete medical history.** The dentist needs each patient's medical history before treatment can begin. Bring a list of all the medications the person you care for is taking and all known allergies.

- **Bring all insurance, billing, and legal information.** Know who is responsible for payment. The dentist may need permission, or legal consent, before treatment can begin. Know who can legally give consent.

- **Be on time.**

Remember

Brushing and flossing every day and seeing the dentist regularly can make a big difference in the quality of life of the person you care for. If you have questions, talk to a dentist.

Chapter 52

Eating Disorders and Oral Health

Dental and oral health are important components of an individual's overall health and well-being. Eating disorders (EDs) can have deleterious consequences for dental and oral health. Individuals with eating disorders may experience several oral manifestations arising from nutritional deficiencies and resulting metabolic impairment. Oral manifestations of EDs may also be caused by drug use, poor personal hygiene, altered nutritional habits, and other psychological disturbances associated with EDs. The tissues usually affected include the oral mucosa, periodontium (the supporting tissues that anchor the teeth to the maxillary and mandibular bones [upper and lower jawbones]), teeth, salivary glands, and perioral area (the soft tissue around the mouth).

General Signs and Symptoms of Dental and Oral Implications of Eating Disorders

- Changes in color, size, and shape of teeth often resulting in brittle, translucent teeth

- Increased sensitivity to extreme temperatures

"Eating Disorders and Oral Health," © 2019 Omnigraphics. Reviewed July 2019.

- Exposed, infected pulp tissue, sometimes, leading to pulpitis (inflammation of dental pulp tissue) and finally to pulp death

Oral Sequelae of Bulimia and Anorexia Nervosa

Chronic self-induced vomiting, a classic symptom of bulimia and anorexia nervosa, is one of the most important etiologies of oral complications associated with the disorders. The severity of oral complications depends largely on the duration of the disease, the frequency of vomiting, and the fundamental quality of the dentition. Tooth erosion, or perimylolysis in medical parlance, is one of the most serious consequences of the binge–purge cycle. At the onset, there is a subtle loss of the tooth enamel—the hard, mineralized outer layer of a tooth that serves as a barrier against food, drinks, and microorganisms. Over time, regular exposure of the dentition to acidic content regurgitated from the stomach during purging begins to wear away the dentine—the dense and calcified bony tissue beneath the enamel.

Tooth erosion may manifest as early as six months following the onset of regular self-induced vomiting, but a definitive diagnosis confirming the lesions associated with EDs may take a year or more. These lesions typically occur in the maxillary teeth. They also occur on the mandibular teeth, albeit to a lesser degree since the tongue protects the lower jaw dentition from acid attack. In addition to acid exposure, mechanical degradation of the dentine is also present, resulting from the abnormal tongue movements and disrupted swallowing patterns characteristic of EDs.

Other oral complications of EDs include tooth decay, gingivitis (nondestructive gum disease), and xerostomia (drying of the oral cavity). Poor oral hygiene and ingestion of high-carbohydrate food and carbonated beverages characteristic of binge-eating episodes cause dental caries (tooth decay). Gum disease results from the exposure of gum tissue to the low-pH gastric content during purging. Volitional purging can also cause enlargement of the salivary glands. This manifests as a swelling of the area between the neck and jaw and is sometimes identifiable by what is commonly described as the "chipmunk cheeks." While this condition may be intermittent during the initial days of purging, it often becomes persistent after a considerable period of purging and results in reduced salivary secretion and xerostomia. While the exact mechanism of salivary-gland enlargement is not clear, this condition presents in over 50 percent of patients with self-induced vomiting, and is seen to regress spontaneously with the cessation of the purging. Rapid ingestion of large amounts of food and forced regurgitation may also injure the oral mucosa (the mucous membranes that line the inside of the mouth) and the pharynx. In some cases, the soft palate may be injured by fingers or other objects used to induce vomiting.

Awareness of the fact that volitional purging strongly associated with bulimia nervosa has serious oral and dental implications is evident, but the fact that anorexia nervosa can be just as detrimental to dental health is less widely known. Individuals suffering from anorexia may also engage in inappropriate compensatory methods, such as self-induced purging to prevent weight gain. In this subtype of anorexia, individuals may purge after binge eating, or even following ingestion of small amounts of food. In addition to purging, most people with an anorexia disorder also engage in restrictive eating in an effort to maintain their abnormally low body weight. Nutritional deficiencies associated with the semi-starvation that is typical of anorexia can also have devastating consequences on health in general. Anorexics may develop osteoporosis and experience weakening of the jawbone, which could lead to the weakening of teeth and subsequent tooth loss. Studies also show a correlation between osteoporosis and progression of periodontal (gum) disease in EDs. Periodontitis is a chronic inflammatory condition involving the soft tissues surrounding the teeth. It usually begins as gingivitis—a mild inflammation of the gums caused by a bacterial infection. Over time, those bacterial toxins work together with the body's natural immune response to infection to break down the bone and connective tissue that hold the teeth in place. This may progress at an accelerated pace if the density of bone affected by periodontitis is already suboptimal as a result of the effect of osteoporosis in EDs.

Dental Management in Eating Disorders

Dentists and dental hygienists are among the first healthcare professionals to detect clinical signs of EDs. If oral healthcare professionals suspect oral manifestations of EDs, it is recommended that they subject their patients to a preliminary screening in a nonconfrontational manner. Discussing the patient's eating habits and recommending weight-management strategies after creating an environment conducive to patient–physician interaction is paramount. This may help open up a line of communication with the patient during subsequent visits and may lead to referrals.

Ideally, individuals with EDs require continuous care and support for managing their oral health. Diagnosis of dental and oral complications are based on external examination and imaging studies of the hard and soft tissues of the oral cavity. Patients should also be encouraged to return for further evaluation and follow-up treatment. Regarding dental treatment involving complex restorative or prosthodontic procedures, clinical authorities recommend that it is initiated only after the cessation of the binge–purge cycle and after the underlying psychiatric components of the disorder have been adequately stabilized. This, however, does not include pain palliation.

Interim measures to arrest further destruction of the tooth structure include:

- Professional dental care on a regular basis and topical fluoride application to reduce thermal hypersensitivity and prevent further erosion

- Rigorous hygiene and home care, including the daily application of fluoride gel or prescription fluoride dental paste to promote remineralization of enamel

- Gum or lozenges to stimulate saliva secretion; or artificial saliva, to treat severe xerostomia

- Mouthwash immediately after vomiting to neutralize acids and protect tooth surfaces

Role of Dental Professionals in Identifying Eating Disorders

Pediatric dentists and orthodontists usually monitor their patients throughout childhood and adolescence and, therefore, play an important role in the early detection of EDs—a crucial factor in aiding recovery and reducing the morbidity and mortality associated with EDs. Hence, it is very important for these dental professionals to pick up clinical clues of EDs from dental examination and radiographs and then utilize them to make referrals for appropriate healthcare services. These service providers can facilitate the management of the underlying psychiatric condition.

It is widely perceived that dental professionals are the first to observe the overt health effects of EDs. Yet studies show that this does not always lead to early diagnosis and intervention for EDs. A lack of knowledge about the scope and severity of EDs among oral-health professionals, lack of skilled training in patient communication, and lack of practice protocol are often seen as barriers to the identification and referral treatment of EDs.

References

1. "Oral Health Fact Sheet for Dental Professionals—Adults with Eating Disorders," University of Washington School of Dentistry (UVSOD), August 17, 2010.

2. "Eating Disorders and Oral Health: A Review of the Literature," *Australian Dental Journal*, 2005.

Chapter 53

Heart Disease and Oral Health

Studies have shown that oral health affects far more than just a person's smile. In fact, it has an impact on many aspects of a person's overall health, including their risk of developing heart disease. More than 80 percent of Americans have some form of periodontal (gum) disease, which is generally related to infrequent brushing of teeth and failure to visit a dentist regularly. Research suggests that those with moderate or advanced forms of gum disease may face a risk of cardiovascular illness that is up to 70 percent higher than people who practice good oral hygiene and brush their teeth at least twice per day.

Scientists believe that the connection between oral health and heart disease centers around bacteria. Periodontal disease is caused by bacteria in the mouth. When these bacteria enter the bloodstream— through a sore in the mouth, for instance, or a gap around a tooth— they may become incorporated into the buildup of fatty deposits or plaques in the lining of artery walls. These plaque deposits can restrict the flow of blood through arteries, leading to serious health problems such as blood clots or atherosclerosis. Bacteria from the mouth may also travel through the bloodstream and attach to damaged areas of the heart, resulting in an infection of the heart lining called "endocarditis." Finally, gum disease bacteria may stimulate the liver and the immune system in ways that produce inflammation. Inflammation

"Heart Disease and Oral Health," © 2017 Omnigraphics. Reviewed July 2019.

causes further narrowing of the blood vessels, which can lead to a heart attack or stroke.

Oral Health Symptoms Linked to Cardiovascular Risk

The risk of developing heart disease is highest for people with advanced periodontal disease or chronic gum conditions such as gingivitis. When these oral health conditions are undiagnosed or untreated, they may cause some of the following symptoms:

- Gums that are red, swollen, or tender

- Gums that bleed frequently while eating, brushing, or flossing

- Gums that appear to be pulling away from teeth

- Bad breath (halitosis) that occurs frequently

- A bad taste in the mouth

- Pus or other signs of infection in the mouth

- Teeth that are loose or appear to be moving away from other teeth

- Changes in the alignment of teeth or bite

Practicing good oral hygiene, such as brushing the teeth at least twice per day and visiting a dentist regularly for examinations and professional cleanings, is the best method of preventing periodontal disease. Although good oral health does not necessarily prevent the development of cardiovascular disease, it can lead to improvements in overall health.

Heart Disease and Dental Treatment

The link between oral health and cardiovascular disease means that some forms of dental care and treatment may pose risks for people with preexisting heart and artery conditions. To reduce the risk of endocarditis from bacteria entering the bloodstream, the American Heart Association (AHA) recommends that people with certain heart conditions take antibiotics before undergoing dental procedures that involve incisions in the gums or manipulation of the tissues surrounding the root of a tooth. Antibiotics are not necessary for routine dental procedures like x-rays, anesthetic injections, adjustment of orthodontic appliances, placement of dentures, or bleeding from injuries to the lips or mouth. Some of the heart conditions that increase the risk of infection from dental procedures include the following:

- Artificial heart valves

- Heart transplants

- A past history of endocarditis

- A heart defect that was not repaired or was repaired with a prosthetic material or device

- Cyanotic heart disease that was not repaired or partially repaired

In addition to these conditions that require pretreatment with antibiotics, other cardiovascular conditions may affect dental treatment in other ways. For instance, some medications that are commonly prescribed to treat high blood pressure, high cholesterol, or angina may have oral effects that the dentist must take into consideration. Blood-thinning medications may cause excessive bleeding following oral surgery, while calcium channel blockers may cause gum overgrowth that requires dental intervention. Some medications prescribed to treat high cholesterol may make patients feel faint when they arise from a reclining dental chair, while some drugs used to treat high blood pressure can cause dry mouth or an altered sense of taste. Electromagnetic devices used in a dentist's office could potentially interfere with a pacemaker.

Because of the many points of interaction between oral health and cardiovascular health, patients with any type of condition affecting the heart or arteries should inform their dentist prior to undergoing treatment. In addition, they should provide their dentist with a complete and up-to-date list of all the medications they take, including prescription drugs, over-the-counter (OTC) medicines, vitamins, and supplements.

References

1. "Cardiovascular Diseases," Colgate Oral Health Center, 2016.

2. "How May Dental Health Be Linked to Cardiovascular Disease?" SimplyHealth, 2012.

Chapter 54

Immune System Disorders and Oral Health

Chapter Contents

Section 54.1

Latex Allergy and Dental Treatment

This section includes text excerpted from "Contact
Dermatitis and Latex Allergy," Centers for Disease
Control and Prevention (CDC), March 3, 2016.

What Is Latex Allergy?

Latex allergy is a reaction to certain proteins in latex rubber. It usually begins within minutes of exposure but can sometimes occur hours later. It produces varied symptoms, which commonly include runny nose, sneezing, itchy eyes, scratchy throat, hives, and itchy burning sensations. However, it can involve more severe symptoms, such as asthma, marked by difficult breathing, coughing spells, and wheezing; cardiovascular and gastrointestinal ailments; and in rare cases, anaphylaxis and death.

What Is Contact Dermatitis?

Contact dermatitis can develop from frequent and repeated use of hand hygiene products, exposure to chemicals, and glove use. Contact dermatitis is classified as either irritant or allergic. Irritant contact dermatitis is common, nonallergic, and develops as dry, itchy, irritated areas on the skin around the area of contact. Allergic contact dermatitis can result from exposure to accelerators and other chemicals used to manufacture rubber gloves or from exposure to other chemicals found in the dental practice setting. Allergic contact dermatitis often causes a rash beginning hours after contact and, like irritant dermatitis, is usually confined to the areas of contact.

What Should Dental Healthcare Personnel Do If They Are Allergic to Latex?

Dental Healthcare Personnel (DHCP) who have contact dermatitis or latex allergy symptoms should see an experienced healthcare professional (e.g., dermatologist, allergist) to determine the diagnosis, treatment, and any necessary work restrictions or accommodations.

The following recommendations are based on those issued by the National Institute for Occupational Safety and Health (NIOSH):

If diagnosed by a medical provider with an allergy to natural rubber latex (NRL) protein:

- Avoid, as far as feasible, subsequent exposure to the protein and use only nonlatex (e.g., nitrile or vinyl) gloves.

- Make sure that other staff in the dental practice wear either nonlatex or reduced-protein, powder-free latex gloves.

- Use only synthetic or powder-free rubber dams.

The following steps will further reduce the risk of latex reactions for DHCP:

- Educate dental staff on the signs and symptoms of latex allergies.

- Frequently change ventilation filters and vacuum bags used in latex-contaminated areas.

- Check ventilation systems to ensure they provide adequate fresh or recirculating air.

- Frequently clean all work areas contaminated with latex dust.

What Should Dental Healthcare Personnel Do When Treating Patients with Latex Allergy?

All patients should be screened for latex allergy (e.g., take a health history and refer for medical consultation when latex allergy is suspected). Patients with a latex allergy should not have direct contact with latex-containing materials and should be treated in a latex-safe environment. Such patients also may be allergic to the chemicals used in manufacturing natural rubber latex gloves, or to metals, plastics, or other materials used to provide dental care.

Dental Healthcare Personnel (DHCP) should take the following precautions for patients with a possible or documented latex allergy:

- Ensure a latex-safe environment in which all latex-containing products have been removed from the vicinity. Any latex-containing devices that cannot be removed from the treatment environment should be adequately covered or isolated.

  - Consider sources of latex other than gloves, such as prophylaxis cups, rubber dams, and orthodontic elastics.

- Be aware that latent allergens in the air can cause respiratory or anaphylactic symptoms among patients with latex hypersensitivity. Schedule patients with latex allergies for the first appointment of the day to minimize their exposure to airborne latex particles.

- Communicate latex allergy procedures (e.g., verbal instructions, written protocols, posted signs) to other personnel to prevent them from bringing latex-containing materials into the treatment area.

- Frequently clean all working areas contaminated with latex powder or dust.

- Have latex-free kits (e.g., dental treatment and emergency kits) available at all times.

Section 54.2

Mouth Problems with Human Immunodeficiency Virus

This section contains text excerpted from the following sources: Text beginning with the heading "Oral Health Problems Are Common among People Living with HIV/AIDS" is excerpted from "Oral Health and HIV," Health Resources and Services Administration (HRSA), n.d.; Text under the heading "Dental Appointments" is excerpted from "Seeing Your Healthcare Provider," HIV.gov, U.S. Department of Health and Human Services (HHS), May 15, 2017.

Oral Health Problems Are Common among People Living with HIV/AIDS

People living with human immunodeficiency virus (HIV)/acquired immunodeficiency syndrome (AIDS) (PLWHA) experience a high incidence of common oral health problems (e.g., dental decay/cavities, gingivitis) as well as other oral health problems that are directly related to HIV infection. Between 32 and 46 percent of PLWHA will have at least one major HIV-related oral health problem—bacterial, viral, and fungal infections as well as cancer and ulcers—in the course of their disease. In addition:

- Poor oral health can impede food intake and nutrition, leading to poor absorption of HIV medications and leaving PLWHA susceptible to the progression of their disease.

- Human immunodeficiency virus (HIV) medications have side effects, such as dry mouth, which predisposes PLWHA to dental decay, periodontal disease, and fungal infections.

- Bacterial infections (i.e., dental decay and periodontal disease) that begin in the mouth can escalate to systemic infections and harm the heart and other organs if not treated, particularly in PLWHA with severely compromised immune systems.

- A history of chronic periodontal disease can disrupt diabetic control and lead to a significant increase in the risk of delivering preterm low-birth-weight babies.

- Poor oral health can adversely affect the quality of life (QOL) and limit career opportunities and social contact as a result of facial appearance and odor.

Many People Living with HIV/AIDS Lack Oral Healthcare

For many years, PLWHA have reported high rates of unmet oral healthcare needs and low utilization of oral health services. When paired with weakened immune systems, lack of dental care puts many PLWHA at high risk for oral diseases and compromised well-being.

- The HIV Cost and Services Utilization Study (HCSUS) found that 58 percent of PLWHA did not receive regular dental care. More recent studies covering specific U.S. regions have reported similar findings. A study in North Carolina, for example, found that 64 percent of PLWHA had unmet dental needs.

- PLWHA have more unmet oral healthcare needs than does the general population. PLWHA also have more unmet oral healthcare needs than unmet medical needs.

- Certain groups of PLWHA, such as people of color (especially women and those without dental insurance) are less likely to receive oral healthcare than others living with HIV.

417

People Living with HIV/AIDS Face Many Barriers to Oral Healthcare

Major factors contributing to unmet oral health needs include the following:

- Lack of dental insurance
- Limited financial resources
- Shortage of dentists trained or willing to treat PLWHA
- Shrinking adult dental Medicaid services
- Patient fear of and discomfort with dentists
- Perceived stigma within healthcare systems
- Lack of awareness of the importance of oral health

Dental Professionals Can Enhance HIV/AIDS Care

- Dentists can control or eliminate a local infection to avoid adverse consequences, such as systemic infections, eliminate pain and discomfort, and restore oral health functions.
- Oral lesions can be the first overt clinical features of HIV infection; therefore, dental professionals are well-positioned to help with early detection and referral. Early detection can improve prognosis and reduce transmission, because infected PLWHA may not know their HIV status.
- Encounters in oral healthcare provide opportunities to prevent disease and address lifestyle behavior practices, such as oral hygiene, smoking cessation assistance, and nutrition counseling.
- A visit to the dentist may be a healthcare milestone for PLWHA. The dental professional can address oral health concerns and play a role in helping engage or reintroduce patients into the healthcare system and coordinate their care with other primary care providers.

How Grantees Can Improve Oral Health Services for People Living with HIV/AIDS

Following are some questions grantees should consider when assessing their oral health services and the kinds of support they may need to successfully meet clients' oral healthcare needs.

Oral Health Services Availability

- What is currently in place?

- What resources are being put toward oral health?

- Are PLWHA in the community receiving routine oral health services through your site? Emergency dental care?

- How are you prioritizing the allocation of funds for oral health services?

- Are efforts being made and agreements in place with private dentists to treat referred patients at reduced fees? How about with community health centers? Are there referral mechanisms between general dental providers and dental specialists?

- What else can be done to expand services?

Integration with Primary Care

- Are there referral mechanisms between medical and dental providers?

- Do dental providers collaborate with the primary medical care providers to obtain information on the medication regimen, immune status, and health of their patients?

- Are dental and primary care services co-located?

- Are dental and medical records electronically linked?

- Do primary care providers perform oral healthcare services, such as oral health screening, oral health education, and referrals?

Quality Management

- Is oral health part of an overall clinical quality management plan?

- Which of the HIV/AIDS Bureau (HAB) oral health performance measures is being monitored?

Dental Appointments

Dental visits are an extremely important part of your care when living with HIV. Many signs of HIV infection can begin in the mouth and throat, and people with HIV are more likely to develop some serious

419

dental problems. For these reasons, it is important to see a dentist regularly.

Tips for your dental visit:

- Make sure you have routine dental visits for cleaning and check-ups. Preventing problems before they occur is always the best approach.

- Tell your dentist you have HIV. That is not because your dentist will need to take additional precautions—all healthcare professionals use "universal precautions" to prevent the transmission of blood-borne diseases to patients and vice versa. Rather, it will help the dentist know to look for particular oral health problems that you might be at risk for.

- Do not wait for problems in your mouth to get out of hand. When you notice something wrong (such as tooth pain or a mouth sore), call your dentist right away.

- Be on time for your dental visit. Try not to miss your appointment, if you can help it—and if you cannot, reschedule it as soon as possible (ASAP).

- Keep a record of your dental visits, just like you do with your visits to your HIV care provider. Keep track of when you had dental x-rays (and what was x-rayed), any procedures or treatments you had, and when your next visit is scheduled.

- Bring copies of your recent test results and lab reports. Your dentist may need to have information about your cluster of differentiation 4 (CD4) count and platelet count to know how best to treat your dental issue. Also, bring a list of any medications you are currently taking, as your dentist needs to know what you are taking to avoid giving you other medications which may have bad interactions.

- Know your rights: Any dentist licensed in the United States should be able to provide at least basic dental care to people living with HIV. If you sense there is discrimination toward you based on your HIV status, there are resources to help you with this.

Chapter 55

Meth (Methamphetamine) Mouth

Methamphetamine—"meth" for short—is a very addictive stimulant drug. It is a powder that can be made into a pill or a shiny rock (called a "crystal"). The powder can be eaten or snorted up the nose. It can also be mixed with liquid and injected into your body with a needle. Crystal meth is smoked in a small glass pipe.

Meth at first causes a rush of good feelings, but then users feel edgy, overly excited, angry, or afraid. Meth use can quickly lead to addiction. It causes medical problems including:

- Making your body temperature so high that you pass out

- Severe itching

- "Meth mouth"—broken teeth and dry mouth

- Thinking and emotional problems

This chapter contains text excerpted from the following sources: Text in this chapter begins with excerpts from "Methamphetamine," MedlinePlus, National Institutes of Health (NIH), May 6, 2016; Text under the heading "Meth Mouth and Crank Bugs" is excerpted from "Meth Mouth and Crank Bugs: Meth-A-Morphosis," National Institute on Drug Abuse (NIDA) for Teens, July 31, 2013. Reviewed July 2019; Text under the heading "Key Findings about Meth Users" is excerpted from "Meth Mouth: Some Ugly Numbers," National Institute on Drug Abuse (NIDA) for Teens, February 29, 2016.

Meth Mouth and Crank Bugs

Meth can mess up your body's chemical structure and even cause problems with your heart and lungs, it also changes your appearance and behavior. Soon, meth users might not even look or act like themselves.

Bad news for teeth and skin. Ever heard of "meth mouth?" It is not pretty. Meth reduces the amount of protective saliva around the teeth. People who use the drug also tend to drink a lot of sugary soda, neglect personal hygiene, grind their teeth, and clench their jaws. The teeth of meth users can eventually fall out—even when doing something as normal as chewing a sandwich. As if that is not bad enough, meth can also cause skin problems—and they are not just talking about regular zits.

No peace of mind. In addition to the "crank bug" hallucinations, long-term meth use leads to problems, such as irritability, fatigue, headaches, anxiety, sleeplessness, confusion, aggressive feelings, violent rages, and depression.

Users may become psychotic and experience paranoia, mood disturbances, and delusions. The paranoia may even make the person think about killing themselves or someone else.

Key Findings about Meth Users

The National Institute on Drug Abuse (NIDA) have described before how using meth can have a lot of really unpleasant effects on the body. One of those effects is "meth mouth," where a meth user's teeth become broken, stained, and rotten, and may eventually fall out.

Well, the news about meth mouth got even worse recently: Turns out it happens to meth users a lot more often than was previously known.

Researchers examined 571 meth users and found that:

- 96 percent of them had cavities (a cavity is a hole or other damage to the outside layers of a tooth—but you probably knew that).

- Adults who said they used meth "moderately" or "heavily" were twice as likely to have untreated cavities as "light" users— "light" users had used the drug for less than 10 days over the previous month. (If a cavity goes untreated, it grows larger and larger, it can cause a really bad toothache, the cavity can become infected, and the tooth may have to be removed.)

- 58 percent of the meth users had untreated tooth decay, compared with 27 percent of the general population in the United States.

- Only 23 percent kept all of their natural teeth, compared to 48 percent of the general population in the United States. That is a lot of additional tooth loss for the people who used meth.

- A significant number of meth users (40%) said they were often self-conscious or embarrassed because of the condition of their teeth or dentures.

So it looks like the question with meth mouth is not really if it will happen to a person who uses meth. The question is more like, how bad will their meth mouth get?

Chapter 56

Organ Transplantation and Oral Health Management

Patient Population

According to the Health Resources and Services Administration (HRSA), nearly 29,000 solid organ transplants and more than 6,300 stem cell transplants from unrelated donors were performed in the United States in 2013. Thousands more patients received stem cell transplants from their family members and far more than that received transplants from their own stem cells. Stem cell transplants are a treatment for life-threatening leukemia, lymphoma, or other diseases.

Of those who received a solid organ transplant in 2013, most (about 17,000) people received a kidney, usually because of end-stage kidney failure resulting from severe diabetes or high blood pressure. About 6,000 livers were transplanted, most often for people with hepatitis C virus or alcoholic liver disease. Other organs transplanted were the heart, lung, pancreas, and intestine.

Because the immune system of a transplant patient is compromised, the patient is at increased risk of oral and systemic infections and other complications and requires specialized dental care delivered by general dentists in collaboration with the medical team. Optimal management

This chapter includes text excerpted from "Dental Management of the Organ or Stem Cell Transplant Patient," National Institute of Dental and Craniofacial Research (NIDCR), July 2016.

of the patient's oral health requires communication between the dentist and the medical team.

Managing Oral Health before Transplantation

Before treating a prospective transplant recipient, obtain and review the patient's medical and dental histories, perform a noninvasive initial oral examination (without periodontal probing), and obtain radiographs. After the examination, discuss with your patient's physician the current status of your patient's overall health and immune system. Decisions about the timing of treatment, the need for antibiotic prophylaxis, precautions to prevent excessive bleeding, and the appropriate medication and dosage should be considered during your discussion.

Whether a patient can tolerate dental treatment is a crucial concern. For some patients, it will be safer to undergo extensive dental treatment after their overall health improves after transplantation.

Preparing for Dental Treatment

Before starting your patient's dental treatment before transplantation, consider several factors:

- **Antibiotic prophylaxis:** Consult with the patient's physician to determine whether antibiotic prophylaxis is required to prevent systemic infection from invasive dental procedures. Unless advised otherwise by the physician, the American Heart Association's (AHA) standard regimen to prevent endocarditis is an accepted option.

- **Oral infection:** If the patient presents with an active oral infection, such as a purulent periodontal infection or an abscessed tooth, antibiotics should be given to the patient before and after dental treatment to prevent systemic infection. Confirm the choice of antibiotic with the patient's physician. Before transplantation, the active oral infection must be eliminated.

- **Excessive bleeding:** Several factors can cause bleeding problems in transplant candidates, such as the disease itself or medications. For example, patients may have a decreased platelet count or be on anticoagulant medications. Patients with end-stage liver disease may have excessive bleeding because the liver is no longer producing sufficient amounts of clotting factors.

Before treatment, assess the patient's bleeding potential with the appropriate laboratory tests and take precautions to limit bleeding.

- Consult with your patient's physician about whether antifibrinolytic drugs, vitamin K, fresh frozen plasma, or other interventions are appropriate for critical dental procedures. The physician also may decide to temporarily decrease the patient's level of anticoagulation before extensive dental surgeries. Because of bleeding risk, some patients are suitable for surgery only in a hospital setting or dental offices designed to handle emergency medical situations.

- Use aggressive suctioning techniques when performing extractions or other invasive procedures to prevent your patient from swallowing blood. In a small number of patients with advanced liver disease, swallowed blood may increase the risk for hepatic coma.

- Manage bleeding sites with careful packing and suturing techniques.

- **Medication considerations:** Patients preparing to undergo organ or stem cell transplantation may be taking multiple medications. These include anticoagulants, beta-blockers, calcium channel blockers, diuretics, and others. Be aware of the side effects of these medications, which range from xerostomia and gingival hyperplasia to orthostatic hypotension and hyperglycemia, and their interactions with drugs that you might prescribe.

Likewise, use caution when prescribing medication to patients with end-stage kidney or liver disease. Many medications commonly used in dental practice, including nonsteroidal anti-inflammatory drugs (NSAIDs), opiates, and some antimicrobials, are metabolized by these organs and are not removed from circulation as quickly in patients with markedly reduced kidney or liver function. Before dental treatment, consult the patient's physician on appropriate drug selection, dosage, and administration intervals.

- **Other medical problems:** Patients with end-stage organ failure may have other major medical conditions. A person with end-stage kidney disease, for example, may have diabetes or significant pulmonary or heart disease. Carefully review your patient's medical history to determine what additional treatment considerations your patient may have.

427

Dental Treatment

Whenever possible, all active dental disease should be eliminated before transplantation, since postoperative immunosuppression decreases a patient's ability to resist systemic infection.

- Eliminate or stabilize sites of oral infection. Patients with active dental disease who can tolerate treatment should receive indicated dental care. Depending on the patient's condition, temporary restoration may be appropriate until her or his health improves.

- Extract nonrestorable teeth.

- Consider removing orthodontic bands or adjusting prostheses if a patient is expected to receive cyclosporine after transplant because some people taking this drug will develop gingival hyperplasia. Overgrowth can be minimized with good plaque control, and removing orthodontic bands may make it easier to maintain good oral hygiene.

- Conduct dental procedures on days that your patient with end-stage renal disease does not undergo hemodialysis.

- Pay special attention to your patient's anxiety and pain tolerance.

- Counsel the patient about oral health. Explain that effective oral hygiene is crucial before and after transplantation. The patient may experience fewer oral and dental problems after transplantation by reducing the number of oral bacteria and inhibiting their proliferation.

- Instruct patients to bring a current list of their medications, including over-the-counter (OTC) drugs, to every appointment and note those medications that may be problematic.

Managing Oral Health after Transplantation

Except for emergency dental care, patients who receive organ or stem cell transplants should avoid dental treatment for at least three months. Dosage of immunosuppressive drugs is highest in the early posttransplant period, and patients are at greatest risk for serious complications, such as rejection of the transplanted organ, during that time. Once the graft has stabilized (which typically occurs within three to six months of the transplant procedure) and the medical team clears the patient for dental treatment, patients can be treated in the dental office with proper precautions.

Preparing for Dental Treatment

Treatment after transplantation requires consultation with your patient's physician. The medical consult can help you understand your patient's general health and ability to tolerate treatment. Posttransplant patients vary widely in their ability to endure dental treatment and heal following invasive procedures. Your discussion needs to address whether your patient requires antibiotic prophylaxis and if the physician will need to adjust other medications before treatment.

- **Infection:** Patients who have had a transplant procedure are at increased risk for serious infection. Bacterial, viral, and fungal infections are more common, especially immediately after the procedure. The decision to premedicate for invasive dental procedures and selection of the appropriate regimen should be done in consultation with the patient's physician.

- **Medication considerations:** Your transplant patient may be taking one or more medications that affect dental treatment. Immunosuppressive drugs can cause gingival hyperplasia, poor healing, and infections and may interact with commonly prescribed medications. Anticoagulant medications may contribute to excessive bleeding problems, whereas a patient taking steroids is at risk for acute adrenal crisis. The patient's physician may want to adjust these medications several days before an invasive dental procedure.

Dental Treatment

All new dental disease should be treated after the patient's transplant has stabilized.

- Check your patient's blood pressure before you begin treatment. Know baseline levels for each patient and call her or his physician immediately if blood pressure exceeds accepted thresholds. Do not treat a patient when this problem is present.

- Know your patient's bleeding potential and take appropriate steps to manage excessive bleeding.

- Prescribe an antimicrobial rinse when appropriate.

- Recommend saliva substitutes and fluoride rinses if your patient has dry mouth.

- Advise your patients to follow a conscientious oral hygiene routine and emphasize the importance of oral health.

- Examine the patient's mouth thoroughly for dental infection, since immunosuppressive drugs can hide signs of a problem. As a result, infections are often more advanced than they appear when detected. Treat all infections aggressively.

- Watch for signs of adrenal insufficiency with surgical stress in patients taking steroids. These patients may require hydrocortisone replacement therapy at the time of extensive dental procedures to avoid adrenal insufficiency syndrome. A person experiencing this condition may become hypertensive, weak, feverish, and nauseated and should be transported immediately to a hospital for treatment.

- Exercise care in prescribing medications to avoid potentiating the renal and hepatic toxicities of immunosuppressant drugs. Consult the patient's physician to ensure proper drug selection and dosing.

Side Effects of Immunosuppressive Drugs

Immunosuppressive drugs are associated with side effects and oral complications. These adverse reactions are among the most frequent oral health problems affecting transplant recipients, and the clinical presentation of oral lesions may differ from that observed in immunocompetent patients.

Several complications associated with immunosuppression manifest in the mouth, including bacterial infections, oral candidiasis, reactivation of herpes simplex virus, uncommon viral and fungal infections, hairy leukoplakia, and aphthous ulcers. Oral ulcers may be caused by herpes simplex virus reactivation or side effects of systemic immunosuppression, and in stem cell transplant patients, oral ulcers may be a sign of graft-versus-host disease. In addition, progressive periodontal disease, delayed wound healing, and excessive bleeding may become problems for these patients.

Notify the patient's physician if you notice signs of marked immunosuppression. In some cases, the dosage of anti-rejection agents prescribed for patients may need to be reduced. This may help control the opportunistic infections and other oral complications. However, there will be patients who must be maintained on high-dose immuno-suppression. Treatment of oral opportunistic infection is necessary in any transplanted patient.

Common immunosuppressive drugs and their side effects include:

- **Cyclosporine:** Changes in liver/kidney function, hypertension, bleeding problems, and poor wound healing are among the adverse effects of this potent agent, which also interacts with a number of other drugs. Gingival hyperplasia occurs in some patients. Calcium channel blockers, for example, may exacerbate the problem. Children tend to be more susceptible to gingival overgrowth than adults. Emphasize conscientious daily oral hygiene to all patients.

- **Tacrolimus:** An immunosuppressive drug used increasingly in place of cyclosporine, tacrolimus causes less gingival overgrowth but is associated with oral ulcerations and numbness or tingling, especially around the mouth.

- **Azathioprine:** Bone marrow suppression and related complications, such as stomatitis and opportunistic infections are significant side effects of this drug. A decrease in white blood cell counts and excessive bleeding may occur.

- **Mycophenolate mofetil:** This immunosuppressive drug is commonly used as an alternative to azathioprine. Adverse effects include decreased white cell counts, opportunistic infections, and gastrointestinal problems.

- **Corticosteroids:** Steroid drugs increase the risk of oral and systemic infection, and at the same time, they may mask the typical signs of infection occurring in the mouth. Hypertension, high blood glucose (steroid-induced diabetes), poor wound healing, and changes in mood are other side effects of these drugs. If your patient has cushingoid facies (moon face), you may find oral lesions resulting from cheek and tongue biting. In addition, adrenal suppression may occur, making invasive dental and medical procedures more difficult for your patient.

- **Sirolimus:** Side effects of this immunosuppressive drug can include hypertension, joint pain, low white blood cell count, and hypercholesterolemia. In addition, because oral ulcers can result from high levels of sirolimus, refer a patient with oral ulcers to the transplant team for drug titration.

431

Chronic Graft versus Host Disease

In patients who receive a stem cell transplant from a donor, an autoimmune-like disease called "chronic graft versus host disease" (cGVHD) may develop, usually within two years of transplantation. cGVHD may affect multiple organ systems, including the mouth, and you should screen stem cell transplant patients at every dental visit because treatment and supportive care for pain, sensitivity, and dry mouth are important. Oral cGVHD has three components: mucosal involvement, sclerotic involvement of the mouth and surrounding tissues, and salivary gland involvement:

- **Mucosa:** The oral mucosa presents with the classic findings in cGVHD, including lichenoid changes, erythema, ulcerations, hyperkeratotic patches, and mucosal atrophy.

- **Musculoskeletal tissue:** Limited mouth opening and limited tongue mobility may be caused by the involvement of the temporomandibular joints or by sclerotic changes in the perioral tissues.

- **Salivary glands:** Salivary gland dysfunction may result from medication, inflammation, and fibrosis of the major and minor salivary glands.

Treatment and supportive care for the oral effects of cGVHD should be coordinated with the patient's medical team. Patients may need artificial saliva for dry mouth; topical immunosuppressive agents, such as steroid rinses, to manage their oral disease; and palliative agents, such as lidobenalox rinse or viscous lidocaine, to manage oral pain.

Oral Cancer

The long-term use of immunosuppressive drugs and other treatments puts transplant patients at risk of developing cancers, including cancers of the oral cavity. Squamous cell carcinoma, especially of the tongue, salivary gland, lip, or throat; oral Kaposi's sarcoma; and lymphoma are among the malignancies that sometimes occur in transplant patients. Because early detection of oral cancer is essential for effective treatment, screen patients at every appointment, and biopsy new oral lesions that lack a clear etiology.

Organ Rejection

If a patient's body begins to reject a transplanted organ, only emergency dental care may be provided. Before dental treatment, talk with the patient's physician about antibiotic prophylaxis or other special needs.

Chapter 57

Osteoporosis Affects Bones and Teeth

Chapter Contents

Section 57.1

Oral Health and Bone Disease

This section includes text excerpted from "Oral Health and Bone Disease," NIH Osteoporosis and Related Bone Diseases—National Resource Center (NIH ORBD—NRC), November 2018.

Skeletal Bone Density and Dental Concerns

The portion of the jawbone that supports our teeth is known as the "alveolar process." Several studies have found a link between the loss of alveolar bone and an increase in loose teeth (tooth mobility) and tooth loss. Women with osteoporosis are three times more likely to experience tooth loss than those who do not have the disease.

Low-bone density in the jaw can result in other dental problems as well. For example, older women with osteoporosis may be more likely to have difficulty with loose or ill-fitting dentures and may have less optimal outcomes from oral surgical procedures.

Periodontal Disease and Bone Health

Periodontitis is a chronic infection that affects the gums and the bones that support the teeth. Bacteria and the body's own immune system break down the bone and connective tissue that hold teeth in place. Teeth may eventually become loose, fall out, or have to be removed.

Although tooth loss is a well-documented consequence of periodontitis, the relationship between periodontitis and skeletal-bone density is less clear. Some studies have found a strong and direct relationship among bone loss, periodontitis, and tooth loss. It is possible that the loss of alveolar bone mineral density leaves bone more susceptible to periodontal bacteria, increasing the risk for periodontitis and tooth loss.

Role of the Dentist and Dental X-Rays

Research supported by the National Institute of Arthritis and Musculoskeletal and Skin Diseases (NIAMS) suggests that dental x-rays may have benefits as a screening tool for osteoporosis. Researchers found that dental x-rays were highly effective in distinguishing people with osteoporosis from those with normal bone density.

Because many people see their dentist more regularly than they see their doctor, dentists are in a unique position to help identify people with low-bone density and to encourage them to talk to their doctors about their bone health. Dental concerns that may indicate low-bone density include loose teeth, gums detaching from the teeth or receding gums, and ill-fitting or loose dentures.

Effects of Osteoporosis Treatments on Oral Health

It is not known whether osteoporosis treatments have the same beneficial effect on oral health as they do on other bones in the skeleton. Additional research is needed to fully clarify the relationship between osteoporosis and oral bone loss; however, scientists are hopeful that efforts to optimize skeletal-bone density will have a favorable impact on dental health.

Bisphosphonates, a group of medications available for the treatment of osteoporosis, have been linked to the development of osteonecrosis of the jaw (ONJ), which is cause for concern. The risk of ONJ has been greatest in patients receiving large doses of intravenous bisphosphonates, a therapy used to treat cancer. The occurrence of ONJ is rare in individuals taking oral forms of the medication for osteoporosis treatment.

Taking Steps for Healthy Bones

A healthy lifestyle can be critically important for keeping bones strong. You can take many important steps to optimize your bone health:

- Eat a well-balanced diet rich in calcium and vitamin D.

- Engage in regular physical activity or exercise. Weight-bearing activities—such as walking, jogging, and dancing—are the best for keeping bones strong. Resistance exercises, such as lifting weights, also can strengthen bones.

- Do not smoke, and limit alcohol intake.

- Report any problems with loose teeth, detached or receding gums, and loose or ill-fitting dentures to your dentist and your doctor.

Section 57.2

Osteogenesis Imperfecta

This section includes text excerpted from "Osteogenesis Imperfecta Overview," NIH Osteoporosis and Related Bone Diseases—National Resource Center (NIH ORBD—NRC), December 2018.

Osteogenesis imperfecta (OI) is a genetic disorder characterized by bones that break easily, often from little or no apparent cause. A classification system of different types of OI is commonly used to help describe how severely a person with OI is affected. For example, a person may have just a few or as many as several hundred fractures in a lifetime.

Prevalence of Osteogenesis Imperfecta

Although the number of people affected with OI in the United States is unknown, the best estimate suggests a minimum of 25,000 and possibly as many as 50,000.

Diagnosis of Osteogenesis Imperfecta

Osteogenesis Imperfecta (OI) is caused by genetic defects that affect the body's ability to make strong bones. Collagen is the major protein of the body's connective tissue and is part of the framework around bones are formed. In dominant (classical) OI, a person has either too little type 1 collagen or poor quality of type 1 collagen caused by a mutation in one of the type 1 collagen genes. In recessive OI, mutations in other genes interfere with collagen production. The result in all cases is weak bones that break easily.

It is often possible to diagnose OI based solely on clinical features. Clinical geneticists can perform biochemical (collagen) or molecular deoxyribonucleic acid (DNA) tests that can help confirm a diagnosis of OI in some situations.

These tests generally require several weeks before results are known. Both the collagen biopsy test and the DNA test are thought to detect nearly 90 percent of all type 1 collagen mutations.

A positive collagen type I test confirms the diagnosis of dominant OI, but a negative result leaves open the possibility that:

- A type 1 collagen mutation is present but was not detected.

- The patient has a form of the disorder that is not associated with type 1 collagen mutations.

- The patient has a recessive form of OI.

Therefore, a negative type 1 collagen study does not rule out OI. When a type 1 collagen mutation is not found, other DNA tests can check for recessive forms.

Clinical Features of Osteogenesis Imperfecta

The characteristic features of OI vary greatly from person to person, even among people with the same type of OI and even within the same family. Not all characteristics are evident in each case. The majority of OI cases (possibly 85 to 90 %) are caused by a dominant mutation in a gene coding for type 1 collagen (Types I, II, III, and IV in the following list). Types V and VI do not have a type 1 collagen mutation, but the genes causing them have not yet been identified. Types VII and VIII are newly discovered forms that are inherited in a recessive manner, and the genes causing these two types have been identified. The general features of each of the known types of OI, which vary in characteristics and severity, are as follows:

Type I Osteogenesis Imperfecta

- Most common and mildest type of OI
- Bones predisposed to fracture (most fractures occur before puberty)
- Normal or near-normal stature
- Loose joints and muscle weakness
- Blue, purple, or gray tint to sclera (whites of the eyes)
- Triangular face
- Tendency toward spinal curvature
- Absent or minimal bone deformity
- Possible brittle teeth
- Possible hearing loss, often beginning in early twenties or thirties
- Normal collagen structure, but less than normal amount

Type II Osteogenesis Imperfecta

- Most severe form of OI

439

- Frequently causes death at birth or shortly after, because of respiratory problems
- Numerous fractures and severe bone deformity
- Small stature with under-developed lungs
- Blue, purple, or gray tinted sclera
- Improperly formed collagen

Type III Osteogenesis Imperfecta

- Most severe type among those who survive the neonatal period
- Easily fractured bones (fractures often present at birth; x-rays may reveal healed fractures that occurred before birth)
- Short stature
- Blue, purple, or gray tinted sclera
- Loose joints and poor muscle development in arms and legs
- Barrel-shaped rib cage
- Triangular face
- Spinal curvature
- Possible respiratory problems
- Often severe bone deformity
- Possible brittle teeth
- Possible hearing loss
- Improperly formed collagen

Type IV Osteogenesis Imperfecta

- Between Type I and Type III OI in severity
- Bones easily fractured (most fractures occur before puberty)
- Shorter than average stature
- Sclera normal in color (i.e., white or near-white)
- Mild to moderate bone deformity
- Tendency toward spinal curvature

- Barrel-shaped rib cage
- Triangular face
- Possible brittle teeth
- Possible hearing loss
- Improperly formed collagen

By studying the appearance of OI bone under the microscope, investigators noticed that some people who are clinically within the Type IV group had a distinct pattern to their bone. When they reviewed the full medical history of these people, they found the groups had other features in common. They named these groups Type V and Type VI OI. The mutations causing these forms of OI have not been identified, but people in these two groups do not have mutations in the type 1 collagen genes.

Type V Osteogenesis Imperfecta

- Clinically similar to Type IV OI in appearance and symptoms
- A dense band seen on x-rays adjacent to the growth plate of the long bones
- Unusually large calluses, called "hypertrophic calluses," at the sites of fractures or surgical procedures. (A callus is an area of new bone that is laid down at the fracture site as part of the healing process.)
- Calcification of the membrane between the radius and ulna (the bones of the forearm), which leads to restriction of forearm rotation
- Sclera normal in color (i.e., white or near-white)
- Normal teeth "mesh-like" appearance to bone when viewed under the microscope
- Dominant inheritance pattern

Type VI Osteogenesis Imperfecta

- Clinically similar to Type IV OI in appearance and symptoms, but is extremely rare
- Slightly elevated activity level of alkaline phosphatase (an enzyme linked to bone formation), which can be determined by a blood test

- Distinctive "fish-scale" appearance to bone when viewed under the microscope

- Diagnosed by bone biopsy

- Unknown whether this form is inherited in a dominant or recessive manner, but researchers believe the mode of inheritance is most likely recessive

New Recessive Forms of Osteogenesis Imperfecta

After years of research, in 2006, scientists discovered two forms of OI that are inherited in a recessive manner. Genes that affect collagen formation cause both types. The discovery of these new forms of OI provides information for people who have severe or moderately severe OI but do not have a primary collagen mutation.

Type VII Osteogenesis Imperfecta

- Resembles Type IV OI in many aspects of appearance and symptoms in the first described cases

- In other instances, similar appearance and symptoms to Type II lethal OI, except infants had white sclera, a small head, and a round face

- Short stature

- Short humerus (arm bone) and short femur (upper leg bone)

- Coxa vara (a deformed hip joint in which the neck of the femur is bent downward) is common; the acutely angled femur head affects the hip socket

- Results from recessive inheritance of a mutation in the CRTAP gene. Partial (10%) expression of CRTAP leads to moderate bone dysplasia. A total absence of the cartilage-associated protein has been lethal in all identified cases

Type VIII Osteogenesis Imperfecta

- Resembles lethal Type II or Type III OI in appearance and symptoms, except that infants have white sclera

- Severe growth deficiency

- Extreme skeletal undermineralization

- Caused by the absence or severe deficiency of prolyl 3-hydroxylase activity due to mutations in the *LEPRE1* gene

Inheritance Factors of Osteogenesis Imperfecta

Most cases of OI (85 to 90%) are caused by a dominant genetic defect. This means that only one copy of the mutation-carrying gene is necessary for the child to have OI. A person with a form of OI caused by a dominant mutation has a 50 percent chance of passing on the disorder to each of her or his children.

Some children who have the dominant form of OI inherit the disorder from a parent. Other children are born with the dominant form of OI even though there is no family history of the disorder. In these children, the genetic defect occurred as a spontaneous mutation.

Approximately 10 to 15 percent of OI cases are the result of a recessive mutation. In this situation, the parents do not have OI, but both carry the mutation in their genes. To inherit recessive OI, the child must receive a copy of the mutation from both parents.

The parents of a child with recessive OI have a 25 percent chance per pregnancy of having another child with OI. Siblings of a person with recessive OI have a 50 percent chance of being a carrier of the recessive gene. DNA testing is available to help parents and siblings determine if they are carriers of this type of gene mutation.

If one parent has OI because of a recessive mutation, 100 percent of their children will be carriers of the recessive OI mutation. Whether any of these children will have OI will depend on the genes inherited from the other parent. Genetic counselors can help people with OI and their family members understand OI genetics and the possibility of recurrence, and they can assist in prenatal diagnosis for those who wish to exercise that option.

Treatment of Osteogenesis Imperfecta

There is not yet a cure for OI. Treatment is directed toward preventing or controlling the symptoms, maximizing independent mobility, and developing optimal bone mass and muscle strength. Care of fractures, extensive surgical and dental procedures, and physical therapy are often recommended for people with OI. Use of wheelchairs, braces, and other mobility aids is common, particularly (although not exclusively) among people with more severe types of OI.

Doctors frequently consider a surgical procedure called "rodding" for people with OI. This treatment involves inserting metal rods through the length of the long bones to strengthen them. The treatment also prevents or corrects deformities.

Scientists are exploring several medications and other treatments for their potential use to treat OI. These include growth hormone treatment, intravenous and oral drugs called "bisphosphonates," an injected drug called "teriparatide" (for adults only), and gene therapies. It is not clear whether people with recessive OI and those with dominant OI will respond to these treatments in the same manner. The OI Foundation can provide current information on research studies and experimental treatments to help individuals with OI decide whether to participate in clinical trials.

People with OI are encouraged to exercise as much as possible to promote muscle and bone strength, which can help prevent fractures. Swimming and water therapy are common exercise choices for people with OI, as water allows independent movement with little risk of fracture. For those who are able, walking (with or without mobility aids) is an excellent exercise. People with OI should consult their doctor or physical therapist to discuss appropriate and safe exercise.

Children and adults with OI will also benefit from maintaining a healthy weight, eating a nutritious diet, and avoiding activities such as smoking, excessive alcohol, and caffeine consumption, and taking steroid medications—all of which may deplete bone and exacerbate bone fragility.

Prognosis of Osteogenesis Imperfecta

The prognosis for a person with OI varies greatly depending on the number and severity of symptoms. Respiratory failure is the most frequent cause of death for people with OI, followed by accidental trauma. Despite numerous fractures, restricted activity, and small stature, most adults and children with OI lead productive and successful lives. They attend school, develop friendships and other relationships, have careers, raise families, participate in sports and other recreational activities, and are active members of their communities.

Chapter 58

Pregnancy and Oral Health

Women have unique oral health concerns. Changing hormone levels during your menstrual cycle, pregnancy, and menopause can raise your risk for problems in your mouth, teeth, or gums. Health issues, such as diabetes can also affect your oral health. Regular brushing, flossing, and dentist visits can help prevent disease in your mouth and the rest of your body.

What Is Oral Health?

Oral health is the health of your mouth, including your teeth, gums, throat, and bones around the mouth. Oral health problems, such as gum disease, might be a sign that you have other health problems. Gum diseases are infections caused by plaque, which is a sticky film of bacteria that forms on your teeth. If left untreated, the bacteria in plaque can destroy the tissue and bone around your teeth, leading to tooth loss. Infections in your mouth can also affect your unborn baby if you are pregnant.

How Often Should I Brush and Floss My Teeth?

Dentists recommend that everyone brush their teeth at least twice a day with fluoride toothpaste and floss once a day. Flossing removes plaque between your teeth, a place that you cannot reach by brushing.

This chapter includes text excerpted from "Oral Health," Office on Women's Health (OWH), U.S. Department of Health and Human Services (HHS), December 5, 2017.

You can also remove this plaque with tools other than floss. These tools, called "interdental cleaners," include wooden or plastic picks and water flossers.

How Do Women's Hormones Affect Oral Health?

Changing hormone levels at different stages of a woman's life can affect oral health. When your hormone levels change, your gums can get swollen and irritated. Your gums may also bleed, especially during pregnancy, when your body's immune system is more sensitive than usual. This can cause inflammation (redness, swelling, and sometimes pain) in the gums. Regular, careful brushing and flossing can lessen gum irritation and bleeding.

Other causes of changing hormone levels that may affect your oral health include:

- Your menstrual cycle

- Hormonal birth control

- Menopause

I Am Pregnant. Is It Safe for Me to Get a Dental Checkup?

Yes. You need to continue your regular dentist visits to help protect your teeth during pregnancy.

- **Tell your doctor you are pregnant.** Because you are pregnant, your dentist might not take routine x-rays. But, the health risk to your unborn baby is very small. If you need emergency treatment or specific dental x-rays to treat a serious problem, your doctor can take extra care to protect your baby.

- **Schedule your dental exam early in your pregnancy.** After your 20th week of pregnancy, you may be uncomfortable sitting in a dental chair.

- **Have all needed dental treatments.** If you avoid treatment, you may risk your own health and your baby's health.

How Can I Prevent Oral Health Problems?

You can help prevent oral health problems by taking the following steps:

- **Visit your dentist once or twice a year.** Your dentist may recommend more or fewer visits depending on your oral health. At most routine visits, the dentist and a dental hygienist (assistant) will treat you. During regular checkups, dentists look for signs of disease, infections, and injuries.

- **Choose healthy foods.** Limit the amount of sugary foods and drinks you have. Lower your risk for tooth decay by brushing after meals and flossing once a day.

- **Do not smoke.** Smoking raises your risk of gum disease and mouth and throat cancers. It can also stain your teeth and cause bad breath.

- **Drink less soda.** Try to replace soda with water. Even diet soda has acids that can erode tooth enamel.

Chapter 59

Tobacco Use-Associated Oral Changes

Chapter Contents

Section 59.1

Tobacco Use and Oral Cancer

This section includes text excerpted from documents published
by three public domain sources. Text under the heading marked
1 is excerpted from "Tobacco," National Cancer Institute (NCI),
January 23, 2017; Text under the headings marked 2 are excerpted
from "Oral Cancer," National Institute of Dental and Craniofacial
Research (NIDCR), July 2018; Text under the heading marked
3 is excerpted from "Oral Cavity, Pharyngeal, and Laryngeal
Cancer Prevention (PDQ®)—Patient Version," National Cancer
Institute (NCI), March 28, 2019.

Tobacco Use[1]

Tobacco use is a leading cause of cancer and of death from cancer. People who use tobacco products or who are regularly around
environmental tobacco smoke (also called "secondhand smoke") have
an increased risk of cancer because tobacco products and secondhand smoke have many chemicals that damage deoxyribonucleic acid
(DNA).

Tobacco use causes many types of cancer, including cancer of the
lung, larynx (voice box), mouth, esophagus, throat, bladder, kidney,
liver, stomach, pancreas, colon and rectum, and cervix, as well as acute
myeloid leukemia. People who use smokeless tobacco (snuff or chewing
tobacco) have increased risks of cancers of the mouth, esophagus, and
pancreas.

There is no safe level of tobacco use. People who use any type of
tobacco product are strongly urged to quit. People who quit smoking,
regardless of their age, have substantial gains in life expectancy compared with those who continue to smoke. Also, quitting smoking at the
time of a cancer diagnosis reduces the risk of death.

Oral Cancer[2]

Oral cancer includes cancers of the mouth and the back of the
throat. Oral cancers develop on the tongue, the tissue lining the mouth
and gums, under the tongue, at the base of the tongue, and the area
of the throat at the back of the mouth.

Oral cancer accounts for roughly three percent of all cancers diagnosed annually in the United States, or about 49,700 new cases each
year.

Oral cancer most often occurs in people over the age of 40 and affects more than twice as many men as women. Most oral cancers are related to tobacco use, alcohol use (or both), or infection by the human papillomavirus (HPV).

Causes[2]

- **Tobacco and alcohol use.** Tobacco use of any kind, including cigarette smoking, can cause oral cancers. Heavy alcohol use also increases the chances of causing oral cancer.

- **HPV.** Infection with the sexually transmitted human papillomavirus (specifically the HPV 16 type) has been linked to oral cancers.

- **Age.** Oral cancers most often occur in people over the age of 40.

- **Sun exposure.** Cancer of the lip can be caused by sun exposure.

- **Diet.** A diet low in fruits and vegetables may play a role in oral cancer development.

Risk Factors[3]

The risk of oral cavity, oropharyngeal, hypopharyngeal, and laryngeal cancer is higher in people who use both tobacco and alcohol than in people who use only tobacco or only alcohol. The risk of oral cavity cancer and oropharyngeal cancer is about 35 times higher in people who smoke 2 or more packs of cigarettes per day and have more than 4 alcoholic drinks per day than it is in people who have never smoked cigarettes or consumed alcohol.

Chewing betel quid or gutka (betel quid mixed with tobacco) has been shown to increase the risk of oral cavity, pharyngeal, and laryngeal cancer. Betel quid contains areca nut, which is a cancer-causing substance. The risk of oral cavity, pharyngeal, and laryngeal cancer increases with how long and how often betel quid or gutka are chewed. The risk for oral cavity, pharyngeal, and laryngeal cancer is higher when chewing gutka than when chewing betel quid alone. Betel quid and gutka chewing is common in many countries in South Asia and Southeast Asia, including China and India.

Symptoms[2]

If you have any of these symptoms for more than two weeks, see a dentist or a doctor.

- A sore, irritation, lump or thick patch in your mouth, lips, or throat

- A white or red patch in your mouth

- A feeling that something is caught in your throat

- Difficulty chewing or swallowing

- Difficulty moving your jaw or tongue

- Swelling in your jaw

- Numbness in your tongue or other areas of your mouth

- Pain in one ear without hearing loss

Diagnosis[2]

Because oral cancer can spread quickly, early detection is important. An oral cancer examination can detect early signs of cancer. The exam is painless and takes only a few minutes. Many dentists will perform the test during your regular dental check-up.

During the exam, your dentist or dental hygienist will check your face, neck, lips, and entire mouth for possible signs of cancer.

Treatment[2]

When oral cancer is detected early, it is treated with surgery or radiation therapy. Oral cancer that is further along when it is diagnosed may use a combination of treatments.

For example, radiation therapy and chemotherapy are often given at the same time. Another treatment option is targeted therapy, which is a newer type of cancer treatment that uses drugs or other substances to precisely identify and attack cancer cells. The choice of treatment depends on your general health, where the cancer began, i.e., in your mouth or throat, the size and type of the tumor, and whether the cancer has spread.

Your doctor may refer you to a specialist. Specialists who treat oral cancer include:

- Head and neck surgeons

- Dentists who specialize in surgery of the mouth, face, and jaw (oral and maxillofacial surgeons)

- Ear, nose, and throat doctors (otolaryngologists)

- Doctors who specifically treat cancer (medical and radiation oncologists)

Other healthcare professionals who may be part of a treatment team include dentists, plastic surgeons, reconstructive surgeons, speech pathologists, oncology nurses, registered dietitians, and mental-health counselors.

Helpful Tips[2]

Oral cancer and its treatment can cause dental problems. It is important that your mouth is in good health before cancer treatment begins.

- See a dentist for a thorough exam one month, if possible, before starting cancer treatment to give your mouth time to heal after any dental work you might need.

- Before, during, and after cancer treatment, ask your healthcare provider for ways to control pain and other symptoms, and to relieve the side effects of therapy.

- Talk to your healthcare team about financial aid, transportation, home care, emotional, and social support for yourself and your family.

Section 59.2

Gum Disease, Tooth Loss, and Smoking

This section includes text excerpted from "Smoking, Gum Disease, and Tooth Loss," Centers for Disease Control and Prevention (CDC), March 22, 2018.

What Is Gum Disease?

Gum (periodontal) disease is an infection of the gums and can affect the bone structure that supports your teeth. In severe cases, it can make your teeth fall out. Smoking is an important cause of severe gum disease in the United States.

Gum disease starts with bacteria (germs) on your teeth that get under your gums. If the germs stay on your teeth for too long, layers of plaque (film) and tartar (hardened plaque) develop. This buildup leads to early gum disease, called "gingivitis."

When gum disease gets worse, your gums can pull away from your teeth and form spaces that get infected. This is severe gum disease, also called "periodontitis." The bone and tissue that hold your teeth in place can break down, and your teeth may loosen and need to be pulled out.

Warning Signs and Symptoms of Gum Disease

• Red or swollen gums

• Tender or bleeding gums

• Painful chewing

• Loose teeth

• Sensitive teeth

• Gums that have pulled away from your teeth

How Is Smoking Related to Gum Disease?

Smoking weakens your body's infection fighters (your immune system). This makes it harder to fight off a gum infection. Once you have gum damage, smoking also makes it harder for your gums to heal.

What does this mean for me if I am a smoker?

• You have twice the risk for gum disease compared with a nonsmoker.

• The more cigarettes you smoke, the greater your risk for gum disease.

• The longer you smoke, the greater your risk for gum disease.

• Treatments for gum disease may not work as well for people who smoke.

Tobacco use in any form—cigarettes, pipes, and smokeless (spit) tobacco—raises your risk for gum disease.

How Can Gum Disease Be Prevented?

You can help avoid gum disease with good dental habits.

- Brush your teeth twice a day
- Floss often to remove plaque
- See a dentist regularly for checkups and professional cleanings
- Do not smoke. If you smoke, quit.

How Is Gum Disease Treated?

Regular cleanings at your dentist's office and daily brushing and flossing can help treat early gum disease (gingivitis).
More severe gum disease may require:

- Deep cleaning below the gum line
- Prescription mouth rinse or medicine
- Surgery to remove tartar deep under the gums
- Surgery to help heal bone or gums lost to periodontitis. Your dentist may use small bits of bone to fill places where bone has been lost. Or your dentist may move tissue from one place in your mouth to cover exposed tooth roots.

If you smoke or use spit tobacco, quitting will help your gums heal after treatment.

Chapter 60

Mouth Microbes: The Helpful and the Harmful

The mouth is home to about 700 species of microbes. These include germs, such as bacteria and fungi. "Everybody has these microbes in their mouth," says Dr. Robert Palmer, an *NIH News in Health* expert on oral microbes. Some microbes are helpful. Others can cause problems, such as tooth decay and gum disease. Troubles begin when microbes form a sticky, colorless film called "plaque" on your teeth. Brushing and flossing help to keep your mouth clean. But, after you brush and floss, germs grow again and more plaque forms. That is why you need to clean your mouth regularly.

Community Growth

Different microbes grow in different places. Some stick to your teeth. Others prefer your tongue. Some lurk in the tiny pockets between tooth and gum. Once they have found their homes, they form diverse communities with the other germs.

Mouth microbes work together to protect themselves with a slimy, sticky material called a "matrix." The matrix in plaque makes it harder to remove it. The communities within the matrix include both helpful

This chapter includes text excerpted from "Mouth Microbes—The Helpful and the Harmful," *NIH News in Health*, National Institutes of Health (NIH), May 2019.

and disease-causing microbes. The good microbes help keep the growth of bad microbes in check. Good microbes also help you digest food and can protect against harmful microbes in food. Certain things you may be doing can help bad microbes grow better than the good ones. Sugary foods and drinks feed some microbes and help them increase in number and spread out.

Some of these sugar-loving microbes can turn sugar into matrix and acid. The acid destroys the surface of your teeth. The more sugar in your diet, the more fuel is available for these microbes to build up plaque and damage teeth. "It is more productive to think about the community than it is to think about the single microbe that causes disease," Palmer explains. You cannot stop tooth decay by getting rid of just one type of acid-making microbe. There are several different types of microbes in the plaque that make acid. The good news is that limiting sweets and brushing and flossing regularly can help prevent bad microbes from growing out of control.

Helpful Neighbors

"Many bacteria in our mouths depend on help from other members of their community to survive and prosper," says Dr. Floyd Dewhirst, a dental expert who studies microbes at the Forsyth Institute. Because microbes grow in communities, it is important to understand how both helpful and harmful microbes work. Dewhirst's team is trying to identify all the different germs living in the mouth and what they do. Before the team can study a microbe, they have to figure out how to grow it. The challenge is that some microbes do not like to grow anywhere but in your mouth. About 30 percent of the 700 species have not been grown in the lab yet.

Dewhirst's team is working on growing those microbes in the lab that no one has grown before. They are using genetic and other information to identify each one and learn more about them. "The question is," he says, "once you know who is there and have a quick way of identifying them, what are all of these bacteria doing?" Dewhirst's studies have shown that some microbes make certain substances that help their neighbors grow. His team is trying to identify what those substances are.

They also want to find out how these microbes may affect people's health. Being able to grow microbes in the lab lets scientists run tests to figure out how they are involved in health and disease. This information could one day help scientists come up with better ways of preventing and treating oral diseases.

Partners in Decay

An important health problem caused by mouth microbes is early childhood tooth decay. "In the United States, about 23 percent of our children between the ages of one and five are affected by this disease," says Dr. Hyun (Michel) Koo, a dental researcher and oral health expert at the University of Pennsylvania. Tooth decay can get worse very fast. The microbe matrix and acid from bacteria are thought to be the main cause of tooth decay in young kids.

Koo's team has found that there is also fungus in the plaque of kids with rampant tooth decay. The fungus partners with the matrix- and acid-making bacteria to worsen tooth decay. "Bacteria by itself can cause tooth decay," Koo explains. "But when fungus is there, it boosts up the entire machinery."

Koo's team has also shown that some fungus can get energy from sugar that bacteria release while making acid. The fungus then releases substances that feed the bacteria's growth. This helps the bacteria form an even tougher matrix and make more acid.

Busting Plaque

Koo's team is looking for new ways to fight plaque buildup and tooth decay. They have developed tiny substances called "nanoparticles" that are small enough to get inside and destroy the matrix that protects microbes. The nanoparticles can also kill the acid-making bacteria without harming good bacteria in the mouth.

Koo's team has shown that these tiny substances can reduce acid damage to the tooth surface. The researchers hope to test the approach in people in the future.

Nanoparticles are just one approach now being studied to prevent or treat mouth diseases. Future technologies may help keep our mouths healthier. But, there are many things you can do to keep bad mouth microbes in check.

Keep Mouth Microbes in Check

These tips can help prevent tooth decay and mouth infections:

- Brush your teeth with a toothpaste that contains fluoride.

- Floss away the plaque between your teeth.
- Do not forget to brush your tongue.
- Limit sugary foods and drinks.
- Drink fluoridated water.
- Get regular dental exams and professional cleanings.

Part Seven

Finding and Financing Oral Health in the United States

Chapter 61

Access to Oral Healthcare

Chapter Contents

Section 61.1

Oral-Health Status and Interventions Programs

This section contains text excerpted from the following sources: Text beginning with the heading "Overview of Oral Health" is excerpted from "Oral Health," Office of Disease Prevention and Health Promotion (ODPHP), U.S. Department of Health and Human Services (HHS), January 1, 2016; Text beginning with the heading "What the CDC's Department of Oral Health Does" is excerpted from "Division of Oral Health at a Glance," Centers for Disease Control and Prevention (CDC), May 25, 2019.

Overview of Oral Health

Oral diseases ranging from dental caries (cavities) to oral cancers cause pain and disability for millions of Americans. The impact of these diseases does not stop at the mouth and teeth. A growing body of evidence has linked oral health, particularly periodontal (gum) disease, to several chronic diseases, including diabetes, heart disease, and stroke. In pregnant women, poor oral health has also been associated with premature births and low birth weight. These conditions may be prevented in part with regular visits to the dentist. In 2007, however, only 44.5 percent (age adjusted) of people aged 2 years and older had a dental visit in the past 12 months, a rate that has remained essentially unchanged over the past decade.

Impact of Oral Health

Oral health is an essential part of staying healthy. Good oral health allows a person to speak, smile, smell, taste, touch, chew, swallow, and make facial expressions to show feelings and emotions. Poor oral health has serious consequences, including painful, disabling, and costly oral diseases. Millions of Americans are living with one or more oral diseases, including:

- Dental caries (cavities)
- Periodontal (gum) disease
- Cleft lip and palate
- Oral and facial pain
- Oral and pharyngeal (mouth and throat) cancers

Gum disease, in particular, is associated with diabetes, heart disease, and stroke. In pregnant women, gum disease is also associated with premature births and low birth weight.

Many of these oral diseases may be prevented with regular dental care.

Oral Health across Life Stages

Poor oral health affects Americans at all life stages, from infancy through older adulthood. For example:

Children and Adolescents

- Tooth decay affects more than 1 in 4 U.S. children aged 2 to 5 years.

- Tooth decay affects 1 in 2 U.S. adolescents aged 12 to 15 years.

Adults

- 1 in 7 adults aged 35 to 44 years has gum disease; among adults older than 65 years, the rate increases to 1 in 4.

Older Adults

- 1 in 4 U.S. adults age 65 years or older has lost all the teeth.

- More than 7,800 people, mostly older Americans, die from oral and pharyngeal (mouth and throat) cancers each year.

Determinants of Oral Health

The ability to access oral healthcare is associated with gender, age, education level, income, race and ethnicity, access to medical insurance, and geographic location. Addressing these determinants is key in reducing health disparities and improving the health of all Americans. Efforts are needed to overcome barriers to access to oral healthcare caused by geographic isolation, poverty, insufficient education, and lack of communication skills.

The Centers for Disease Control and Preventions (CDC's) Division of Oral Health (DOH) promotes proven interventions, such as community water fluoridation and dental sealants, to reduce the rate of cavities, especially for populations at highest risk. The DOH supports state oral-health programs, collects surveillance data on oral diseases, and develops and promotes adherence to infection prevention and control guidelines for dental healthcare personnel. The division supports the integration of medical and dental care to address other chronic diseases associated with poor oral health. The DOH also strengthens the dental public-health workforce with a residency training program.

What the CDC's Department of Oral Health Does

With fiscal year 2019 budget of $19 million, the DOH focuses on improving oral health and reducing disparities, which are differences in oral-health status and access to preventive treatments across different geographic, racial, ethnic, and socioeconomic groups. To meet these goals, the DOH works to:

- Measure how cavities and other oral diseases affect populations in the United States

- Study interventions to find out and promote what works best to prevent cavities and gum disease

- Fund and guide states to maintain oral-health infrastructure, use proven interventions, and evaluate programs

- Share information to help all Americans have better oral health and keep their natural teeth longer

Why the CDC's Department of Oral Health Does This

Oral health affects our ability to speak, smile, eat, and show emotions. It also affects self-esteem, school performance, and attendance at work and at school. Oral diseases—which range from cavities to gum disease to oral cancers—cause pain and disability to millions of Americans. 1 in 5 U.S. children aged 6 to 11 years has at least one untreated cavity. 1 in 4 adults has untreated cavities, and more than 40 percent have felt pain in their mouth in the last year. On average, 34 million school hours are lost each year because of unplanned (emergency) dental care, and over $45 billion is lost in productivity. About 100 million Americans do not have access to fluoridated tap water, and 6 in 10 children do not get dental sealants.

How the CDC's Department of Oral Health Does It
Collecting Data to Monitor Progress in Oral Health

The CDC is the lead federal agency that analyzes data to monitor progress in meeting the oral-health objectives of Healthy People 2020, the nation's agenda for improving the health of all Americans. One of these objectives is to increase the percentage of children, adolescents, and adults who received oral healthcare in the past year. This objective is also one of the 12 high-priority Healthy People 2020 objectives called "Leading Health Indicators." The CDC uses a web-based system called "Oral Health Data" to bring together data from the National Oral Health Surveillance System (NOHSS) and various state sources, including state oral health surveys, Behavioral Risk Factor Surveillance System (BRFSS) surveys, and biennial water fluoridation surveys. Users can export information into several formats to create tables, charts, and maps.

The CDC also helps state health departments collect, interpret, and share local and state data on oral health and the use of preventive services. States and communities use the data to monitor their progress in meeting their oral-health objectives and set program priorities to reach people with the greatest needs.

Promoting Community Water Fluoridation to Reduce Cavities

Community water fluoridation is recognized as one of the 10 great public-health achievements of the 20th century. Even with the widespread use of products with added fluoride, such as toothpaste, studies have found that people living in communities with water fluoridation have 25 percent fewer cavities than those living in communities without fluoridation.

The CDC works with state and national partners to improve water fluoridation quality by training state drinking-water system engineers and oral-health and other public-health staff. In 2019, DOH will release a new web-based, interactive training called "Fluoridation Learning Online" (FLO).

The CDC also manages a web-based reporting system that helps states monitor the quality of their water fluoridation programs. The public component of this database, My Water's Fluoride (MWF), allows residents in participating states to learn the fluoride content of their public water system.

In 2018, the CDC and the National Association of County and City Health Officials (NACCHO) developed a fluoridation communications toolkit to help public-health professionals, water-system operators, and civic leaders educate community members about the benefits of community water fluoridation.

Promoting School Sealant Programs to Prevent Cavities

1 in 5 children aged 6 to 11 years has at least one untreated cavity, which can lead to problems eating, speaking, and learning. Dental sealants protect against 80 percent of cavities for 2 years and continue to protect against 50 percent of cavities for up to 4 years. Children aged 6 to 11 years without sealants have almost 3 times more first molar cavities than children with sealants.

Sealant use increased by about 70 percent among low-income children and 23 percent among higher-income children from 1999 to 2004 and from 2011 to 2014. However, this effective intervention remains underused; less than half of the children aged 6 to 11 years have dental sealants.

School sealant programs provide dental sealants at no charge to children who are less likely to receive private dental care. These programs provide sealants at school during the school day using mobile dental equipment. The CDC provides guidance to state and community programs to help them plan, set up, and evaluate school sealant programs and to complement the services provided by private dentists.

Preventing Infections in Dental Care Settings through Guidelines and Training

Dental healthcare settings must meet the same high standards for infection prevention and control as any medical setting. To help reduce the risk of disease transmission, the CDC develops recommendations to guide infection prevention and control practices in all settings in which dental treatment is provided.

In 2016, the CDC published the *Summary of Infection Prevention Practices in Dental Settings: Basic Expectations for Safe Care.* This resource includes current recommendations from the CDC and a checklist to measure compliance. The recommendations guide infection-prevention practices in dental offices nationally and globally and provide direction for dental healthcare personnel.

In 2017, the CDC released a new mobile app called "CDC DentalCheck" to support the implementation of these recommendations. Dental healthcare personnel can use the app to assess practices in their facility and make sure they are providing safe care. In 2018, the CDC created a complementary 10-module training slide series called "Basic Expectations for Safe Care Training Modules."

Supporting Programs and Partners to Improve Oral Health

The CDC provides 20 states with funds, technical assistance, and training to build strong oral-health programs. This support helps states promote oral health, monitor oral-health behaviors and problems, and conduct and evaluate prevention programs. It also helps states better coordinate and manage community water fluoridation programs and school dental sealant programs and develop ways to better integrate dental and medical care.

The CDC funds two national partners to support these efforts— the Association for State and Territorial Dental Directors (ASTDD) and the National Association of Chronic Disease Directors (NACDD). The ASTDD provides assistance and resources to states, assesses state programs, and provides assistance to territorial programs. NACDD supports the integration of oral-health programs with other chronic-disease programs.

The DOH also works with other chronic disease programs to promote prevention strategies designed to reduce risk factors associated with multiple chronic conditions, including gum disease. In addition, the CDC works to produce skilled specialists in dental public health through its Dental Public Health Residency Program.

Section 61.2

Disparities in Oral Health

This section includes text excerpted from "Disparities in Oral Health," Centers for Disease Control and Prevention (CDC), May 17, 2016.

Oral-health disparities are profound in the United States. Despite major improvements in oral health for the population as a whole, oral-health disparities still exist in many racial and ethnic groups, by socioeconomic status, gender, age, and geographic location.

Some social factors that can contribute to these differences are lifestyle behaviors, such as tobacco use, frequency of alcohol use, and poor dietary choices. Just as they affect general health, these behaviors can affect oral health. The economic factors that often relate to poor oral health include access to health services and an individual's ability to get and keep dental insurance.

Some of the oral-health disparities that exist include the following:

- **Overall.** Non-Hispanic Blacks, Hispanics, and American Indians and Alaska Natives generally have the poorest oral health of any racial and ethnic groups in the United States.

- **Children and tooth decay.** The greatest racial and ethnic disparity among children aged 2 to 4 years and aged 6 to 8 years is seen in Mexican American and Black, non-Hispanic children.

- **Adults and untreated tooth decay.** Blacks, non-Hispanics, and Mexican Americans aged 35 to 44 years experience untreated tooth decay nearly twice as much as White, non-Hispanics.

- **Tooth decay and education.** Adults aged 35 to 44 years with less than a high school education experience untreated tooth decay nearly three times that of adults with at least some college education.

  - In addition, adults aged 35 to 44 years with less than a high school education experience destructive periodontal (gum) disease nearly three times that of adults with a least some college education.

- **Adults and oral cancer.** The 5-year survival rate is lower for oral pharyngeal (throat) cancers among Black men than among Whites (36% versus 61%).

- **Adults and periodontitis.** 47.2 percent of U.S. adults have some form of periodontal disease. In adults aged 65 and older, 70.1 percent have periodontal disease.

  - Periodontal disease is higher in men than in women, and greatest among Mexican Americans and non-Hispanic Blacks, and those with less than a high school education.

Healthy People 2020 Works to Eliminate Oral-Health Disparities

Healthy People 2020 is the nation's framework for improving the health of all Americans. The overarching goals of Healthy People 2020 are to increase quality and years of healthy life and eliminate health disparities. Interventions, such as community water fluoridation and school-based dental sealant programs can help achieve this goal.

Community water fluoridation reduces and aids in preventing tooth decay among different socioeconomic, racial, and ethnic groups. Currently, this Healthy People 2020 objective is moving toward its target of 79.6 percent of community water having fluoride.

School sealant programs provide sealants to children who may not receive routine dental care. This includes children at highest risk for tooth decay: those from low-income families and certain racial and ethnic groups. Sealants are thin plastic coatings applied to the tiny grooves on the chewing surfaces of the teeth.

Chapter 62

Expenditures and Financing of Oral Healthcare

Chapter Contents

Section 62.1

Health-Related Expenditures: An Overview

This section includes text excerpted from "National Health
Expenditures 2017 Highlights," Centers for Medicare and Medicaid
Services (CMS), December 7, 2018.

Healthcare spending in the United States increased 3.9 percent to
reach $3.5 trillion, or $10,739 per person, in 2017. Healthcare spending
growth in 2017 was similar to average growth from 2008 to 2013, which
preceded the faster growth experienced during the 2014 to 2015 period
that was marked by insurance-coverage expansion and high rates of
growth in retail prescription-drug spending. The overall share of the
gross domestic product (GDP) related to healthcare spending was 17.9
percent in 2017, similar to that in 2016 (18%).

Healthcare Spending by Type of Service or Product

- **Dental services (4% share):** Spending for dental services
  increased 3.2 percent in 2017 to $129.1 billion, decelerating from
  5.2 percent growth in 2016. Private health insurance (which
  accounted for 45% of dental spending) increased 2.8 percent in
  2017—a slowdown from growth of 5.3 percent in 2016. Out-of-
  pocket spending for dental services (which accounted for 41% of
  dental spending) also slowed, growing 2.5 percent in 2017, after
  growth of 5 percent in 2016.

- **Hospital care (33% share):** Spending for hospital care
  increased 4.6 percent to $1.1 trillion in 2017, which was slower
  than the 5.6 percent growth in 2016. The slower growth in 2017
  was driven by slower growth in the use and intensity of services.
  Hospital care expenditures slowed among the major payers—
  private health insurance, Medicare, and Medicaid.

- **Physician and clinical services (20% share):** Spending on
  physician and clinical services increased 4.2 percent to $694.3
  billion in 2017. Growth for physician and clinical services slowed in
  2017 and was driven by growth in nonprice factors, such as use and
  intensity of services. Although slowing, growth in clinical services
  continued to outpace the growth in physician services in 2017.

- **Retail prescription drugs (10% share):** Growth in retail
  prescription drug spending slowed in 2017, increasing 0.4

percent to $333.4 billion. The slower growth in 2017 followed 2.3 percent growth in 2016 and was the lowest growth in retail prescription drug spending since 2012, when several blockbuster drugs lost patent protection. The key drivers of the slower growth were a continued shift to lower-cost generic drugs and slower growth in the sales volume of some high-cost drugs.

- **Other health, residential, and personal care services (5% share):** Spending for other health, residential, and personal care services grew 5.6 percent in 2017 to $183.1 billion after increasing 5.3 percent in 2016. The slight acceleration was driven by faster growth in residential mental health and substance abuse facilities and ambulance services. This category includes expenditures for medical services that are generally delivered by providers in nontraditional settings, such as schools, community centers, and the workplace; as well as by ambulance providers and residential mental health and substance abuse facilities.

- **Nursing care facilities and continuing care retirement communities (5% share):** Growth in spending for freestanding nursing care facilities and continuing care retirement communities decelerated in 2017, growing 2 percent to $166.3 billion compared to 3.1 percent growth in 2016. The slower growth in 2017 is largely attributable to slower spending growth in both out-of-pocket and private health insurance spending.

- **Home healthcare (3% share):** Spending for freestanding home healthcare agencies increased 4.3 percent in 2017, the same rate as 2016, to $97 billion. Slower growth in Medicaid spending and private health insurance spending was offset by faster Medicare spending and out-of-pocket spending. Medicare and Medicaid together made up 76 percent of home health spending in 2017.

- **Other professional services (3% share):** Spending for other professional services reached $96.6 billion in 2017 and increased 4.6 percent, a slower rate of growth compared to the increase of 5.1 percent in 2016. Spending in this category includes establishments of independent health practitioners (except physicians and dentists) that primarily provide services, such as physical therapy, optometry, podiatry, or chiropractic medicine.

- **Other nondurable medical products (2% share):** Retail spending for other nondurable medical products, such as over-the-counter (OTC) medicines, medical instruments, and surgical dressings, grew 2.2 percent (slower than the rate of growth in 2016 of 4.1%) to $64.1 billion in 2017.

- **Durable medical equipment (2% share):** Retail spending for durable medical equipment, which includes items, such as contact lenses, eyeglasses, and hearing aids, reached $54.4 billion in 2017 and increased 6.8 percent, which was faster than the 4.9 percent growth in 2016. The faster growth was driven by an acceleration in Medicare spending as well as continued strong growth in private health insurance and out-of-pocket spending which accounted for almost 70 percent of total durable medical equipment spending.

Health Spending by Major Sources of Funds

- **Private health insurance (34% share):** Private health insurance spending increased 4.2 percent to $1.2 trillion in 2017, which was slower than 6.2 percent growth in 2016. The deceleration was driven in part by slower growth in medical benefits and a decline in fees and taxes resulting from the Consolidated Appropriations Act of 2016, which suspended collection of the health insurance plan fee in 2017.

- **Medicare (20% share):** Medicare spending grew 4.2 percent to $705.9 billion in 2017, which was similar to the rate of growth in 2016 of 4.3 percent. The growth in 2017 reflected slower growth in spending for Medicare fee-for-service (2.6% in 2016 to 1.4% in 2017) that was almost entirely offset by faster growth in Medicare spending for private health plans (8.1% in 2016 to 10% in 2017).

- **Medicaid (17% share):** Total Medicaid spending decelerated in 2017, increasing 2.9 percent to $581.9 billion compared to growth of 4.2 percent in 2016. The slower growth in 2017 was influenced by slower growth in enrollment and a reduction in the Medicaid net cost of health insurance. State and local Medicaid expenditures grew 6.4 percent, while federal Medicaid expenditures increased 0.8 percent in 2017.

- **Out-of-pocket spending (10% share):** Out-of-pocket spending grew 2.6 percent in 2017 to $365.5 billion, which was slower than 4.4 percent growth in 2016.

Section 62.2

Dental Coverage in the Marketplace

This section includes text excerpted from "Dental Coverage in the Marketplace," Centers for Medicare and Medicaid Services (CMS), February 2, 2017.

In the health insurance Marketplace, you can get dental coverage in two ways: as part of a health plan, or by itself through a separate, stand-alone dental plan.

Dental Coverage Is Available Two Ways

- **Health plans that include dental coverage.** Dental coverage is included in some Marketplace health plans. You can see which plans include dental coverage when you compare them.

If a health plan includes dental, the premium covers both health and dental coverage.

- **Separate, stand-alone dental plans.** In some cases, separate, stand-alone plans are offered. You can see them when you shop for plans in the Marketplace.

If you choose a separate dental plan, you will pay a separate, additional premium.

Dental Plan Categories: High and Low

There are two categories of Marketplace dental plans: high and low.

- The high coverage level has higher premiums but lower copayments and deductibles. So you will pay more every month, but less when you use dental services.

- The low coverage level has lower premiums but higher copayments and deductibles. So you will pay less every month, but more when you use dental services.

When you compare dental plans in the Marketplace, you will find details about each plan's costs, copayments, deductibles, and services covered.

Adult and Child Dental Insurance in the Marketplace

Under the healthcare law, dental insurance is treated differently for adults and children 18 and under.

- **Dental coverage is an essential health benefit for children.** This means if you are getting health coverage for someone 18 or younger, dental coverage must be available for your child either as part of a health plan or as a stand-alone plan. Note: While dental coverage for children must be available to you, you do not have to buy it.

- **Dental coverage is not an essential health benefit for adults.** Insurers do not have to offer adult dental coverage.

Do I Have to Pay a Penalty If I Do Not Have Dental Coverage?

No. Dental coverage is optional, even for children. So you do not need it to avoid the penalty for being uncovered.

Can I Cancel My Marketplace Dental Coverage and Still Keep My Health Coverage?

It depends.

- If you have a separate, stand-alone dental plan, you can cancel any time. Learn how to cancel a stand-alone dental plan while keeping your health plan.

- If you are enrolled in a health plan with dental benefits, you can change health plans only if you have a life event that qualifies you for a special enrollment period. If you qualify, you can choose a new health plan with or without dental coverage. But you cannot get dental coverage by itself.

Chapter 63

Head Start Programs

Overview of Head Start and Early Head Start

Head Start is a federal program that promotes the school readiness of children from birth to age five from low-income families by enhancing their cognitive, social, and emotional development. Head Start programs provide a learning environment that supports children's growth in many areas, such as language, literacy, and social and emotional development. Head Start emphasizes the role of parents as their child's first and most important teacher. These programs help build relationships with families that support family well-being and many other important areas.

Many Head Start programs also provide Early Head Start, which serves infants, toddlers, and pregnant women and their families who have incomes below the federal poverty level.

Requirements of Head Start and Early Head Start

Children from birth to age five from families with low income, according to the poverty guidelines published by the federal government, are eligible for Head Start and Early Head Start services.

This chapter contains text excerpted from the following sources: Text beginning with the heading "Overview of Head Start and Early Head Start" is excerpted from "Head Start and Early Head Start," Benefits.gov, USA.gov, n.d.; Text under the heading "How Head Start Programs Work" is excerpted from "Head Start Programs," Office of Head Start (OHS), U.S. Department of Health and Human Services (HHS), February 11, 2019; Text under the heading "Tips for Choosing This Type of Care" is excerpted from "Head Start and Early Head Start," Child-Care.gov, Administration for Children and Families (ACF), October 19, 2017.

Children in foster care, homeless children, and children from families receiving public assistance (Temporary Assistance for Needy Families (TANF) or Supplemental Security Income (SSI)) are categorically eligible for Head Start and Early Head Start services regardless of income.

Head Start programs may enroll up to 10 percent of children from families that have incomes above the poverty guidelines. Programs may also serve up to an additional 35 percent of children from families whose incomes are above the poverty guidelines, but below 130 percent of the poverty line if the program can ensure that certain conditions have been met.

Pregnant women may also be eligible for Early Head Start.

Because many programs offer services to families that may qualify them under other local criteria, they strongly recommend you contact the program in your community for more information and guidance.

How Head Start Programs Work

Head Start programs promote school readiness of children ages birth to five from low-income families by supporting the development of the whole child.

Head Start and Early Head Start programs offer a variety of service models, depending on the needs of the local community. Many Head Start and Early Head Start programs are based in centers and schools. Other programs are located in child care centers and family child care homes. Some programs offer home-based services that assign dedicated staff who conduct weekly visits to children in their own home and work with the parent.

Head Start programs support children's growth and development in a positive learning environment through a variety of services, which include:

- **Early learning:** Children's readiness for school and beyond is fostered through individualized learning experiences. Through relationships with adults, play, and planned and spontaneous instruction, children grow in many aspects of development. Children progress in social skills and emotional well-being, along with language and literacy learning, and concept development.

- **Health:** Each child's perceptual, motor, and physical development is supported to permit them to fully explore and function in their environment. All children receive health and development screenings, nutritious meals, oral health and mental health support. Programs connect families with medical, dental, and mental health services to ensure that children are receiving the services they need.

- **Family well-being:** Parents and families are supported in achieving their own goals, such as housing stability, continued education, and financial security. Programs support and strengthen parent–child relationships and engage families around children's learning and development.

Delivered through 1,700 agencies in local communities, Head Start and Early Head Start programs provide services to over a million children every year, in every U.S. state and territory, in farmworker camps, and in over 155 tribal communities. Head Start programming is responsive to the ethnic, cultural, and linguistic heritage of each child and family. More than 80 percent of children served by Head Start programs are 3- and 4-year-olds. Infants, toddlers, and pregnant women makeup just under 20 percent of Head Start enrollment, and are served through Early Head Start programs. Early Head Start programs are available to the family until the child turns 3 years old and is ready to transition into Head Start or another pre-K program.

Tips for Choosing This Type of Care

- Ask whether your family qualifies for Head Start services and if your local program has any openings for children your child's age.

- Ask about the programs hours and if the program is available in the summer. Make sure that the program is open when you need care. If you need full-day or full-year care and the Head Start program does not offer this, ask about partnerships with other child care providers that can care for your child when Head Start is not open.

- Ask about what types of services you and your child will receive and whether there are any other requirements.

- Ask about the program's staff turnover rate (how frequently staff leave). If a program experiences a large amount of turnover, your child could experience many transitions to new teachers. A high turnover rate could also mean that there are issues that could affect the quality of the program.

- Ask what curriculum is used. Also ask the provider to explain the types of daily activities planned for the children, and how those activities will support your child's learning.

- Ask about information and activities provided for parents. Ask if the program provides opportunities for parents to learn about how their children are doing or talk about their children's progress.

- Print a list of questions and things to look for that you can take with you when visiting a potential child care program.

Chapter 64

Dental Sealants at School-Based Services

What Are Dental Sealants?

Dental sealants are thin coatings that when painted on the chewing surfaces of the back teeth (molars) can prevent cavities (tooth decay) for many years. Sealants protect the chewing surfaces from cavities by covering them with a protective shield that blocks out germs and food. Once applied, sealants protect against 80 percent of cavities for two years and continue to protect against 50 percent of cavities for up to 4 years. Children aged 6 to 11 years without sealants have almost three times more first molar cavities than children with sealants.

Depending on state law and regulations, sealants can be applied by a dentist, dental hygienist, or other qualified dental professional. This can be done in dental offices or using portable dental equipment in community settings, such as a school.

School Sealant Programs

School sealant programs are an effective way to reach millions of children with dental sealants to prevent cavities. The Community

This chapter contains text excerpted from the following sources: Text under the heading "What Are Dental Sealants?" is excerpted from "Dental Sealants," Centers for Disease Control and Prevention (CDC), May 3, 2019; Text beginning with the heading "School Sealant Programs" is excerpted from "School Sealant Programs," Centers for Disease Control and Prevention (CDC), March 1, 2018.

Preventive Services Task Force (CPSTF) strongly recommends using school-based sealant delivery programs to prevent cavities among children. In addition, school sealant programs can be cost-saving within two years of placing sealants, and delivering sealants to children at high risk for cavities can be cost-saving to Medicaid.

School sealant programs provide pit and fissure sealants to children using portable equipment in a school setting. Although each state-coordinated program may be different in how they structure their program, generally speaking, school sealant programs focus on providing sealants to children aged 6 to 11 years or in grades 3 through 5. A typical sealant program will visit an individual school over the course of 1 to 3 days. A licensed dental professional will screen children for oral disease. They also check to see if the children already have sealants, and if so, how well those sealants are being retained. Children with a signed permission slip from their parents or guardians who do not have dental sealants will get them applied, typically at no cost. Any child that needs additional follow-up care will get a referral to a local dentist.

School sealant programs are especially important for reaching children who are at greater risk for developing cavities and less likely to receive private dental care. Programs generally target schools with a higher percentage of children eligible for federal free or reduced-cost meal programs.

Compared with children from higher-income families, children from low-income families are more likely to:

- Have untreated tooth decay
- Have few or no dental sealants
- Not have had yearly dental visits

Ways to Increase Sealant Use

There are many actions that states, dental providers, schools, and parents can take to increase sealant prevalence.

The federal government is:

- Classifying pediatric dental services as an essential health benefit to be covered by dental insurance as part of the Affordable Care Act (ACA)

- Matching state costs for applying dental sealants for all children enrolled in Medicaid/Children's Health Insurance Program (CHIP) and tracking program performance

- Encouraging community health centers with dental programs to start or expand school-based sealant programs to help more low-income children

- Helping fund states to increase the number of dental sealant programs

- Providing incentives for dentists to practice in underserved areas to increase access to dental services

State officials can:

- Target school-based sealant programs to the areas of greatest need

- Track the number of schools and children participating in sealant programs

- Implement policies that deliver school-based sealant programs in the most cost-effective manner

- Help schools connect to Medicaid and CHIP, local health department clinics, community health centers, and dental providers in the community to encourage more use of sealants and reimbursement of services

Dental care providers can:

- Apply sealants to children at highest risk of cavities, including those covered by Medicaid/CHIP. Donate time and resources to a school-based dental sealant program

- Learn about school-based dental sealant programs and their effectiveness

- Accept children into their practice who are identified as needing more services when they receive sealants in schools

School administrators can:

- Work with the local or state public-health programs and local dental providers to start school-based sealant programs

- Support having sealant programs in schools and promote its benefits to teachers, staff, and parents. Help children enroll in sealant programs by putting information for parents in registration packets in the beginning of the school year

- Encourage schools to develop relationships with local dental offices and community dental clinics to help children get dental care

Parents can:

- Ask your child's dentist to apply sealants when appropriate
- Sign your child up to participate in a school-based sealant program. If your school does not have sealant program, ask them to start one
- Find a dentist if your child needs one

Chapter 65

Finding Low-Cost Dental Care

Role of the National Institute of Dental and Craniofacial Research Toward Dental Care

The National Institute of Dental and Craniofacial Research (NIDCR), one of the federal government's National Institutes of Health (NIH), leads the nation in conducting and supporting research to improve oral health. As a research organization, the NIDCR does not provide financial assistance for dental treatment but invites participants in dental research. You can contact the NIDCR's National Oral Health Information Clearinghouse (NOHIC) at 866-232-4528 or nidcrinfo@mail.nih.gov if you have questions.

Clinical Trials

The NIDCR seeks volunteers with specific dental, oral, and craniofacial conditions to participate in research studies, also known as "clinical trials." Researchers may provide study participants with limited free or low-cost dental treatment for the particular condition they are studying. To find a clinical trial, contact:

This chapter includes text excerpted from "Finding Low-Cost Dental Care," National Institute of Dental and Craniofacial Research (NIDCR), September 2015. Reviewed July 2019.

- ClinicalTrials.gov (www.clinicaltrials.gov)—a database of government and private clinical trials in the United States and around the world.

- National Institutes of Health (NIH) Clinical Research Studies (www.clinicalstudies.info.nih.gov/)—a database of clinical trials at the NIH Clinical Center in Bethesda, Maryland; to talk with someone about studies at the Clinical Center, call 800-411-1222.

Dental Schools and Dental Hygiene Schools

Dental schools can be a good source of quality, reduced-cost dental treatment. Most of these teaching facilities have clinics that allow dental students to gain experience treating patients while providing care at a reduced cost. Experienced, licensed dentists closely supervise the students. At most schools, there are also clinics where graduate students and faculty members provide care.

Dental hygiene schools may offer supervised, low-cost preventive dental care as part of the training experience for dental hygiene students. To find a dental or dental hygiene school in your area, contact:

- **Dental schools**—American Dental Association (ADA) (www.ada.org/en/coda/find-aprogram/search-dental-programs/dds-dmd-programs)

- **Dental hygiene schools**—American Dental Hygienists' Association (ADHA) (www.adha.org/dental-hygiene-programs)

Community Health Centers

The federal government's Health Resources and Services Administration (HRSA) runs federally funded community health centers across the country that provide free or reduced-cost health services, including dental care. To find a health center in your area, visit:

- HRSA.gov (www.hrsa.gov) and type your location in the "Find a Health Center" box.

Medicaid and Children's Health Insurance Program

- Medicaid is a state-run program that provides medical benefits—and in some cases dental benefits—to eligible individuals and families. States are required to provide dental benefits for children covered by Medicaid, but states can choose whether to provide dental benefits for adults. Most states provide only limited dental services for adults, while some offer extensive services.

- The Children's Health Insurance Program (CHIP) is a state-run program for children whose families earn too much to qualify for Medicaid but cannot afford private insurance. CHIP provides dental services to children up to age 19. Dental services covered under this program vary from state to state.

Medicare

Medicare is a federal health insurance program for people 65 and older and for people under 65 with specific disabilities. Medicare only covers dental services related to certain medical conditions or treatments. It does not cover dentures or most routine care, such as check-ups, cleanings, or fillings.

State and Local Resources

Your state or local health department may know of programs in your area that offer free or reduced-cost dental care. To find state and local resources:

- Call your local or state health department to learn more about their financial assistance programs.
- Call 211 to find services in your area.

United Way

The United Way may be able to direct you to free or reduced-cost dental services in your community. To find the United Way in your area, visit:

- United Way (www.unitedway.org) and type your zip code in the top right box next to "Find Your United Way."

Part Eight

Additional Help and Information

Chapter 66

Glossary of Terms Related to Dental Care and Oral Health

absorption: The process of taking in. For a person or an animal, absorption is the process of a substance getting into the body through the eyes, skin, stomach, intestines, or lungs.

adverse effect: An unexpected medical problem that happens during treatment with a drug or other therapy. Adverse effects may be mild, moderate, or severe, and may be caused by something other than the drug or therapy being given. Also called adverse event.

aerosol: Particles of respirable size (<10 μm) generated by both humans and environmental sources that can remain viable and air-borne for extended periods in the indoor environment; commonly generated in dentistry during use of handpieces, ultrasonic scalers, and air/water syringes.

alcohol: A chemical substance found in drinks such as beer, wine, and liquor. It is also found in some medicines, mouthwashes, household products, and essential oils (scented liquid taken from certain plants). It is made by a chemical process called "fermentation" that uses sugars and yeast.

anesthetic: A drug that causes insensitivity to pain and is used for surgeries and other medical procedures.

This glossary contains terms excerpted from documents produced by several sources deemed reliable.

antibiotic: A drug used to treat infections caused by bacteria and other microorganisms.

antigen: Any substance that causes the body to make an immune response against that substance. Antigens include toxins, chemicals, bacteria, viruses, or other substances that come from outside the body.

antiseptic: A germicide that is used on skin or living tissue for the purpose of inhibiting or destroying microorganisms.

anxiety: Feelings of fear, dread, and uneasiness that may occur as a reaction to stress. A person with anxiety may sweat, feel restless and tense, and have a rapid heart beat.

arthritis: A term used to describe more than 100 rheumatic diseases and conditions that affect joints, the tissues which surround the joint and other connective tissue.

aspiration: The removal of fluid or tissue through a needle. Also, the accidental breathing in of food or fluid into the lungs.

assessment: The process of gathering evidence and documentation of a student's learning.

bacteria: A large group of single-cell microorganisms. Some cause infections and disease in animals and humans.

blood: A tissue with red blood cells (RBCs), white blood cells (WBCs), platelets, and other substances suspended in fluid called plasma. Blood takes oxygen and nutrients to the tissues, and carries away wastes.

bone: A living, growing tissue made mostly of collagen.

calcium: A mineral that is an essential nutrient for bone health. It is also needed for the heart, muscles, and nerves to function properly and for blood to clot.

cancer: A term for diseases in which abnormal cells in the body divide without control. Cancer cells can invade nearby tissues and can spread to other parts of the body through the blood and lymphatic system, which is a network of tissues that clears infections and keeps body fluids in balance.

candidiasis (oral): Yeast or fungal infection that occurs in the oral cavity or pharynx or both.

central nervous system (CNS): Comprised of the nerves in the brain and spinal cord. These nerves are used to send electrical impulses throughout the body, resulting in voluntary and reflexive movement.

Information about the environment is received by the senses and sent to the central nervous system, which causes the body to respond appropriately.

cervix: The lower, narrow part of the uterus (womb). The cervix forms a canal that opens into the vagina, which leads to the outside of the body.

chemotherapy: Treatment with anticancer drugs.

chronic disease: A disease that has one or more of the following characteristics: is permanent; leaves residual disability; is caused by nonreversible pathological alteration; requires special training of the patient for rehabilitation; or may be expected to require a long period of supervision, observation, or care.

chronic pain: Pain that can range from mild to severe, and persists or progresses over a long period of time.

cigarette: A tube-shaped tobacco product that is made of finely cut, cured tobacco leaves wrapped in thin paper. It may also have other ingredients, including substances to add different flavors.

cleft lip or palate: A congenital opening or fissure occurring in the lip or palate.

clinical trial: A research study in which one or more human subjects are prospectively assigned to one or more interventions (which may include placebo or other control) to evaluate the effects of those interventions on health-related biomedical or behavioral outcomes.

computed tomography (CT): A procedure for taking x-ray images from many different angles and then assembling them into a cross-section of the body. This technique is generally used to visualize bone.

contaminated: State of having been in contact with microorganisms.

corticosteroids: Steroid-type hormones that have antitumor activity in lymphomas and lymphoid leukemias. In addition, corticosteroids may be used for hormone replacement and for the management of some of the complications of cancer and its treatment.

dental caries (dental decay or cavities): An infectious disease that results in demineralization and ultimately cavitation of the tooth surface if not controlled or remineralized. Dental decay may be either treated (filled) or untreated (unfilled).

dental implant: A metal device that is surgically placed in the jawbone. It acts as an anchor for an artificial tooth or teeth.

dental plaque: A sticky film of bacteria can build up on teeth. Plaque produces acids that, over time, eat away at the tooth's hard outer surface and create a cavity.

dental sealants: Thin plastic coatings that protect the chewing surfaces of children's back teeth from tooth decay.

dental visits: Regular use of the oral healthcare delivery system leads to better oral health by providing an opportunity for clinical preventive services and early detection of oral diseases.

dentures: False teeth made to replace teeth you have lost. Dentures can be complete or partial. Complete dentures cover your entire upper or lower jaw. Partials replace one or a few teeth.

deoxyribonucleic acid (DNA): The double-helix molecule that provides the basis of genetic heredity, about two nanometers in diameter but often several millimeters in length.

diet: What a person eats and drinks. Any type of eating plan.

e-cigarette: A device that has the shape of a cigarette, cigar, or pen and does not contain tobacco. It uses a battery and contains a solution of nicotine, flavorings, and other chemicals, some of which may be harmful.

enzyme: A protein that speeds up chemical reactions in the body.

epidemiology: The branch of medical science that investigates all the factors that determine the presence or absence of diseases and disorders in a population.

exercise: A type of physical activity that involves planned, structured, and repetitive bodily movement done to maintain or improve one or more components of physical fitness.

fetus: A developing unborn offspring in the uterus (womb). This stage of pregnancy begins 8 weeks after conception and lasts until birth.

fluoridation status: Status of a community water system in regards to water fluoridation level. Most water contains some amount of natural fluoride. Fluoridation involves adjusting fluoride in the water to the level optimal for the prevention of dental caries.

fracture: Broken bone. People with osteoporosis, osteogenesis imperfecta, and Paget disease are at greater risk for bone fracture.

genetics: The study of particular genes, deoxyribonucleic acid (DNA), and heredity.

gingivitis: An inflammatory condition of the gum tissue, which can appear reddened and swollen and frequently bleeds easily.

hand hygiene: A general term that applies to handwashing, antiseptic handwash, antiseptic hand rub, and surgical hand antisepsis.

hoarseness: Abnormally rough or harsh-sounding voice caused by vocal abuse and other disorders, such as gastroesophageal reflux, thyroid problems, or trauma to the larynx (voice box).

hormone: Substance produced by one tissue and conveyed by the bloodstream to another to affect a function of the body, such as growth or metabolism.

human immunodeficiency virus (HIV): A virus that infects and destroys the body's immune cells and causes a disease called AIDS, or acquired immunodeficiency syndrome.

immune system: A complex system of cellular and molecular components having the primary function of distinguishing self from not self and defense against foreign organisms or substances.

intestines: The long, tube-like organ in the human body that completes digestion or the breaking down of food. They consist of the small intestine and the large intestine. Also known as the bowels.

laryngeal cancer: Cancer that forms in tissues of the larynx (area of the throat that contains the vocal cords and is used for breathing, swallowing, and talking). Most laryngeal cancers are squamous cell carcinomas (cancer that begins in flat cells lining the larynx).

larynx: The area of the throat containing the vocal cords and used for breathing, swallowing, and talking. Also called voice box.

latex: A milky white fluid extracted from the rubber tree Hevea brasiliensis that contains the rubber material cis-1,4 polyisoprene.

latex allergy: A type I or immediate anaphylactic hypersensitivity reaction to the proteins found in natural rubber latex.

magnetic resonance imaging (MRI): A noninvasive procedure that uses magnetic fields and radio waves to produce three-dimensional computerized images of areas inside the body.

menopause: The cessation of menstruation in women. Bone health in women often deteriorates after menopause due to a decrease in the female hormone estrogen.

metabolism: The chemical changes that take place in a cell or an organism. These changes make energy and the materials cells and organisms need to grow, reproduce, and stay healthy. Metabolism also helps get rid of toxic substances.

migraine: A medical condition that usually involves a very painful headache, usually felt on one side of the head. Besides intense pain, migraine also can cause nausea and vomiting and sensitivity to light and sound. Some people also may see spots or flashing lights or have a temporary loss of vision.

nicotine: Chemical in tobacco that causes and maintains the powerful addicting effects of tobacco products.

nutrition: The taking in and use of food and other nourishing material by the body. Nutrition is a 3-part process. First, food or drink is consumed. Second, the body breaks down the food or drink into nutrients.

obesity: Excess body fat. Because body fat is usually not measured directly, a ratio of body weight to height is often used instead.

opportunistic infection: An infection caused by a microorganism that does not ordinarily cause disease but is capable of doing so, under certain host conditions.

organ: A part of the body that performs a specific function. For example, the heart is an organ.

oropharyngeal cancer: Cancer that forms in tissues of the oropharynx (the part of the throat at the back of the mouth, including the soft palate, the base of the tongue, and the tonsils). Most oropharyngeal cancers are squamous cell carcinomas (cancer that begins in flat cells lining the oropharynx).

oropharynx: The part of the throat at the back of the mouth behind the oral cavity. It includes the back third of the tongue, the soft palate, the side and back walls of the throat, and the tonsils.

osteoporosis: Literally means "porous bone." This disease is characterized by too little bone formation, excessive bone loss, or a combination of both, leading to bone fragility and an increased risk of fractures of the hip, spine, and wrist.

otolaryngologist: Physician/surgeon who specializes in diseases of the ears, nose, throat, and head and neck.

over-the-counter (OTC): Diseases, including ulcerative colitis (UC) and Crohn disease, that cause swelling in the intestine and/or digestive tract, which may result in diarrhea, abdominal pain, fever, and weight loss. People with inflammatory bowel disease (IBD) are at an increased risk for osteoporosis.

panic: Sudden extreme anxiety or fear that may cause irrational thoughts or actions. Panic may include rapid heart rate, flushing (a hot, red face), sweating, and trouble breathing.

papillomavirus: Group of viruses that can cause noncancerous wart-like tumors to grow on the surface of skin and internal organs, such as the respiratory tract; can be life-threatening.

parts per million (PPM): A measure of concentration in solution.

periodontal diseases: The diseases including gingivitis and periodontitis. Both are inflammatory conditions of the gingival tissues.

physical activity: Any bodily movement that is produced by the contraction of skeletal muscle and that substantially increases energy expenditure.

pregnancy: The condition between conception (fertilization of an egg by a sperm) and birth, during which the fertilized egg develops in the uterus. In humans, pregnancy lasts about 288 days.

prevalence: The number of disease cases (new and existing) within a population at a given time.

prevention: Actions that reduce exposure or other risks, keep people from getting sick, or keep disease from getting worse.

prognosis: The likely outcome or course of a disease; the chance of recovery or recurrence.

protein: A molecule made up of amino acids. Proteins are needed for the body to function properly. They are the basis of body structures, such as skin and hair, and of other substances such as enzymes, cytokines, and antibodies.

radiation: Energy moving in the form of particles or waves. Familiar radiations are heat, light, radio, and microwaves.

smell: To perceive odor or scent through stimuli affecting the olfactory nerves.

spina bifida: A condition that affects the spine and is usually apparent at birth. It is a type of neural tube defect (NTD).

stroke: Caused by a lack of blood to the brain, resulting in the sudden loss of speech, language, or the ability to move a body part, and, if severe enough, death. Also known as a cerebrovascular accident (CVA).

taste: Sensation produced by a stimulus applied to the gustatory nerve endings in the tongue. The four tastes are salt, sour, sweet, and bitter. Some scientists indicate the existence of a fifth taste, described as savory.

taste buds: Groups of cells located on the tongue that enable one to recognize different tastes.

taste disorder: Inability to perceive different flavors. Taste disorders may result from poor oral hygiene, gum disease, hepatitis, or medicines and chemotherapeutic drugs. Taste disorders may also be neurological.

tobacco: A plant with leaves that have high levels of the addictive chemical nicotine. After harvesting, tobacco leaves are cured, aged, and processed in various ways. The resulting products may be smoked (in cigarettes, cigars, and pipes), applied to the gums (as dipping and chewing tobacco), or inhaled (as snuff).

tongue: Large muscle on the floor of the mouth that manipulates food for chewing and swallowing. It is the main organ of taste, and assists in forming speech sounds.

tooth decay: A commonly known term for dental caries, an infectious, transmissible, disease caused by bacteria.

toxic: Causing temporary or permanent effects detrimental to the functioning of a body organ or group of organs.

virus: A small organism that can infect a person and cause illness or disease.

vitamin D: A nutrient that the body needs to absorb calcium.

voice: Sound produced by air passing out through the larynx and upper respiratory tract.

x-ray: A type of high-energy radiation. In low doses, x-rays are used to diagnose diseases by making pictures of the inside of the body.

xerostomia/salivary gland dysfunction: Dryness of the mouth because of thickened, reduced, or absent salivary flow; increases the risk for infection and compromises speaking, chewing, and swallowing.

Chapter 67

Directory of Local Dental Schools

Alabama

*University of Alabama
(UAB) School of Dentistry*
1720 Second Ave. S.
SDB 125
Birmingham, AL 35294-0007
Phone: 205-934-3387
Fax: 205-934-0209
Website: www.uab.edu/
dentistry/home
E-mail: dentaladmissions@uab.
edu

Arizona

*Arizona School of Dentistry
and Oral Health (ASDOH)*
A.T. Still University (ATSU)
5855 E. Still Cir.
Mesa, AZ 85206
Phone: 480-248-8100
Website: www.atsu.edu/asdoh

ASDOH Dental Care West
Arizona School of Dentistry &
Oral Health (ASDOH)
5855 E. Still Cir.
Mesa, AZ 85206
Phone: 480-248-8100
Website: www.atsu.edu/asdoh

Resources in this chapter were compiled from several sources deemed reliable;
all contact information was verified and updated in July 2019.

*College of Dental
Medicine-Arizona*
Midwestern University
19555 N. 59th Ave.
Glendale, AZ 85308
Toll-Free: 888-247-9277
Phone: 623-572-3215
Website: www.midwestern.edu/
course_catalog_home/glendale_
az_campus_/college_of_dental_
medicine-arizona.html
E-mail: admissaz@midwestern.
edu

California

*Herman Ostrow School of
Dentistry*
University of Southern
California (USC)
925 W. 34th St.
Los Angeles, CA 90089-0641
Phone: 213-740-2800
Website: dentistry.usc.edu/
patient-care/contact
E-mail: patientfeedback@usc.edu

*Loma Linda University
(LLU)*
School of Dentistry
11092 Anderson St.
Loma Linda, CA 92350
Phone: 909-558-4222
Website: dentistry.llu.edu

*University of California at
Los Angeles (UCLA) School
of Dentistry*
10833 Le Conte Ave.
CHS-Box 951668
Los Angeles, CA 90095-1668
Phone: 310-206-3904
Fax: 310-825-2951
Website: www.dentistry.ucla.
edu/patient-care

*University of California
at San Francisco (UCSF)
School of Dentistry*
UCSF Dental Center
707 Parnassus Ave.
San Francisco, CA 94143
Phone: 415-502-5800
Website: dentistry.ucsf.edu/
about/contact

*University of the Pacific
Arthur A. Dugoni School of
Dentistry*
155 Fifth St.
San Francisco, CA 94103
Phone: 415-929-6400
Fax: 415-929-6654
Website: dental.pacific.edu/
Dental_Services.html

Colorado

University of Colorado School of Dental Medicine (UCSDM)
Anschutz Medical Campus
13065 E. 17th Ave.
MS F833 Rm. 310
Aurora, CO 80045
Phone: 303-724-6900
Website: www.ucdenver.
edu/academics/colleges/
dentalmedicine/PatientCare/
Pages/BecomeaPatient.aspx

Connecticut

University of Connecticut School of Dental Medicine (SDM)
263 Farmington Ave.
Farmington, CT 06030
Phone: 860-679-2000
Website: dentalmedicine.uconn.
edu

District of Columbia

Howard University (HU) College of Dentistry
Howard University Hospital
600 W. St. N.W.
Rm. 126
Washington, DC 20059
Phone: 202-806-0400
Fax: 202-806-0303
Website: healthsciences.howard.
edu/education/colleges/dentistry
E-mail: HUCDAdmit@howard.
edu

Florida

Nova Southeastern University (NSU) College of Dental Medicine
3301 College Ave.
Fort Lauderdale, FL 33314-7796
Toll-Free: 800-541-6682
Website: dental.nova.edu/index.
html

University of Florida (UF) College of Dentistry
1395 Center Dr.
P.O. Box 100405
Gainesville, FL 32610
Phone: 352-273-5800
Fax: 352-392-3070
Website: dental.ufl.edu

Georgia

The Dental College of Georgia (DCG) at Augusta University
1430 John Wesley Gilbert Dr.
Augusta, GA 30912
Phone: 706-721-3587
Website: www.augusta.edu/
dentalmedicine

Illinois

Southern Illinois University School of Dental Medicine (SIU-SDM)
2800 College Ave.
Alton, IL 62002
Phone: 618-474-7000
Website: www.siue.edu/dental

503

University of Illinois at Chicago (UIC) College of Dentistry
801 S. Paulina St.
Chicago, IL 60612
Phone: 312-996-7555
Website: dentistry.uic.edu
E-mail: dentalclinics@uic.edu

Indiana

Indiana University (IU) School of Dentistry
1121 W. Michigan St.
Indianapolis, IN 46202
Phone: 317-274-7957
Website: dentistry.iu.edu
E-mail: dswww@iu.edu

Iowa

University of Iowa College of Dentistry
Dental Sciences Bldg.
801 Newton Rd.
Iowa City, IA 52242
Phone: 319-335-7499
Website: www.dentistry.uiowa.edu

Kentucky

University of Kentucky (UK) College of Dentistry
Dental Sciences Bldg.
800 Rose St.
Lexington, KY 40536-0297
Phone: 859-323-DENT
(859-323-3368)
Website: dentistry.uky.edu

University of Louisville (UofL) School of Dentistry
501 S. Preston St.
Louisville, KY 40202
Phone: 502-852-5096
Website: louisville.edu/dentistry

Louisiana

Louisiana State University Health Sciences Center (LSUHSC) School of Dentistry
1100 Florida Ave.
New Orleans, LA 70119
Phone: 504-619-8700
Website: www.lsusd.lsuhsc.edu/Patients.html

Maryland

University of Maryland School of Dentistry (UMSOD)
650 W. Baltimore St., Ste. 6410
Baltimore, MD 21201
Phone: 410-706-7472
Fax: 410-706-0945
Website: www.dental.umaryland.edu
E-mail: ddsadmissions@umaryland.edu

Massachusetts

Boston University Henry M. Goldman School of Dental Medicine (GDSM)
635 Albany St.
Boston, MA 02118
Phone: 617-358-8300
Website: www.bu.edu/dental/about/contact
E-mail: gsdmcomm@bu.edu

Harvard School of Dental Medicine (HSDM)
188 Longwood Ave.
Boston, MA 02115
Phone: 617-432-1434
Website: hsdm.harvard.edu
E-mail: hsdm_dean@hsdm.harvard.edu

Tufts University School of Dental Medicine (TUSDM)
One Kneeland St.
Boston, MA 02111
Phone: 617-636-6828
Website: dental.tufts.edu

Michigan

University of Detroit Mercy (UDM) School of Dentistry
2700 Martin Luther King Jr. Blvd.
Detroit, MI 48208-2576
Phone: 313-494-6700
Website: dental.udmercy.edu/index.php

University of Michigan (UM) School of Dentistry
1011 N. University Ave.
Ann Arbor, MI 48109
Toll-Free: 888-707-2500
Phone: 734-763-6933
Website: dent.umich.edu

Minnesota

University of Minnesota School of Dentistry
515 Delaware St. S.E.
Moos Tower
Minneapolis, MN 55455
Phone: 612-625-2495
Website: www.dentistry.umn.edu
E-mail: umdentcl@umn.edu

Mississippi

University of Mississippi School of Dentistry
University of Mississippi Medical Center (UMMC)
2500 N. State St.
Jackson, MS 39216
Phone: 601-984-6155
Website: www.umc.edu/sod/SOD_Home.html

Missouri

University of Missouri-Kansas City (UMKC) School of Dentistry
University of Missouri-Kansas City (UMKC)
650 E. 25th St.
Kansas City, MO 64108
Phone: 816-235-2100
Website: dentistry.umkc.edu
E-mail: dentistry@umkc.edu

Nebraska

Creighton University School of Dentistry
2500 California Plaza
Omaha, NE 68178
Phone: 402-280-2700
Website: dentistry.creighton.edu

University of Nebraska Medical Center (UNMC) College of Dentistry
4000 E. Campus Loop S.
Box 830740
Lincoln, NE 68583-0740
Phone: 402-472-1333
Website: www.unmc.edu/
dentistry

Nevada

University of Nevada, Las Vegas (UNLV) School of Dental Medicine
1001 Shadow Ln.
MS 7410
Las Vegas, NV 89106-4124
Phone: 702-774-2400
Fax: 702-774-2521
Website: www.unlv.edu/dental
E-mail: unlvdentsch@unlv.edu

New Jersey

University of Medicine and Dentistry of New Jersey (UMDNJ)
110 Bergen St.
Las Vegas, NV 89106
Toll-Free: 877-895-2794
Phone: 973-972-7370

New York

Columbia University College of Dental Medicine (CDM)
630 W. 168th St.
New York, NY 10032
Phone: 212-305-6100
Website: www.dental.columbia.
edu

New York University (NYU) College of Dentistry
345 E. 24th St.
Corner of First Ave.
New York, NY 10010
Phone: 212-998-9800
Website: dental.nyu.edu

Stony Brook School of Dental Medicine (SDM)
S. Dr.
Stony Brook, NY 11794-8700
Phone: 631-632-8989
Website: dentistry.
stonybrookmedicine.edu

University at Buffalo School of Dental Medicine (UBSDM)
University at Buffalo, South Campus
Squire Hall
Buffalo, NY 14215
Phone: 716-829-2836
Website: dental.buffalo.edu

North Carolina

University of North Carolina at Chapel Hill (UNC-CH) Adams School of Dentistry
CB 7450
Chapel Hill, NC 27599-7450
Phone: 919-537-3737
Website: www.dentistry.unc.edu

Ohio

Case Western Reserve University (CWRU) School of Dental Medicine
10900 Euclid Ave.
Cleveland, OH 44106-4905
Phone: 216-368-2000
Website: case.edu/dental

The Ohio State University College of Dentistry
Postle Hall
305 W. 12th Ave.
Columbus, OH 43210-1267
Phone: 614-292-2751
Website: dent.osu.edu

Oklahoma

University of Oklahoma (OU) College of Dentistry
1201 N. Stonewall Ave.
Oklahoma City, OK 73117
Phone: 405-271-7744
Website: dentistry.ouhsc.edu

Oregon

Oregon Health and Science University (OHSU) School of Dentistry
2730 S.W. Moody Ave.
Portland, OR 97201
Phone: 503-494-8867
Website: www.ohsu.edu/school-of-dentistry
E-mail: sodcontactus@ohsu.edu

Pennsylvania

Maurice H. Kornberg School Of Dentistry
Temple University
3223 N. Broad St.
Philadelphia, PA 19140
Phone: 215-707-2900
Website: dentistry.temple.edu

Penn Dental Medicine
The Robert Schattner Center,
University of Pennsylvania
240 S. 40th St.
Philadelphia, PA 19104-6030
Phone: 215-898-8965
Website: www.dental.upenn.edu

University of Pittsburgh
School of Dental Medicine
3501 Terr. St.
Pittsburgh, PA 15261
Phone: 412-648-8616
Website: www.dental.pitt.edu/patients/index.php

Puerto Rico

James B. Edwards College of Dental Medicine
Medical University of South Carolina (MUSC)
173 Ashley Ave.
MSC Code 507
Charleston, SC 29425
Phone: 843-792-2101
Website: education.musc.edu/colleges/dental

University of Puerto Rico-School of Dental Medicine (SDM)
Medical Sciences Campus
P.O. Box 365067
San Juan, PR 00936-5067
Phone: 787-758-2525
Website: dental.rcm.upr.edu

Tennessee

Meharry Medical College (MMC) School of Dentistry
1005 D.B. Todd Jr. Blvd.
Nashville, TN 37208
Phone: 615-327-6207
Fax: 615-327-6213
Website: home.mmc.edu/school-of-dentistry

University of Tennessee Health Science Center (UTHSC) College of Dentistry
875 Union Ave.
Memphis, TN 38163
Phone: 901-448-6200
Fax: 901-448-1625
Website: www.uthsc.edu/dentistry

Texas

Texas A&M College of Dentistry
3302 Gaston Ave.
Dallas, TX 75246
Phone: 214-828-8100
Website: dentistry.tamhsc.edu

The University of Texas School of Dentistry (UTSD)
7500 Cambridge St.
Houston, TX 77054
Phone: 713-486-4000
Website: dentistry.uth.edu

University of Texas (UT) Health San Antonio Dentistry
8210 Floyd Curl Dr.
San Antonio, TX 78229
Phone: 210-450-3700
Website: www.uthscsa.edu/patient-care/dental

Virginia

Virginia Commonwealth University (VCU) School of Dentistry
Lyons Dental Bldg.
520 N. 12th St.
Fourth Fl. P.O. Box 980566
Richmond, VA 23298-0566
Phone: 804-828-9190
Website: dentistry.vcu.edu

Washington

University of Washington (UW) School of Dentistry
1959 N.E. Pacific St. B-307
P.O. Box 356365
Seattle, WA 98195-6365
Phone: 206-616-6996
Website: dental.washington.edu
E-mail: askuwsod@uw.edu

West Virginia

West Virginia University (WVU) School of Dentistry
Robert C. Byrd Health Sciences Center
P.O. Box 9400
Morgantown, WV 26506-9400
Phone: 304-293-2521
Fax: 304-293-2859
Website: dentistry.hsc.wvu.edu

Wisconsin

Marquette University School of Dentistry
1801 W. Wisconsin Ave.
Milwaukee, WI 53233
Toll-Free: 800-445-5385
Phone: 414-288-6790
Website: www.marquette.edu/dentistry

Chapter 68

Directory of Organizations That Provide Information about Dental Care and Oral Health Resources

Government Agencies That Provide Information about Dental and Oral Health

Agency for Healthcare Research and Quality (AHRQ)
5600 Fishers Ln.
Rockville, MD 20857
Phone: 301-427-1364
Website: www.ahrq.gov

Centers for Disease Control and Prevention (CDC)
1600 Clifton Rd.
Atlanta, GA 30329-4027
Toll-Free: 800-CDC-INFO
(800-232-4636)
Toll-Free TTY: 888-232-6348
Website: www.cdc.gov

Resources in this chapter were compiled from several sources deemed reliable; all contact information was verified and updated in July 2019.

Centers for Medicare and Medicaid Services (CMS)
7500 Security Blvd.
Baltimore, MD 21244
Toll-Free: 877-267-2323
Phone: 410-786-3000
TTY: 410-786-0727
Toll-Free TTY: 866-226-1819
Website: www.cms.gov

ChildCare.gov
Office of Child Care (OCC)
Mary E. Switzer Bldg.
330 C St. S.W., Fourth Fl.
Washington, DC 20201
Phone: 202-690-6782
Website: childcare.gov

Clinical Center
National Institutes of Health (NIH)
10 Center Dr.
Bethesda, MD 20892
Phone: 301-496-2563
Fax: 301-402-2984
Website: clinicalcenter.nih.gov

Effective Health Care Program
Agency for Healthcare Research and Quality (AHRQ)
5600 Fishers Ln.
Rockville, MD 20857
Phone: 301-427-1364
Website: effectivehealthcare.ahrq.gov

Eunice Kennedy Shriver National Institute of Child Health and Human Development (NICHD)
P.O. Box 3006
Rockville, MD 20847
Toll-Free: 800-370-2943
Toll-Free TTY: 888-320-6942
Toll-Free Fax: 866-760-5947
Website: www.nichd.nih.gov
E-mail: NICHDInformation ResourceCenter@mail.nih.gov

Genetic and Rare Diseases Information Center (GARD)
P.O. Box 8126
Gaithersburg, MD 20898-8126
Toll-Free: 888-205-2311
Phone: 301-251-4925
Toll-Free TTY: 888-205-3223
Fax: 301-251-4911
Website: rarediseases.info.nih.gov

Head Start
Early Childhood Learning and Knowledge Center (ECLKC)
Toll-Free: 866-763-6481
Website: eclkc.ohs.acf.hhs.gov/hslc/hs
E-mail: HeadStart@eclkc.info

Health Resources and Services Administration (HRSA)
5600 Fishers Ln.
Rockville, MD 20857
Website: www.hrsa.gov

Medicaid-CHIP State Dental Association (MSDA)
4411 Connecticut Ave. N.W.
Ste. 401
Washington, DC 20008
Phone: 508-322-0557
Fax: 202-248-2315
Website: www.medicaiddental.
org

National Cancer Institute (NCI)
NCI Public Inquiries Office
9609 Medical Center Dr.
BG 9609 MSC 9760
Bethesda, MD 20892-9760
Toll-Free: 800-4-CANCER
(800-422-6237)
Website: www.cancer.gov
E-mail: NCIinfo@nih.gov

National Diabetes Education Program (NDEP)
National Institute of Diabetes
and Digestive and Kidney
Diseases (NIDDK)
Toll-Free: 800-860-8747
Toll-Free TTY: 866-569-1162
Website: www.celiac.nih.gov
E-mail: healthinfo@niddk.nih.gov

National Diabetes Information Clearinghouse (NDIC)
National Institute of Diabetes
and Digestive and Kidney
Diseases (NIDDK)
Toll-Free: 800-860-8747
Toll-Free TTY: 866-569-1162
Website: www.celiac.nih.gov
E-mail: healthinfo@niddk.nih.
gov

National Digestive Diseases Information Clearinghouse (NDDIC)
National Institute of Diabetes
and Digestive and Kidney
Diseases (NIDDK)
Toll-Free: 800-860-8747
Toll-Free TTY: 866-569-1162
Website: www.celiac.nih.gov
E-mail: healthinfo@niddk.nih.
gov

National Institute of Dental and Craniofacial Research (NIDCR)
Toll-Free: 866-232-4528
Website: www.nidcr.nih.gov
E-mail: nidcrinfo@mail.nih.gov

National Institute of Diabetes and Digestive and Kidney Diseases (NIDDK)
Toll-Free: 800-860-8747
Toll-Free TTY: 866-569-1162
Website: www2.niddk.nih.gov
E-mail: healthinfo@niddk.nih.
gov

National Institute of Neurological Disorders and Stroke (NINDS)
NIH Neurological Institute
P.O. Box 5801
Bethesda, MD 20824
Toll-Free: 800-352-9424
Website: www.ninds.nih.gov

513

National Institute on Aging (NIA)
31 Center Dr. MSC 2292
Bldg. 31 Rm. 5C27
Bethesda, MD 20892
Toll-Free: 800-222-2225
Toll-Free TTY: 800-222-4225
Website: www.nia.nih.gov
E-mail: niaic@nia.nih.gov

National Institute on Deafness and Other Communication Disorders (NIDCD)
31 Center Dr.
MSC 2320
Bethesda, MD 20892-2320
Toll-Free: 800-241-1044
Phone: 301-827-8183
Toll-Free TTY: 800-241-1055
Website: www.nidcd.nih.gov
E-mail: nidcdinfo@nidcd.nih.gov

National Institute on Drug Abuse (NIDA) for Teens
Website: teens.drugabuse.gov
E-mail: drugfacts@nida.nih.gov

National Institutes of Health (NIH)
9000 Rockville Pike
Bethesda, MD 20892
Phone: 301-496-4000
TTY: 301-402-9612
Website: www.nih.gov
E-mail: NIHinfo@od.nih.gov

National Oral Health Information Clearinghouse (NOHIC)
National Institute of Dental and Craniofacial Research (NIDCR)
One NOHIC Way
Bethesda, MD 20892
Toll-Free: 866-232-4528
Fax: 301-907-8830
Website: www.nidcr.nih.gov
E-mail: nohic@nidcr.nih.gov

NIH News in Health
NIH Office of Communications and Public Liaison (OCPL)
Bldg. 31, Rm. 5B52
Bethesda, MD 20892-2094
Phone: 301-451-8224
Website: newsinhealth.nih.gov
E-mail: nihnewsinhealth@od.nih.gov

NIH Osteoporosis and Related Bone Diseases— National Resource Center (NIH ORBD—NRC)
Toll-Free: 800-624-BONE (800-624-2663)
Phone: 202-223-0344
TTY: 202-466-4315
Fax: 202-293-2356
Website: www.bones.nih.gov
E-mail: NIHBoneInfo@mail.nih.gov

Office of Disease Prevention and Health Promotion (ODPHP)
Office of the Assistant Secretary for Health, Office of the Secretary
1101 Wootton Pkwy
Ste. LL100
Rockville, MD 20852
Fax: 240-453-8281
Website: health.gov
E-mail: odphpinfo@hhs.gov

Office of Head Start (OHS)
Administration for Children and Families (ACF)
330 C St. S.W.
Fourth Fl.
Washington, DC 20201
Toll-Free: 866-763-6481
Fax: 202-205-9721
Website: www.acf.hhs.gov/office-of-head-start

Office on Women's Health (OWH)
U.S. Department of Health and Human Services (HHS)
200 Independence Ave. S.W.
Rm. 712E
Washington, DC 20201
Toll-Free: 800-994-9662
Phone: 202-690-7650
Fax: 202-205-2631
Website: www.womenshealth.gov

U.S. Department of Health and Human Services (HHS)
200 Independence Ave. S.W.
Washington, DC 20201
Toll-Free: 877-696-6775
Website: www.hhs.gov

U.S. Environmental Protection Agency (EPA)
1200 Pennsylvania Ave. N.W. (2310A)
Washington, DC 20460
Phone: 202-564-8040
Fax: 202-564-1778
Website: www.epa.gov

U.S. Food and Drug Administration (FDA)
10903 New Hampshire Ave.
Silver Spring, MD 20993
Toll-Free: 888-INFO-FDA (888-463-6332)
Website: www.fda.gov

Private Agencies That Provide Information about Dental and Oral Health

Academy of General Dentistry (AGD)
560 W. Lake St.
Sixth Fl.
Chicago, IL 60661
Toll-Free: 888-AGD-DENT
(888-243-3368)
Fax: 312-335-3443
Website: www.agd.org

American Academy of Cosmetic Dentistry (AACD)
402 W. Wilson St.
Madison, WI 53703
Toll-Free: 800-543-9220
Phone: 608-222-8583
Fax: 608-222-9540
Website: www.aacd.com

American Academy of Implant Dentistry (AAID)
211 E. Chicago Ave.
Ste. 750
Chicago, IL 60611
Toll-Free: 877-335-AAID
(877-335-2243)
Phone: 312-335-1550
Fax: 312-335-9090
Website: www.aaid-implant.org
E-mail: info@aaid.com

American Academy of Oral Medicine (AAOM)
2150 N. 107th St., Ste. 205
Seattle, WA 98133
Phone: 206-209-5279
Website: www.aaom.com/
patients
E-mail: info@aaom.com

American Academy of Pediatric Dentistry (AAPD)
211 E. Chicago Ave.
Ste. 1600
Chicago, IL 60611-2637
Phone: 312-337-2169
Fax: 312-337-6329
Website: www.aapd.org

American Academy of Periodontology (AAP)
737 N. Michigan Ave.
Ste. 800
Chicago, IL 60611
Phone: 312-787-5518
Website: www.perio.org

American Association of Endodontists (AAE)
180 N. Stetson Ave.
Ste. 1500
Chicago, IL 60601
Toll-Free: 800-872-3636
Phone: 312-266-7255
Toll-Free Fax: 866-451-9020
Website: www.aae.org
E-mail: info@aae.org

American Association of Oral and Maxillofacial Surgeons (AAOMS)
9700 W. Bryn Mawr Ave.
Rosemont, IL 60018-5701
Toll-Free: 800-822-6637
Phone: 847-678-6200
Fax: 847-678-6286
Website: www.aaoms.org

American Association of Orthodontists (AAO)
401 N. Lindbergh Blvd.
St. Louis, MO 63141
Toll-Free: 800-424-2841
Phone: 314-993-1700
Fax: 314-997-1745
Website: www.aaomembers.org
E-mail: info@aaortho.org

American Dental Assistants Association (ADAA)
140 N. Bloomingdale Rd.
Bloomingdale, IL 60108
Toll-Free: 877-874-3785
Phone: 630-994-4247
Fax: 630-351-8490
Website: www.dentalassistant.org

American Dental Association (ADA)
211 E. Chicago Ave.
Chicago, IL 60611
Toll-Free: 800-621-8099
Phone: 312-440-2500
Website: www.ada.org

American Dental Hygienists Association (ADHA)
444 N. Michigan Ave., Ste. 3400
Chicago, IL 60611
Phone: 312-449-8900
Website: www.adha.org

American Diabetes Association (ADA)
2451 Crystal Dr.
Ste. 900
Arlington, VA 22202
Toll-Free: 800-DIABETES
(800-342-2383)
Website: www.diabetes.org

American Head and Neck Society (AHNS)
11300 W. Olympic Blvd.
Ste. 600
Los Angeles, CA 90064
Phone: 310-437-0559
Fax: 310-437-0585
Website: www.ahns.info

Children's Dental Health Project (CDHP)
2021 L. St. N.W.
Ste. 101-269
Washington, DC 20036
Phone: 202-833-8288
Fax: 202-833-8288
Website: www.cdhp.org
E-mail: info@cdhp.org

Cleft Palate Foundation (CPF)
1504 E. Franklin St.
Ste. 102
Chapel Hill, NC 27514-2820
Toll-Free: 800-242-5338
Phone: 919-933-9044
Fax: 919-933-9604
Website: www.cleftline.org

Cleveland Clinic
9500 Euclid Ave.
Cleveland, OH 44195
Toll-Free: 800-223-2273
Website: www.clevelandclinic.org

FACES: The National Craniofacial Association
P.O. Box 11082
Chattanooga, TN 37401
Toll-Free: 800-332-2373
Phone: 423-266-1632
Website: www.faces-cranio.org
E-mail: faces@faces-cranio.org

Health Physics Society (HPS)
950 Herndon Pkwy
Ste. 450
Herndon, VA 20170
Phone: 703-790-1745
Website: www.hps.org
E-mail: hps@BurkInc.com

Hispanic Dental Association (HDA)
401 Penn St.
Third Fl. Washington Ste.
Reading, PA 19601
Toll-Free: 855-337-9992
Phone: 217-529-6517
Website: www.hdassoc.org
E-mail: support@hdassoc.org

Juvenile Diabetes Research Foundation International (JDRF)
26 Bdwy.
14th Fl.
New York, NY 10004
Toll-Free: 800-533-CURE
(800-533-2873)
Fax: 212-785-9595
Website: www.jdrf.org
E-mail: info@jdrf.org

National Academy of Sciences (NAS)
500 Fifth St. N.W.
Washington, DC 20001
Phone: 202-334-2000
Website: www.nationalacademies.org

National Dental Association (NDA)
6411 Ivy Ln.
Ste. 703
Greenbelt, MD 20770
Phone: 240-241-4448
Fax: 240-297-9181
Website: www.ndaonline.org

National Eating Disorders Association (NEDA)
1500 Bdwy.
Ste. 1101
New York, NY 10036
Toll-Free: 800-931-2237
Phone: 212-575-6200
Fax: 212-575-1650
Website: www.nationaleatingdisorders.org
E-mail: info@NationalEatingDisorders.org

National Maternal and Child Oral Health Resource Center (OHRC)
Georgetown University
3300 Whitehaven St. N.W.
Washington, DC 20007
Phone: 202-784-9771
Fax: 202-784-9777
Website: www.mchoralhealth.org
E-mail: OHRCinfo@georgetown.edu

The Nemours Foundation /
KidsHealth®
1600 Rockland Rd.
Wilmington, DE 19803
Phone: 302-651-4000
Website: www.kidshealth.org

Sjögren's Syndrome
Foundation (SSF)
10701 Parkridge Blvd.
Ste. 170
Reston, VA 20191
Toll-Free: 800-475-6473
Phone: 301-530-4420
Fax: 301-530-4415
Website: www.sjogrens.org

Special Care Dentistry
Association (SCDA)
2800 W. Higgins Rd.
Hoffman Estates, IL 60169
Phone: 312-527-6764
Fax: 847-885-8393
Website: scdaonline.org
E-mail: SCDA@SCDAonline.org

Support for People with
Head and Neck Cancer
(SPOHNC)
P.O. Box 53
Locust Valley, NY 11560-0053
Toll-Free: 800-377-0928
Fax: 516-671-8794
Website: www.spohnc.org
E-mail: info@spohnc.org

TNA Facial Pain Association
22 S.E. Fifth Ave.
Ste. D
Gainesville, FL 32601
Toll-Free: 800-923-3608
Phone: 352-384-3600
Fax: 352-384-3600
Website: www.fpa-support.org

Index

Index

Page numbers followed by 'n' indicate a footnote. Page numbers in *italics* indicate a table or illustration.